DIFFERE
DIAGN
OF COMMON
COMPLAINTS

Sixth Edition

ROBERT H. SELLER, MD

Emeritus Professor of Family Medicine and Medicine
Former Chairman, Department of Family Medicine
State University of New York at Buffalo
School of Medicine and Biomedical Science
Buffalo, New York

ANDREW B. SYMONS, MD, MS

Assistant Professor and Vice Chair for Medical Student Education
Department of Family Medicine
Course Director, Clinical Practice of Medicine
State University of New York at Buffalo
Medical Staff, Mercy Hospital of Buffalo
Buffalo, New York
Medical Staff, Millard Fillmore Suburban Hospital
Williamsville, New York

ELSEVIER
SAUNDERS

ELSEVIER
SAUNDERS

1600 John F. Kennedy Blvd.
Ste 1800
Philadelphia, PA 19103-2899

DIFFERENTIAL DIAGNOSIS OF COMMON COMPLAINTS   ISBN: 978-1-4557-0772-0
Copyright © 2012, 2007, 2000, 1996, 1993, 1986 by Saunders, an imprint of Elsevier Inc.

Notice

Knowledge and best practice in this field are constantly changing. As new research and experience broaden our understanding, changes in research methods, professional practices, or medical treatment may become necessary.

Practitioners and researchers must always rely on their own experience and knowledge in evaluating and using any information, methods, compounds, or experiments described herein. In using such information or methods they should be mindful of their own safety and the safety of others, including parties for whom they have a professional responsibility.

With respect to any drug or pharmaceutical products identified, readers are advised to check the most current information provided (i) on procedures featured or (ii) by the manufacturer of each product to be administered, to verify the recommended dose or formula, the method and duration of administration, and contraindications. It is the responsibility of practitioners, relying on their own experience and knowledge of their patients, to make diagnoses, to determine dosages and the best treatment for each individual patient, and to take all appropriate safety precautions.

To the fullest extent of the law, neither the Publisher nor the authors, contributors, or editors assume any liability for any injury and/or damage to persons or property as a matter of products liability, negligence or otherwise, or from any use or operation of any methods, products, instructions, or ideas contained in the material herein.

Previous editions copyrighted 2007, 2000, 1996, 1993, 1986

Library of Congress Cataloging-in-Publication Data
Seller, Robert H., 1931-
   Differential diagnosis of common complaints.—6th ed. / Robert H. Seller, Andrew B. Symons.
     p. ; cm.
   Includes bibliographical references and index.
   ISBN 978-1-4557-0772-0 (pbk. : alk. paper) 1. Diagnosis, Differential. I. Symons, Andrew B. II. Title.
   [DNLM: 1. Diagnosis, Differential. WB 141.5]
   RC71.5.S45 2013
   616.07'5—dc23   2011022111

Acquisitions Editor: James Merritt
Developmental Editor: Barbara Cicalese
Publishing Services Manager: Anne Altepeter
Project Manager: Deepthi Unni, Louise King
Designer: Steven Stave

Printed in China
Last digit is the print number 9 8 7 6 5 4 3

Working together to grow
libraries in developing countries

www.elsevier.com | www.bookaid.org | www.sabre.org

ELSEVIER   BOOK AID International   Sabre Foundation

To my sons,
Michael, Adam, and Stuart

RHS

To my wife, Einav,
who supports me in all my endeavors

ABS

Preface

The purpose of the sixth edition of *Differential Diagnosis of Common Complaints* remains the same as the first—to help physicians accurately and efficiently diagnose common complaints. This book emphasizes a clinical approach to diagnosis rather than one that relies largely on diagnostic studies. Most medical school curricula, texts, and continuing education courses deal with diseases. However, patients usually come to their physicians complaining of headache, backache, or fatigue—not migraine, spinal stenosis, or depression. To address this reality, this book is organized around common presenting complaints— the patients' symptoms rather than the disease. The 36 symptoms reviewed account for more than 80% of the chief complaints with which physicians are confronted. The physician who has mastered the differential diagnosis of these symptoms will be able to diagnose accurately almost all the problems seen in a typical medical practice.

Each chapter deals with different common complaints, which are presented alphabetically. The chapters are organized to approximate the problem-solving process that most physicians use to make a diagnosis. Initially, the presenting symptom suggests several diagnostic possibilities. Then, this diagnostic list is further refined and reduced by additional, more specific, historical findings; by the patient's physical findings; and then by the results of diagnostic studies. The index lists all complaints, symptoms, and diagnoses noted in the text.

As with prior editions, this sixth edition has been revised to include suggestions by colleagues and students who appreciate the book's clinical orientation and practical approach to differential diagnosis. Each chapter has been revised to include new information, with an emphasis on the latest clinical and diagnostic studies.

The text does not deal extensively with pathophysiology or therapy except in situations in which this information is particularly useful in the diagnostic process. The most useful and up-to-date diagnostic studies for differential diagnosis are reviewed. When available, evidence-based information is included. The text concentrates on the most likely diagnoses and common illnesses that include many serious illnesses. It also notes when the physician must rule out extremely serious diagnostic possibilities.

The format of each chapter has remained the same:

Introduction. Includes relevant definitions as well as a list of the most common causes of the symptoms.

Nature of patient. Identifies those conditions that are most prevalent within a particular subgroup (e.g., children, the elderly, and premenopausal, diabetic, hypertensive, and immunocompromised individuals).

Nature of symptoms. Further identifies conditions by amplifying additional characteristics of the symptoms (how, when, where, radiation, acute/chronic, and others).

Associated symptoms.

Precipitating and aggravating factors.

Ameliorating factors.

Physical findings.

Diagnostic studies.

Less common diagnostic considerations.

Differential diagnosis table. A concise table located at the end of each chapter summarizes the salient differential diagnostic features of the most common clinical entities that cause a particular complaint.

Selected references. Most articles represent an approach to the differential diagnosis of problems rather than a review of a specific disease.

Clinicians and students may use this book for general information about the many causes of common chief complaints. They can also use it as a reference text when treating a patient who is complaining of a specific symptom (e.g., facial pain, shortness of breath, fever) when the diagnosis is not apparent.

Differential Diagnosis of Common Complaints was written to be useful. We hope you find it so. Remember the adage: "If you don't think about it, you will never diagnose it."

Robert H. Seller
Andrew B. Symons

Acknowledgments

Carolyn Doueck, CGF Health Sciences Libraries, provided invaluable assistance with the literature reviews. We also wish to thank two editors: Lisette Bralow, who, as the initial acquisitions editor, saw the potential of what became the first edition of this book, and Jim Merritt, senior acquisitions editor at Elsevier, who encouraged us to write this sixth edition.

RHS
ABS

Contents

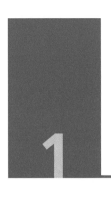

Abdominal Pain in Adults

1

Abdominal pain is the most common complaint seen in emergency departments in the United States and one of the 10 most common complaints in family medicine outpatient settings. The most common causes of abdominal pain are discussed here, with special attention given to the acute abdomen and recurrent abdominal pain. The term *acute abdomen* is medical jargon that refers to any acute condition within the abdomen that requires immediate medical or surgical attention. Acute abdominal pain may be of nonabdominal origin and does not always require surgery. The majority of patients who consult a physician about abdominal pain do not have an acute abdomen, although the chief complaint may have a sudden onset. In studies involving analysis of large series of patients presenting to emergency departments with acute abdominal pain, nonspecific abdominal pain (NSAP) was the most common diagnosis. Most patients with this symptom probably have gastroenteritis.

The common causes of abdominal pain are *gastroenteritis, gastritis, peptic ulcer disease, gastroesophageal reflux disease (GERD), irritable bowel syndrome (IBS), dysmenorrhea, salpingitis, appendicitis, cholecystitis, cholelithiasis, intestinal obstruction, mesenteric adenitis, diverticulitis, pancreatitis, ureterolithiasis, incarcerated hernias, gas entrapment syndromes,* and *ischemic bowel disease* (particularly in the elderly). All of these conditions can manifest as an acute or sudden onset of abdominal pain, many can cause recurrent abdominal pain, and a few require surgical intervention. Any acute abdominal condition requires the physician to make an early, precise diagnosis, because prognosis often depends on prompt initiation of therapy, particularly surgical treatment. The more serious the problem, the more urgent the need for an accurate diagnosis.

The examiner can best establish a complete and accurate diagnosis by carefully noting the patient's age, gender, and past medical history; precipitating factors; location of the pain and of radiating discomfort; associated vomiting; altered bowel habits; chills and fever; and findings of the physical examination, particularly of the abdomen. **Abdominal pain without other symptoms or signs is rarely a serious problem. The presence of alarm signs (weight loss, gastrointestinal [GI] bleeding, anemia, fever, frequent nocturnal symptoms, or onset of symptoms in patients older than 50 years) suggests a serious problem.**

1

The physician must be especially aware of the conditions that cause abdominal pain and usually require surgical intervention. According to one large study, the most common conditions requiring surgical intervention are *appendicitis, cholecystitis,* and *perforated peptic ulcer.* Others are *acute intestinal obstruction, torsion* or *perforation of a viscus, ovarian torsion, tumors, ectopic pregnancy, dissecting* or *ruptured aneurysms, mesenteric occlusion, bowel embolization,* and *bowel infarction.*

Several authorities warn against the practice of *pattern matching* in the diagnosis of acute abdominal surgical conditions; they have discovered that there are typical findings in only 60% to 70% of patients. This means that if physicians attempt to match acute problems with patterns or stereotypes of the disease, they will fail to make the correct diagnosis in 30% to 40% of cases. Therefore, to improve diagnostic accuracy, physicians must know the standard and typical presentations and must also be aware of the subtleties involved in the differential diagnosis. The *best-test* method is more accurate than pattern matching in establishing the diagnosis.

The best-test method involves elicitation of specific information that correlates well with the correct diagnosis. This method suggests that when a specific symptom or physical sign is noted, its presence is highly useful in establishing the correct diagnosis. For instance, the finding of pain in the right upper quadrant (RUQ) most frequently suggests *cholecystitis.* Likewise, if pain is aggravated by movement, it most frequently indicates *appendicitis* but also suggests *perforated peptic ulcer* to a lesser degree. A best-test question used to differentiate the most common causes of abdominal pain—NSAP and appendicitis—is whether the pain is aggravated by coughing or movement. The pain of appendicitis is aggravated by movement or coughing, whereas the pain of NSAP is not. Abdominal pain that is aggravated by movement or coughing is probably caused by peritoneal inflammation. Best-test signs that are helpful in differential diagnosis include the presence of a *palpable mass* in diverticular disease, *hyperactive bowel sounds* in small-bowel obstruction, *reduced bowel sounds* in perforation, and *involuntary guarding* in the right lower quadrant (RLQ) in appendicitis. The validity of best-test findings has been supported by retrospective studies in which the diagnosis is known.

NATURE OF PATIENT

It is often difficult for the physician to elicit an accurate description of the nature of the pain in elderly patients. They may be unable to distinguish new symptoms from preexisting complaints and concomitant illnesses. Many elderly patients present late in their illnesses, often after treating themselves for indigestion or constipation. In contrast to the high frequency of appendicitis, cholecystitis, and perforated ulcers in most general surgical series, the most common causes of acute surgical abdomen in patients older than 70 years are *strangulated hernias* (45%) and other forms of *intestinal obstruction* (25%).

In several studies, both the primary diagnosis and the discharge diagnosis in elderly patients with acute abdominal pain were less reliable than those in younger patients. Elderly patients are found to have organic disease more often than younger patients, possibly justifying more liberal use of radiologic studies in the older population.

The physician must remember that cancer is a common cause of abdominal pain in the elderly. In a study of patients older than 50 years with NSAP, 10% had cancer, the majority of whom had large-bowel cancer. *Colon cancer* is almost as common as perforated peptic ulcer, pancreatitis, and renal colic in patients over age 50. Cancer should be strongly suspected if the patient is older than 50 years and has had previous bouts of unexplained abdominal pain, if the present abdominal pain has lasted at least 4 days, and if constipation is present.

Elderly patients also have a higher frequency of uncommon causes of surgical abdomen, including *ruptured aortic aneurysm, acute mesenteric infarction,* and *inflammatory diverticular disease.*

The person's age also offers clues to diagnosis in other groups of patients. *Appendicitis* has its peak incidence in the second decade, although it can occur in patients older than 60 years as well as in infants. The incidence of *cholecystitis* increases with age and is the most frequent cause of acute abdominal pain in patients older than 50 years.

Cholecystitis is more common in whites than in blacks, more prevalent in females than in males, and more common in women who take oral contraceptives or estrogens than in those who do not. Drugs that increase cholesterol saturation also increase the incidence of *cholelithiasis*. They include gemfibrozil, fenofibrate conjugated estrogens, and estrogen-progestin combinations.

NSAP is an imprecise diagnosis, yet it is the most common diagnosis given to patients presenting to an emergency department with abdominal pain as the chief complaint. This diagnosis is most common in patients younger than of 40 years.

Irritable bowel syndrome seems to be most common in young women, particularly those who have young children. This frequency has been attributed to the life pressures to which these women are subjected. Symptoms of irritable bowel are also more frequent in others under stress, including children. The abdominal pain from an irritable bowel may be a vague discomfort or pain in the left lower quadrant (LLQ), RLQ, or midabdomen. It occasionally radiates to the back. This pain may be relieved by defecation and may be associated with other well-recognized symptoms of irritable bowel: mucus in the stool, constipation alternating with diarrhea, and small marble-like stools.

Lower abdominal or pelvic pain in women is often difficult to evaluate. *Ectopic pregnancy, ovarian torsion, ruptured ovarian cyst, pelvic inflammatory disease, endometriosis,* and *mittelschmerz* must always be kept in mind. It has been suggested that all young women with lower abdominal pain be tested for *Chlamydia*. Surgical emergencies of gynecologic origin are more common in women of reproductive age and include *pelvic inflammatory disease with abscess, ectopic pregnancy, hemorrhage from an ovarian cyst,* and *adnexal* or *ovarian torsion.*

Peptic ulcer pain is most common between ages 30 and 50 years but may occur in teenagers and, rarely, in young children. It is considerably more common in men than in women. However, this diagnosis should not be entirely disregarded in women because a significant incidence of perforated peptic ulcer among women may be a result of physicians' failure to consider peptic ulcer in the diagnosis. Although only 15% of patients with ulcer symptoms are older than 60 years, 80% of deaths from ulcers occur in this group, because ulcer disease in elderly patients is more likely to run a virulent course.

Acute intestinal obstruction occurs in all age groups. In the elderly, intestinal obstruction is usually caused by *strangulated hernias* or *cancer*. However, in any patient with severe abdominal pain and a history of abdominal surgery, adhesions constitute the most likely cause of intestinal obstruction.

Pancreatitis occurs most frequently in alcoholic patients and patients with gallstones. *Sigmoid volvulus* is more common in males, patients with cognitive disabilities, and patients with parkinsonism; *cecal volvulus* is more common in females. *Gallstone ileus* causes small-bowel obstruction more often in the elderly and in women. *Mesenteric adenitis* is more common in children. *Peptic esophagitis* is more common in obese patients. The incidence of *diverticulitis* increases with age; this disorder is more common after age 60.

NATURE OF PAIN

There are three types of visceral pain:

Tension—often colicky owing to increased force of peristalsis

Inflammatory—localized due to involvement of the parietal peritoneum, as in appendicitis

Ischemic—sudden, intense, progressive, and unrelieved by analgesics (See table "Differential Diagnosis of Abdominal Pain in Adults" at end of chapter).

Classically, *biliary colic* develops in the evening and is usually a steady midepigastric or RUQ pain. Colicky or crampy pain that begins in the midabdomen and progresses to a constant pain in the RLQ suggests *appendicitis*. Other conditions that may begin in a crampy or colicky manner and progress to a more constant pain include *cholelithiasis* and *cholecystitis* (which tend to localize in the RUQ), *intestinal obstruction,* and *ureterolithiasis* (which involves excruciating pain that frequently radiates to the groin, testes, or medial thigh).

A constant, often annoying burning or gnawing pain located in the midepigastrium and occasionally associated with posterior radiation is seen with *peptic ulcer*. Peptic ulcer pain may be worse at night, although this pattern is unusual. The pain is not ordinarily made worse by recumbency. The pain of peptic ulcer in elderly patients may be vague and poorly localized. Because of a lack of classic symptoms, an occasional absence of prior symptoms, and a confusing picture of abdominal pain, perforation associated with peritonitis is more common in older patients. It is particularly important to note that pain induced by percussion in the epigastrium may be the only physical finding to suggest ulcer disease in a person complaining of typical peptic ulcer pain. Likewise, severe exacerbation of pain that occurs when the physician percusses over the RUQ strongly suggests the presence of an *inflamed gallbladder.*

The *Rome II* criteria (12 weeks of symptoms in the preceding year; a change in the frequency or form of the stool, bloating, and pain that is usually dull, crampy, and recurrent) suggest *irritable bowel syndrome.* It is often associated with constipation that alternates with diarrhea, small stools, and mucus in the stools. In addition, moderate pain may be elicited when the physician palpates the colon. However, in elderly patients, severe diverticulitis may exist with similar symptoms.

Most abdominal pain, even when severe, usually develops over several hours. When the onset of severe abdominal pain is abrupt, it suggests *perforation, strangulation, torsion, dissecting aneurysms,* or *ureterolithiasis.* The most severe abdominal pain occurs with dissecting aneurysms and ureterolithiasis. The pain of a dissecting aneurysm is often described as a *tearing* or *ripping* sensation and frequently radiates into the legs and through the torso to the back. Such pain usually manifests in patients who are in profound shock. Individuals with the excruciating pain of ureterolithiasis may be writhing in agony but do not experience cardiovascular collapse. The pain of ureterolithiasis is usually unilateral in the flank, groin, or testicle and is often associated with nausea and occasional vomiting.

LOCATION OF PAIN

The location of the pain is one of the best tests for determination of a diagnosis (Fig. 1-1). RUQ pain is most frequently seen in *cholecystitis, cholelithiasis,* and leaking *duodenal ulcer* (Fig. 1-2). Another clue to gallbladder disease is the radiation of RUQ pain to the inferior angle of the right scapula. RUQ pain is also seen in patients with *hepatitis* or *congestive heart failure.* In the latter group the pain is thought to be caused by swelling of the liver, which results in distention of Glisson's capsule. Myocardial infarction may manifest as RUQ pain. Less severe RUQ pain may be seen in patients with *hepatic flexure syndrome* (gas entrapment in the hepatic flexure of the colon). If questioned carefully, these patients will admit to experiencing relief with the passage of flatus.

A gnawing, burning, midabdominal to upper abdominal pain suggests a condition with a peptic etiology—*ulcer, gastritis,* or *esophagitis.* Burning epigastric pain that radiates to the jaw is frequently seen in patients with peptic esophagitis. Severe upper abdominal pain that radiates into the back and is associated with nausea and vomiting suggests *pancreatitis.* Typically, this pain is worse when the patient lies down and improves when s/he leans forward.

Left upper quadrant (LUQ) pain is most frequently seen in patients with *gastroenteritis* or *irritable bowel* and less often in those with splenic flexure syndrome, splenic infarction, or pancreatitis. The pain from splenic flexure syndrome may be located in the LUQ or in the chest; therefore, it is also part of the differential diagnosis of chest pain. These pains tend to arise when the individual bends over or wears a tight garment, and they are frequently relieved by the passage of flatus.

Diffuse pain

Peritonitis
Pancreatitis
Leukemia
Sickle cell crisis
Early appendicitis
Mesenteric adenitis
Mesenteric thrombosis
Gastroenteritis
Aneurysm
Colitis
Intestinal obstruction
Metabolic, toxic, and
  bacterial causes

A

Right upper quadrant pain

Gall bladder and biliary tract
Hepatitis
Hepatic abscess
Hepatomegaly due to
  congestive failure
Peptic ulcer
Pancreatitis
Retrocecal appendicitis
Renal pain
Herpes zoster
Myocardial ischemia
Pericarditis
Pneumonia
Empyema

B

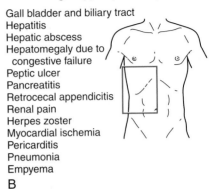

Right lower quadrant pain

Appendicitis
Intestinal obstruction
Regional enteritis
Diverticulitis
Cholecystitis
Perforated ulcer
Leaking aneurysm
Abdominal wall
  hematoma
Ectopic pregnancy
Ovarian cyst or torsion
Salpingitis
Mittelschmerz
Endometriosis
Ureteral calculi
Renal pain
Seminal vesiculitis
Psoas abscess

C

Left lower quadrant pain

Diverticulitis
Intestinal obstruction
Appendicitis
Leaking aneurysm
Abdominal wall
  hematoma
Ectopic pregnancy
Mittelschmerz
Ovarian cyst or torsion
Salpingitis
Endometriosis
Ureteral calculi
Renal pain
Seminal vesiculitis
Psoas abscess

D

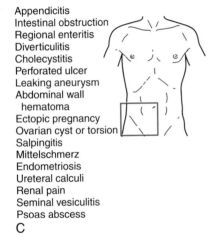

Left upper quadrant pain

Gastritis
Pancreatitis
Splenic enlargement,
  rupture, infarction,
  aneurysm
Renal pain
Herpes zoster
Myocardial ischemia
Pneumonia
Empyema

E

Figure 1-1. Characteristic location of abdominal pain associated with various diseases. (From Schwartz S: Principles of Surgery, 2nd ed. New York, McGraw-Hill, 1974, p 972.)

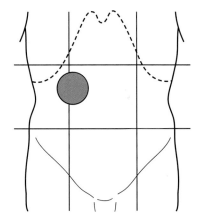

Figure 1-2. Tenderness and rigidity in right hypochondrium. (From Cope Z: Early Diagnosis of the Acute Abdomen, 13th ed. London, Oxford University Press, 1968, p 43.)

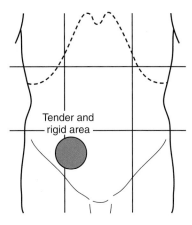

Figure 1-3. Tenderness and rigidity in right iliac region. (From Cope Z: Early Diagnosis of the Acute Abdomen, 13th ed. London, Oxford University Press, 1968, p 45.)

Other causes of both RUQ and LUQ pain include supradiaphragmatic conditions with inflammation of the diaphragm, such as pneumonia, pulmonary embolism, pleurisy, and pericarditis.

RLQ pain is most often seen with *muscle strain, appendicitis, salpingitis,* and *diverticulitis* (Fig. 1-3). However, pain associated with diverticulitis is more common in the LLQ. Less common causes of RLQ pain include ileitis, terminal ileitis (Crohn's disease), pyelonephritis, obturator hernia, carcinoma of the cecum, and colonic obstruction in patients with a competent ileocecal valve.

Other causes of RLQ or LLQ pain are *ureterolithiasis, salpingitis, endometriosis, ruptured ovarian cyst, ovarian torsion, ectopic pregnancy,* and *obturator hernia.* The pain of salpingitis is usually unilateral, although it may manifest bilaterally.

LLQ pain suggests irritable bowel and diverticulitis.

Common causes of central abdominal pain include early *appendicitis, small-bowel obstruction, gastritis,* and *colic* (Fig. 1-4).

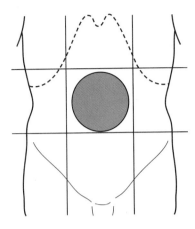

Figure 1-4. Acute central abdominal pain without any other symptom. (From Cope Z: Early Diagnosis of the Acute Abdomen, 13th ed. London, Oxford University Press, 1968, p 38.)

ASSOCIATED SYMPTOMS

Red flags include new onset of pain, change in pain or altered bowel habits in the elderly, weight loss, blood in stools or melena, anemia, enlarged supraclavicular lymph nodes, family history of serious bowel disease, or nocturnal pain. The abdominal pain seen with a truly *acute abdomen* is usually of such severity that patients overlook any associated symptoms they might have. Thus, it can be said that any additional complaint (e.g., headache) contradicts the diagnosis of an acute abdomen.

The timing of vomiting in relation to the onset of abdominal pain and associated symptoms may help the physician establish a precise diagnosis. The earlier the vomiting occurs in relation to the onset of abdominal pain, the less the abdominal distention. Patients with lower intestinal obstruction experience less vomiting and greater distention. Vomiting that precedes the onset of pain reduces the probability of an acute abdomen. Vomiting that begins after the onset of pain is more consistent with the diagnosis of an acute abdomen and is frequently seen in patients with *appendicitis*. However, the absence of vomiting does not preclude the diagnosis of an acute abdomen.

If vomiting occurs soon after the onset of pain and the vomitus is light in color, it probably consists of digestive juices and bile; this suggests *gastritis, cholecystitis,* or *obstruction.*

Jaundice, dark urine, and light to acholic stools may be seen in patients with abdominal pain caused by *cholecystitis.* These symptoms suggest an obstructive etiology of the jaundice, and complete biliary obstruction should be suspected. **A history of occasional silver-colored stools alternating with normal or light-colored stools is virtually pathognomonic of** *carcinoma of the ampulla of Vater.* The production of silver-colored stools is a result of mixing of upper gastrointestinal blood from the ampullary carcinoma with acholic stools.

Examination of vomitus from patients with acute abdominal obstruction may provide a clue to the location of the obstruction. Undigested food in the vomitus suggests that the obstruction is proximal to the stomach; this may result from *achalasia* or *peptic esophagitis*. Occasionally, undigested food may be seen in vomitus from patients with *pyloric obstruction*. This diagnosis is most likely if the vomiting persists and does not contain bile.

Brown vomitus with a fecal odor suggests mechanical or paralytic *bowel obstruction*. The more proximal the obstruction, the more frequent the vomiting.

Constipation with small, dry stools—sometimes alternating with diarrhea or mucus in the stool—is frequently seen in patients experiencing increasing stress and suggests an *irritable bowel syndrome*. When diarrhea and constant abdominal pain occur in patients older than 40 years, a cause requiring surgical intervention is likely.

PRECIPITATING AND AGGRAVATING FACTORS

The pain of *appendicitis* is aggravated by motion or coughing, as is the pain of *peritonitis*, regardless of its cause. The pain of *gastritis* is worsened by the ingestion of most foods, particularly alcoholic beverages. *Peptic ulcer* pain usually begins an hour or so after eating and is generally relieved by eating. If epigastric pain occurs primarily or is worsened in the recumbent position, *peptic esophagitis* should be suspected. Lower abdominal pain may be precipitated or aggravated by laxatives, particularly in instances of intestinal obstruction or constipation.

The pain of *salpingitis* and *endometriosis* is often worse during or before menstruation. Although patients may find that this pain is not exacerbated by limited movement in bed, more strenuous activity, such as descending a flight of stairs, frequently increases the severity of the discomfort. The symptoms of NSAP are precipitated and exacerbated by problems in the individual's environment. They may also be part of a long-term psychiatric illness.

AMELIORATING FACTORS

If the patient experiences relief after eating or taking antacids, *peptic ulcer* or *peptic esophagitis* is the probable cause of pain. The pain of *gastritis*, though worsened by the ingestion of food and alcoholic beverages, may be relieved by antacids. The pain of peptic esophagitis is often lessened when the patient is in an upright position.

Pain relieved by defecation or the passage of flatus suggests an *irritable bowel* or *gas entrapment* in the large bowel, whereas pain relieved by belching suggests *gaseous distention* of the stomach or esophagus. The pain of *gastroenteritis* is occasionally relieved by vomiting or diarrhea. Pelvic pain relieved by urination and associated with urinary frequency and dyspareunia suggests *interstitial cystitis*, which occurs most frequently in young women.

PHYSICAL FINDINGS

Physical examination of the abdomen in patients with abdominal pain should include inspection, auscultation, palpation, and percussion as well as rectal and pelvic examinations. The physical examination should begin with inspection of the abdomen, with the physician standing at the foot of the patient's bed. This part of the examination can often provide major clues to the diagnosis because it allows the physician to note distention, abnormal pulsations, and abdominal movement with respiration. The second part of the examination should always consist of auscultation; it is preferable for the physician to listen to bowel sounds before beginning a manual investigation. In all patients with abdominal pain, the physician should begin palpation away from the painful area and gradually move toward palpation over the most painful spot.

When palpating the abdomen and vaginal area, the physician should be particularly attentive to lymph node enlargements or hernias and to the quality of femoral pulses.

Abdominal wall pain can be diagnosed by the positive result of *Carnett's test*—palpation of the tender abdominal wall spot while the patient tenses the abdominal wall by raising the head and trunk or lower extremities off the examining table. If the pain persists or gets worse, the result is positive and pain is originating in the abdominal wall, not intra-abdominally.

Specific physical findings in *appendicitis, cholecystitis, diverticulitis, and bowel perforation or infarction* vary with the disease. However, if peritonitis is present, certain physical findings are common, regardless of the disease. The pain of peritonitis is severe, generalized, continuous, and of acute or gradual onset. The patient usually has abdominal tenderness with guarding, stabbing pain with gentle coughing, deep inspiration/expiration, and pain on percussion. Abdominal rigidity is occasionally present. Decreased movement of the abdominal wall occurs with respiration. If rebound pain is present, it is usually found over the area of primary disease. Patients with *peritonitis* are often in shock, have fever or chills, and present with decreased or absent bowel sounds. The patient usually lies relatively motionless because movement aggravates the pain. Depending on the severity of the peritonitis and the prior cardiovascular status of the patient, hypotension, tachycardia, pallor, and sweating may also be present. Younger, healthier patients are relatively resistant to hypotension but easily experience tachycardia. In contrast, elderly patients with a decreased cardiovascular reserve more readily become hypotensive. The presence of cardiac disease may impair the development of tachycardia.

Appendicitis

Patients with acute *appendicitis* almost always have tenderness over the inflamed appendix, often with involuntary guarding as well as rebound tenderness over McBurney's point. Classically, a disproportionate rise in the pulse rate occurs with respect to the severity of fever. **Too much emphasis on pain and tenderness and too little attention to the duration of symptoms and objective signs of inflammation may lead to negative exploration results in patients with suspected appendicitis.**

Cholecystitis

Guarding in the RUQ and tenderness on palpation and percussion suggest *cholecystitis*. When gallbladder disease is suspected in patients with RUQ pain, the examiner should begin palpation very gently in other parts of the abdomen and end gently over the gallbladder. The goal of this careful palpation is detection of an enlarged (hydrops) gallbladder. An enlarged gallbladder may not be detected by deep palpation or percussion, because such aggressive examination may result in involuntary guarding, which prevents detection of the enlarged gallbladder.

Peptic Ulcer

Patients with symptoms of *peptic ulcer disease* may show no abnormal physical findings except pain on gentle percussion over the midepigastrium or duodenal sweep. When peritonitis develops in patients with peptic ulcer disease, it is secondary to perforation of the involved viscus. If the viscus penetrates anteriorly, extreme rigidity of the abdominal wall results. If the viscus penetrates posteriorly, back pain is a major symptom, and the symptoms of peritonitis are minimal. In the early stages of a penetrating or perforated peptic ulcer, bowel sounds may be increased or normal, but as the condition progresses, bowel sounds become diminished or absent.

Intestinal Obstruction

Auscultation of the abdomen may help the physician to diagnose *obstruction*. Classically, rushes of high-pitched, tinkling peristalsis are heard. These rushes are often associated with recurring crampy, colicky pain. The physician must listen for a succussion splash in all patients who complain of vomiting. This examination requires the examiner to place the stethoscope over the stomach and to shake the abdomen gently. A succussion splash may be heard over a stomach that is dilated or distended with air and fluid. This finding is normal in infants and adults immediately after eating. By 30 minutes after eating, the sound should not be heard unless an obstruction exists with an air-fluid level. Impaired gastric emptying occurs most often in patients with *pyloric obstruction* (congenital or acquired); it also occurs in patients with gastric tumors or gastric atony. Atonic gastric dilatation is most frequently seen in postoperative patients and in patients who have severe hyperkalemia or diabetic ketoacidosis.

The classic triad of physical findings in patients with acute intestinal obstruction is as follows:
1. Sudden onset of colicky abdominal pain.
2. Vomiting.
3. Obstipation.

Bowel sounds are generally hyperactive and high pitched and occur in rushes; if perforation or peritonitis occurs, the bowel sounds become reduced. When the obstruction is in the large intestine, abdominal distention and general or local intestinal distention may occur. With *volvulus*, gross distention of the entire abdomen may occur early in the disease.

Salpingitis

The physical findings in salpingitis include unilateral or bilateral tenderness on palpation in the lower abdomen and increased bowel sounds. Involuntary guarding and rigidity are rare findings. Pelvic examination often elicits pain, particularly with lateral movement of the cervix and adnexal palpation. The patient frequently has a purulent cervical discharge.

Irritable Bowel

Although most patients with an irritable bowel have no significant physical findings (the diagnosis is made by careful history), a tender ascending or descending colon may be palpable. Diagnosis of IBS is best made using elements of history as suggested by the Rome II criteria (see page 5).

Acute Diverticulitis

The classic triad for acute diverticulitis is as follows:
1. Abdominal tenderness.
2. A palpable mass in the LLQ.
3. Fever.

The mass or tenderness may be occasionally detected only by rectal examination. Diarrhea and rectal bleeding are uncommon, and bowel sounds are usually decreased.

Ureterolithiasis

Tenderness on percussion in the costovertebral angle and ileus may be the only physical finding in patients with ureterolithiasis. This diagnosis is usually confirmed by the presence of hematuria.

DIAGNOSTIC STUDIES

Although plain or flat abdominal radiographs (often with chest radiographs) are frequently ordered in patients with acute abdominal pain, they are diagnostic in less than 50% of cases. They are useful in identifying free air in the case of a *perforated viscous* or dilated loops of bowel in an *intestinal obstruction*. Abdominal computed tomography (CT) scans and abdominal ultrasonography are often helpful, especially when *gallbladder, pancreatic,* or *pelvic disease* is suspected. CT scans provide information concerning the bowel wall, mesentery, and intraperitoneal and retroperitoneal structures and are useful in surgical decision making. Non-contrast CT scanning is useful in diagnosing *ureterolithiasis*. In pregnant women with abdominal pain and negative ultrasound findings, most academic radiology departments prefer CT, particularly in the second and third trimesters, although the role of magnetic resonance imaging (MRI) is increasing, particularly in the first trimester.

If an acute surgical abdomen is suspected but the diagnosis is unknown or dubious, the physician should obtain an electrocardiogram, chest and abdominal radiographs, complete blood count (CBC) with differential, measurements of electrolytes, blood urea nitrogen, serum amylase (if pancreatitis is suspected), and cardiac enzymes, and urine and stool tests.

Specific laboratory tests may be ordered when particular diagnoses are suspected, as follows:

Appendicitis—CBC with differential and C-reactive protein measurement (a normal C-reactive protein level and leukocyte count mitigates against appendicitis)

Cholecystitis—CBC with differential and complete metabolic profile

Ureterolithiasis—microscopic urinalysis

Pancreatitis—serum amylase and lipase measurements

Laparotomy is rarely necessary in patients with recurrent abdominal pain if the diagnosis is not apparent. In one series of 27 laparotomies for unexplained abdominal pain, carcinoma was found in 50% of patients. Laparoscopy has been recommended for all women of reproductive age in whom appendicitis is suspected. Laparoscopy and peritoneal cytology are helpful when surgical intervention is being considered. Recent studies have suggested the routine use of laparoscopy in patients with an acute abdomen. In most situations it has replaced laparotomy. In equivocal cases of abdominal pain, laparoscopy may prevent unnecessary surgery. In patients older than 50 years with *recurrent nonspecific acute abdominal pain,* stool examination for occult blood and colonoscopy should be done to check for cancer.

In one series, 7.4% of patients presenting with abdominal pain with colonic wall thickening on CT had colorectal carcinoma on colonoscopy, and 74% had clinically significant pathology, suggesting the value of colonoscopy for following up colonic wall thickening found on CT. Endoscopic ultrasonography is useful in evaluating esophageal, gastric, and particularly pancreatic lesions.

Despite a more than doubling of the use of CT use in the emergency department in recent years, there has been no increase in detection rates for appendicitis, diverticulitis, and gallbladder disease. Nor was there a reduction in hospital admissions for these conditions. **These data reinforce the principle of the importance of history and physical examination in the diagnosis of abdominal pain.**

LESS COMMON DIAGNOSTIC CONSIDERATIONS

Abdominal pain may result from *pneumonia,* particularly in a lower lobe. Abdominal pain and vomiting may be the presenting symptoms in diabetes. RUQ pain can be caused by *congestive heart failure* resulting from stretching of Glisson's capsule. RUQ pain, jaundice, and anorexia may be the presenting symptoms of *hepatitis.*

RLQ pain from *cecal epiploic appendagitis* can mimic appendicitis. In women of childbearing age, with RUQ pain, *Fitz-Hugh–Curtis syndrome* should be considered.

Amebiasis can mimic appendicitis, diverticulitis, or both. Abdominal or flank pain or both, when associated with nausea and vomiting, may be the presenting symptoms of *hydronephrosis*.

Hereditary angioedema should be suspected in young adults with recurrent abdominal pain when more common causes have been excluded. Angiotensin-converting enzyme inhibitor–related angioedema may also manifest as abdominal pain due to edema of the small bowel.

Cocaine usage can cause gastric ulcers, visceral infarction, intestinal ischemia, and ischemic colitis.

Eosinophilic enteritis, a rare cause of abdominal pain, can cause recurrent abdominal pain associated with vomiting, loose stools, and weight loss.

An acute abdomen in a young black patient classically suggests the possibility of *sickle cell crisis.* Recurrent episodes of abdominal pain may be caused by *familial Mediterranean fever,* which occurs in people of Jewish, Arabic, Turkish, and Armenian ancestry. Severe abdominal wall tenderness can result from a spider bite. Rarely, diffuse abdominal pain can be secondary to marked *gaseous distention.*

When abdominal pain is triggered by spinal movement, *spinal pathology* may be the origin of abdominal pain. Severe pain in the back or flank or vague, poorly localized abdominal pain may be the first presenting symptom in patients with *carcinoma of the pancreas.* If abdominal pain is associated with thrombophlebitis (in the absence of trauma), migratory thrombophlebitis, or the development of diabetes, pancreatic carcinoma should be suspected. Carcinoma of the head of the pancreas usually manifests as jaundice or abdominal pain early in the course of illness.

Abdominal pain, sometimes associated with vomiting, that occurs in the middle of the menstrual cycle is called *mittelschmerz.* It represents pain associated with the physiologic rupture of an ovarian follicle.

If a female of childbearing age suddenly experiences severe, generalized abdominal pain, often associated with syncope or persistent dizziness, *ectopic pregnancy* must be considered. This is more common in younger women, in women of low parity, and in those with a history of pelvic sepsis or infertility. Physical findings include acute abdominal pain with guarding and rigidity, especially in the lower abdomen. Extreme tenderness to cervical manipulation has been reported in 85% of patients with an ectopic pregnancy. Laparoscopy, human chorionic gonadotropin measurement, and ultrasonography may help the physician establish the diagnosis.

Vascular causes of abdominal pain include *mesenteric thrombosis* and *acute mesenteric occlusion* by embolism or torsion. The latter may have no associated signs or symptoms—only severe abdominal pain, with bloody stools occurring later. *Aortic aneurysm* may cause constant low back pain, which may worsen with recumbency; dissection is characterized by severe, excruciating pain.

Purcell (1989) reviews other uncommon conditions simulating an acute abdomen.

Differential Diagnosis of Abdominal Pain in Adults

CAUSE	NATURE OF PATIENT	NATURE OF PAIN	LOCATION OF PAIN	ASSOCIATED SYMPTOMS	PRECIPITATING AND AGGRAVATING FACTORS	AMELIORATING FACTORS	PHYSICAL FINDINGS	DIAGNOSTIC STUDIES
Gastroenteritis	Any age	Crampy	Diffuse	Nausea, vomiting Diarrhea Fever	Food	Occasional relief with vomiting or diarrhea	Hyperactive peristalsis	
Gastritis	Especially alcoholic patients	Constant burning	Epigastrium	Hemorrhage Nausea, vomiting Diarrhea Fever	Alcohol NSAIDs Salicylates Food (occasionally)			Gastroscopy
Appendicitis	Any age: peak age 10–20 yr M > F	Colicky Progressing to constant	Early: epigastrium, periumbilicus Later: RLQ	Vomiting (after pain has started) Constipation Fever	Pain worse with movement and coughing	Lying still	RLQ involuntary guarding Rebound to RLQ	CBC with differential count Ultrasonography Laparoscopy, especially in fertile women CT scan
Cholecystitis, cholelithiasis	Adults F > M	Colicky Progressing to constant	RUQ Radiates to inferior angle of right scapula	Nausea, vomiting Dark urine, light stool Jaundice	Fatty foods Drugs, oral contraceptives Cholestyramine		Tenderness on palpation or percussion in RUQ	Liver function tests CBC, amylase Ultrasonography Isotopic gallbladder scan Limited MRI
Diverticulitis	More common in elderly	Intermittent cramping	LLQ	Constipation Diarrhea			Palpable mass in LLQ	Laparoscopy, especially in women

Continued

Differential Diagnosis of Abdominal Pain in Adults—cont'd

CAUSE	NATURE OF PATIENT	NATURE OF PAIN	LOCATION OF PAIN	ASSOCIATED SYMPTOMS	PRECIPITATING AND AGGRAVATING FACTORS	AMELIORATING FACTORS	PHYSICAL FINDINGS	DIAGNOSTIC STUDIES
Pancreatitis	More common in alcoholic patients and patients with cholelithiasis	Steady Mild to sever	LUQ, epigastric Radiates to back	Nausea, vomiting Prostration Diaphoresis	Lying supine	Leaning forward	Abdominal distention Decreased bowel sounds Diffuse rebound	Amylase measurement Ultrasonography CT scan Abdominal radiographs
Intestinal obstruction	Elderly Prior abdominal surgery	Colicky Sudden onset		Vomiting Obstipation			Hyperactive peristalsis in small-bowel obstruction	CT scan
Intestinal perforation	Elderly F > M	Sudden onset Severe	Diffuse	Guarding Rebound	Pain worse with movement or coughing	Lying still	Decreased bowel sounds Guarding	Abdominal radiographs CT Scan
Peritonitis		Sudden or gradual onset					Diffuse rebound	
Salpingitis	Menstruating females	Cramplike	RLQ LLQ Nonradiating	Chandelier sign	Pain worse while descending stairs and around time of menstruation		Adnexa and cervix tender on manipulation	hCG measurement to rule out ectopic pregnancy Laparoscopy

Differential Diagnosis of Abdominal Pain in Adults—cont'd

CAUSE	NATURE OF PATIENT	NATURE OF PAIN	LOCATION OF PAIN	ASSOCIATED SYMPTOMS	PRECIPITATING AND AGGRAVATING FACTORS	AMELIORATING FACTORS	PHYSICAL FINDINGS	DIAGNOSTIC STUDIES
Ectopic pregnancy	Fertile female with history of menstrual irregularity	Sudden onset Persistent pain	Lower quadrant	Tender adnexal mass (vaginal bleeding)				hCG measurement Ultrasonography
Peptic ulcer with perforation	30-50 yr M > F	Gnawing Burning Sudden onset	Epigastric radiating to sides, back, or right shoulder		Empty stomach Stress Alcohol	Food Alkali	Epigastric tenderness on palpation or percussion	Endoscopy Radiography
Mesenteric adenitis	Children Adolescents After respiratory infection	Constant	RLQ	Vomiting Rebound Constipation Diarrhea Fever				CBC with differential count
Ureterolithiasis		Colicky Occasionally progresses to constant Severe Sudden onset	Lower abdomen Flank Radiating to groin	Nausea, vomiting Abdominal distention Chills, fever			Costovertebral angle tenderness Hematuria	Urinalysis Intravenous pyelography Nonenhanced helical CT
Dissection or rupture of aortic aneurysm	Elderly Hypertensive 40-70 yr	Unbearable Sudden onset	Chest or abdomen May radiate to back and legs	Shock			Shock Decrease or difference in femoral pulses	Radiography Ultrasonography CT scan

Continued

Differential Diagnosis of Abdominal Pain in Adults—cont'd

CAUSE	NATURE OF PATIENT	NATURE OF PAIN	LOCATION OF PAIN	ASSOCIATED SYMPTOMS	PRECIPITATING AND AGGRAVATING FACTORS	AMELIORATING FACTORS	PHYSICAL FINDINGS	DIAGNOSTIC STUDIES
Reflux (peptic) esophagitis		Burning Gnawing	Midepigastrium Occasionally radiating to jaw		Recumbency	Antacids		Upper GI radiographs Endoscopy
Irritable bowel syndrome	More common in young women	Crampy Recurrent	Most common in LLQ	Mucus in stools Rome II criteria		Pain occasionally relieved by defecation	Colon tender on palpation	
Incarcerated hernia	More common in elderly	Constant	RLQ LLQ		Coughing Straining		Hernia or mass	Upper GI radiographs
Mesenteric infarction	Elderly	May be severe	Diffuse	Tachycardia Hypotension			Decreased bowel sounds Blood in stools	Abdominal radiographs CT scan

CBC, Complete blood count; *CT,* computed tomography; *F,* females; *GI,* gastrointestinal; *hCG,* human chorionic gonadotropin; *LLQ,* left lower quadrant; *LUQ,* left upper quadrant; *M,* males; *NSAIDs,* nonsteroidal anti-inflammatory drugs; *RLQ,* right lower quadrant; *RUQ,* right upper quadrant.

Selected References

Andersson RE, Hugander AP, Ghazi SH, et al: Why does the clinical diagnosis fail in suspected appendicitis? *Eur J Surg* 166:796-802, 2000.

Angelini DJ: Obstetric triage revisited: update on non-obstetric surgical conditions in pregnancy, *J Midwifery Women's Health* 48:111-118, 2003.

Cope Z: *Cope's Early Diagnosis of the Acute Abdomen*, New York, 1987, Oxford University Press.

De Dombal FT: Picking the best tests in acute abdominal pain, *J R Coll Physicians [Lond]* 13: 203-208, 1979.

Gaitan HG, Eslava-Schmalbach J, Gómez PI: Cost effectiveness of diagnostic laparoscopy in reproductive aged females suffering from non-specific acute low abdominal pain, *Revista de Salud Publica (Bogota)* 7:166-179, 2005.

Holten KB, Wetherington A: Diagnosing the patient with abdominal pain and altered bowel habits: is it irritable bowel syndrome? *Am Fam Physician* 67:2157-2162, 2003.

Kamin RA, Nowicki TA, Courtney DS, et al: Pearls and pitfalls in the emergency department evaluation of abdominal pain, *Emerg Med Clin North Am* 21:61-72, 2003.

Laurell H, Hansson LE, Gunnarsson U: Acute abdominal pain among elderly patients, *Gerontology* 52:339-344, 2006.

Martinez JP, Mattu A: Abdominal pain in the elderly, *Emerg Med Clin North Am* 24:371-388, 2006.

Mayer IE, Hussain H: Abdominal pain during pregnancy, *Gastroenterol Clin North Am* 27:1-33, 1998.

Miller SK, Alpert PT: Assessment and differential diagnosis of abdominal pain, *Nurse Pract* 31: 38-45, 2006.

Nino-Murcia M, Jeffrey RB: Imaging the patient with right upper quadrant pain, *Semin Roentgenol* 36:81-91, 2001.

Old JL, Dusing RW, Yap W, et al: Imaging for suspected appendicitis, *Am Fam Physician* 71:71-78, 2005.

Pedrosa I, Zeikus EA, Levine D, et al: MR imaging of acute right lower quadrant pain in pregnant and nonpregnant patients, *Radiographics* 27:721-743, 2007:discussion 743-753.

Purcell TB: Nonsurgical and extraperitoneal causes of abdominal pain, *Emerg Med Clin North Am* 7:721-740, 1989.

Spiro HM: An internist's approach to acute abdominal pain, *Med Clin North Am* 77:963-972, 1993.

Abdominal Pain in Children

2

Because functional abdominal pain (previously called *chronic* or *recurrent* abdominal pain) is uncommon in children, the main emphasis of this chapter is the differential diagnosis of acute and recurrent abdominal pain. Abdominal pain in children has many potential causes, so a detailed history and a very careful physical examination are necessary. A small number of selected laboratory studies may also be required. Accurate diagnosis is essential because abdominal pain may be a manifestation of a surgical emergency, which must be identified promptly. Whenever significant concern exists about the presence of a surgical condition, the patient should be hospitalized to permit serial abdominal examinations and laboratory studies.

Red flags for chronic abdominal pain in children include: age less than 5 years, nocturnal pain, blood in stool, dysphagia, arthritis, family history of inflammatory bowel disease, unexplained fever, persistent vomiting (especially bilious) or diarrhea, and weight loss or growth failure.

Gastroenteritis is the most common cause of acute abdominal pain in children, and appendicitis is the second most common. *Constipation,* another common cause of abdominal pain, may be acute but is more often recurrent. Other common nonsurgical causes of acute abdominal pain are *mesenteric adenitis, urinary tract infection, sickle cell disease, poisoning,* and *diabetes. Functional abdominal pain* is defined as weekly episodes of abdominal pain occurring over 2 or more months. It is quite common in children older than 5 years and usually has a psychosomatic cause (Table 2-1). Irritable bowel syndrome is similar, but in addition, there is a change in frequency or form of stool and/or the pain is relieved by defecation.

The most common surgical causes of acute abdominal pain are *appendicitis, hernia strangulation,* and *intussusception.*

NATURE OF PATIENT

Presentation and causes of abdominal pain vary according to three age groups, as follows:
1. Children younger than 5 years
2. Patients between 5 and 12 years of age
3. Adolescents (Table 2-2)

20

TABLE 2-1.   Causes of Acute Abdominal Pain in Children

Gastrointestinal causes	Gastroenteritis Appendicitis Mesenteric lymphadenitis Constipation Abdominal trauma Intestinal obstruction Peritonitis Food poisoning Peptic ulcer Meckel's diverticulum Inflammatory bowel disease Lactose intolerance
Genitourinary causes	Urinary tract infection Urinary calculi Dysmenorrhea Mittelschmerz Pelvic inflammatory disease Threatened abortion Ectopic pregnancy Ovarian/testicular torsion Endometriosis Hematocolpos
Drugs and toxins	Erythromycin Salicylates Lead poisoning Venoms
Pulmonary causes	Pneumonia Diaphragmatic pleurisy Pharyngitis Angioneurotic edema
Metabolic disorders	Diabetic ketoacidosis Hypoglycemia Familial Mediterranean fever Porphyria Acute adrenal insufficiency
Liver, spleen, and biliary tract disorders	Hepatitis Cholecystitis Cholelithiasis Splenic infarction Rupture of the spleen Pancreatitis
Hematologic disorders	Sickle cell anemia Henoch-Schönlein purpura Hemolytic uremic syndrome
Miscellaneous	Infantile colic Functional pain

From Leung AK, Sigalet DL: Acute abdominal pain in children. Am Fam Physician 67:2321-2326, 2003.

TABLE 2-2.   Differential Diagnosis of Acute Abdominal Pain
by Predominant Age

Birth to 1 year	Infantile colic Gastroenteritis Constipation Urinary tract infection Intussusception Volvulus Incarcerated hernia Hirschsprung's disease
2 to 5 years	Gastroenteritis Appendicitis Constipation Urinary tract infection Intussusception Volvulus Trauma Pharyngitis Sickle cell crisis Henoch-Schönlein purpura Mesenteric lymphadenitis
6 to 11 years	Gastroenteritis Appendicitis Constipation Functional pain Urinary tract infection Trauma Pharyngitis Pneumonia Sickle cell crisis Henoch-Schönlein purpura
12 to 18 years	Appendicitis Gastroenteritis Constipation Dysmenorrhea Mittelschmerz Pelvic inflammatory disease Threatened abortion Ectopic pregnancy Ovarian/testicular torsion Mesenteric lymphadenitis

From Leung AK, Sigalet DL: Acute abdominal pain in children. Am Fam Physician 67:2321-2326, 2003.

When otherwise healthy and well-fed infants cry for more than 3 hours a day, for more than 3 days a week, and for more than 3 weeks, the probable cause is *infantile colic*. The cause of abdominal pain in very young children is difficult to determine unless abdominal tenderness, guarding, doubling up, or vomiting is present. **With the exception of infantile colic, when children less than 3 years old complain of abdominal pain, it is usually organic in origin.** Physical examination is particularly important in this age group. *Intussusception* is likely when signs of intestinal obstruction are found in infants (peak incidence, 6 months). A lead point such as Meckel's diverticulum is seldom found.

Appendicitis is uncommon in infants and children up to age 5 years, **but it is the most common condition causing abdominal pain that requires surgery in this age group.** Because appendicitis is seldom considered, the diagnosis is often missed or delayed. Perforation is therefore more common, and a disproportionately high percentage of deaths due to appendicitis occurs in children younger than 5 years. *Poisoning,* most common in children ages 1 to 4 years, is another frequent cause of abdominal pain.

In children between 5 and 12 years, the major dilemma involves *functional abdominal pain,* which is usually of psychosomatic origin, though it may be due to organic disease. Children with functional abdominal pain have a high incidence of behavioral and personality disorders. These patients tend to be *high-strung* perfectionists and are often apprehensive. Many have histories of colic and feeding problems in infancy and stressful family and school situations. Unexplained episodes of recurrent abdominal pain occur in 10% of school-aged children, but an organic cause is found in less than 10% of these cases.

In female adolescents with abdominal pain, dysmenorrhea, endometriosis, pelvic inflammatory disease (PID), ovarian cysts, corpus luteal cysts, and müllerian abnormalities must be considered. *Inflammatory bowel disease* frequently begins during adolescence and can be a cause of acute or recurrent abdominal pain, especially when associated with growth failure. Growth failure may also indicate *gluten-sensitive enteropathy. Sickle cell crises* occur almost exclusively in black patients but occasionally in people of Mediterranean descent. *Acute appendicitis* is most common in children ages 5 to 15 years, with a peak incidence between 10 and 15 years.

NATURE OF PAIN

The timing of the first occurrence of abdominal pain in children may help identify *psychological stress* as the cause. For example, abdominal pain that develops at a time of school problems, peer pressure, the birth of a sibling, family discord, moving, or parental disease or disability suggests a psychological cause. *Functional abdominal pain* is usually central and nonradiating and rarely awakens the patient at night. It is rarely associated with recurrent vomiting or diarrhea but is often associated with vagueness and multiple symptoms, particularly headache and extremity pains. Functional abdominal pain is one of the four functional gastrointestinal disorders described by the Rome III criteria (the others being functional dyspepsia, irritable bowel syndrome, and abdominal migraine).

In addition to observing the severity, duration, and location of abdominal pain, the examiner must note whether the onset is gradual or sudden. A gradual onset of cramping pain often suggests an intestinal cause, such as *appendicitis,* whereas a sudden onset of constant noncramping pain suggests *torsion of a viscus, intussusception,* or *perforation.* The pain of appendicitis classically precedes the development of vomiting and anorexia, begins gradually as a crampy epigastric or periumbilical pain, and progresses to a constant pain in the right lower quadrant (RLQ). In young children this pain may be mild, discontinuous, or both. Because of frequent atypical presentations and a decreased incidence in young children, this diagnosis is often missed.

The pain of *mesenteric adenitis* often mimics that of appendicitis, although a child with adenitis is not quite as sick and is not necessarily anorexic. Mesenteric adenitis usually occurs after a viral or bacterial infection. The associated pain may be colicky in younger children and severe and episodic in older children. **The child has tenderness and guarding when the pain is present and usually shows no guarding when the pain is absent.** This pattern is in contrast to that in appendicitis, in which the guarding persists despite the absence of pain. Guarding and abdominal tenderness are the symptoms most frequently associated with a surgical diagnosis.

Diffuse cramping abdominal pain that follows or coincides with the onset of diarrhea, nausea, or vomiting suggests *gastroenteritis.* Cramping pain occurring primarily after meals, especially if it is relieved by defecation, is often due to *constipation.* This diagnosis should be accepted only when an enema yields a large amount of feces and relieves pain. Sudden onset of severe, crampy, spasmodic pain that causes an infant to scream and draw up the legs should suggest *intussusception.* This spasmodic pain often recurs at 15- to 30-minute intervals, and the child may be normal, lethargic, or sleeping between attacks.

When abdominal pain is severe and colicky and radiates to the groin or flank, *urolithiasis* should be considered. Hematuria may confirm this diagnosis. Hematuria may also be noted when an inflamed retrocecal appendix overlies the ureter. Abdominal pain associated with tenderness on percussion in the region of the costovertebral angle may indicate *pyelonephritis.*

When the abdominal pain is relatively constant, located in the midepigastrium, and exacerbated by eating, *chronic gastritis* caused by *Helicobacter pylori* must be considered. Likewise, *H. pylori* infections should be considered in children with duodenal ulcers and recurrent abdominal pain.

The abdominal pain of *diabetic acidosis* is often generalized, and ketosis is usually present. The abdominal pain of a *sickle cell crisis* is severe and usually associated with ileus. This diagnosis should be considered in all black children with severe abdominal pain. Every black child in whom the diagnosis of appendicitis is considered should undergo a sickle cell test before surgery. When appendicitis is suspected in the patient with a positive sickle cell test result, an appendectomy should not be performed until the patient is clearly not showing response to medical therapy for sickle cell crisis or shows progressive manifestations of sepsis. Recurrent episodes of severe abdominal pain suggest *sickle cell disease, inflammatory bowel disease, cystic fibrosis,* and *constipation.*

LOCATION OF PAIN

Periumbilical pain is most common in functional abdominal pain, though in children less than 8 years of age, it may be due to organic disease. Epigastric pain can come from esophageal, gastric, or duodenal pathology or from functional dyspepsia of the upper gastrointestinal system. Substernal pain usually emanates from the esophagus. The pain of *gastroenteritis* is poorly localized, whereas the pain of gas and constipation is usually located in the RLQ. The presumed mechanism of RLQ pain in *constipation* involves gaseous distention of the cecum. **Increasing localized tenderness in the RLQ associated with rebound to the RLQ is the most helpful finding favoring the diagnosis of appendicitis.** Subsequent to this localization of pain in the RLQ, paralytic ileus may develop. Classic findings often occur with the appendix in its usual location, but atypical symptomatology may result from an unusually located inflamed appendix. It is critical for the physician to perform a rectal examination because pain in the right upper quadrant may be due to retrocecal appendicitis. Left lower quadrant pain suggests proctitis, colitis, or irritable bowel syndrome.

ASSOCIATED SYMPTOMS

A detailed evaluation of associated symptoms often helps establish the diagnosis. Some generally applicable rules concerning the differential diagnosis of acute abdominal pain are as follows:
1. When significant diarrhea is associated with abdominal pain, a surgical lesion is rare.
2. When abdominal distention, particularly with acidosis, is associated with abdominal pain, a surgical emergency is more likely.
3. When vomiting precedes abdominal pain, an extra-abdominal cause is suggested; when abdominal pain precedes vomiting, an abdominal cause is likely.

When abdominal pain is diffuse and no localizing physical signs are found, associated diarrhea, nausea, or vomiting suggests *gastroenteritis.* Viral diarrhea of the small bowel often manifests as midabdominal cramping, pain, and large amounts of watery diarrhea, whereas bacterial diarrhea affects the colon and manifests as lower abdominal pain and smaller amounts of bloody, mucoid diarrhea. A preceding upper respiratory infection (e.g., pharyngitis, tonsillitis, otitis media), a high fever, nausea or vomiting, and a good appetite suggest *mesenteric adenitis.*

Abdominal pain without systemic signs (e.g., fever, leukocytosis) or localized abdominal findings, especially with intense stress at home or school, suggests a *psychosomatic cause.* Some children with such findings also have nausea, vomiting, headaches, and diarrhea. Their pain is poorly localized, and they show no peritoneal signs.

A history of polyuria, polydipsia, weight loss, or diabetes in the patient or the family suggests that the abdominal pain may be caused by *diabetic ketoacidosis.* Growth failure, particularly during adolescence, is an important clue suggesting *inflammatory bowel disease* or *gluten-sensitive enteropathy.*

Other warning signs suggesting an organic cause of recurrent abdominal pain are weight loss, anemia, anorexia, change in bowel habits, rectal bleeding, fever, pain relieved by eating, pain that disturbs sleep or prevents normal activity, and history of significant familial disease.

PRECIPITATING AND AGGRAVATING FACTORS

If a viral infection precedes abdominal pain, mesenteric adenitis is suggested. If eating precipitates crampy lower abdominal pain, constipation is suggested. Eating may also worsen midepigastric pain that is caused by gastritis from drugs or *H. pylori* viral infections. If lactose-containing foods cause pain, a lactase deficiency is possible.

AMELIORATING FACTORS

When recurrent abdominal pain is relieved by defecation, constipation is the likely diagnosis. If triptan medication relieves abdominal pain, then abdominal migraine is the probable cause. When pain is relieved by eating or antacids, then peptic disease is probable.

PHYSICAL FINDINGS

Jones (1979) and Gryskiewicz and Huseby (1980) provide excellent reviews of special techniques useful in pediatric abdominal examination. Physical examination should include general observation of the child and inspection of the abdomen for distention, masses, or abnormal pulsations. Serial examinations by the same doctor are often helpful. The abdomen should be auscultated before palpation or percussion. Diffuse and generalized hyperperistalsis suggests *gastroenteritis,* whereas rushes of high-pitched peristalsis associated with crampy pains suggest an *obstructive process.*

Patients with *appendicitis* have tenderness over the inflamed appendix. Peritoneal inflammation, present in 97% of children with acute appendicitis, usually results in muscle guarding and cough/percussion/hopping tenderness (the elicitation of rebound tenderness should be avoided, as it often causes too much pain). Other signs of peritonitis include shallow breathing, absence of peristalsis, low-grade fever with a disproportionate rise in the pulse rate, and leukocytosis (which may be absent during the first 24 hours). The child may lie quite still or may move cautiously and often prefers to lie on the left side with the right thigh flexed. With a retrocecal appendix, the child may limp and demonstrate a positive psoas or obturator sign, although these signs are difficult to elicit in very young children. The following features of acute appendicitis apply distinctly to children:

1. Surgery should be performed within 24 hours of symptom onset; otherwise, perforation is likely.
2. The pain may be mild and discontinuous.
3. The pain may be atypically located when the appendix is not located in the right iliac area.

Both *mesenteric adenitis* and *nonspecific acute abdominal pain* can mimic appendicitis. It is very difficult for the physician to distinguish mesenteric adenitis from acute appendicitis by physical examination alone. **The value of serial abdominal examinations and serial laboratory tests, often performed in the hospital, cannot be overemphasized, particularly when the diagnosis is unclear.** With early inflammatory processes, irritation may be sufficient to make the abdomen diffusely tender but insufficient to produce peritoneal irritation. Patients with such processes may have no muscle guarding or rebound tenderness. In mesenteric adenitis, the white blood cell count is usually not elevated, the temperature may be high (even higher than in acute appendicitis), and the history or physical findings often reveal a previous viral or bacterial respiratory infection. Mesenteric adenitis may also follow viral gastroenteritis. Diffuse, crampy abdominal pain with nausea, vomiting, or diarrhea gradually changes to constant RLQ pain.

One long-term study of patients with *recurrent abdominal pain* revealed organic causes in only 2%, a finding that is not encouraging to the physician who is considering the possibility of early appendicitis. If the patient has a history of similar pain episodes and the current episode subsides within 24 hours, the diagnosis of functional abdominal pain is more likely. Until the diagnosis is clear, active serial observations are essential. Continued pain, tachycardia, anorexia, diarrhea, pain on movement, and especially rebound tenderness all warn the physician that the pain is *not* nonspecific and that surgical intervention must be seriously considered. When the temperature, blood count, erythrocyte sedimentation rate, and findings of urinalysis and stool examination for occult blood and ova and parasites are normal, functional abdominal pain is most likely.

A bulge in the inguinal area or the presence of an undescended testicle suggests an *inguinal hernia*. A lump may be palpated either rectally or abdominally in infants with *intussusception*. When intussusception is ileocecal (most common), a lump may be palpated in the right upper quadrant or the epigastrium. Rectal examination classically reveals bloody mucus on the examining finger. The "currant jelly" stool of dark blood is a late sign of intussusception. A barium enema not only may reveal the intussusception but also may alleviate it.

Palpation of fecal material in the colon and tenderness over the course of the colon suggest pain from *obstipation*. A firm inspissated stool may be palpated rectally. This diagnosis is confirmed if an enema yields a large amount of stool and relieves the pain. Occasionally an enlarged kidney is detected by palpation, suggesting hydronephrosis as the cause of abdominal pain.

Physical findings associated with abdominal pain from *diabetic ketoacidosis* include Kussmaul's respiration; diffuse abdominal pain; and sweet, fruity breath. The presence of Kussmaul's respiration and the absence of shallow respiration (which is usually seen with peritonitis) also suggest diabetic ketoacidosis.

DIAGNOSTIC STUDIES

Many indications for diagnostic studies have already been reviewed. Studies useful in the differential diagnosis of abdominal pain include complete blood count with differential, measurement of the erythrocyte sedimentation rate, abdominal radiographs, ultrasonography, computed tomography (CT), stool examination for occult blood, urinalysis, and urine culture and sensitivity testing. **Every child should undergo a blood glucose test and urinalysis before abdominal surgery. All black patients should undergo a sickle cell test.** Frequent serial tests may be necessary with acute pain. With recurrent abdominal pain, the tests should be repeated but less frequently. **When chronic or recurrent abdominal pain is the chief complaint, no additional symptoms suggest organic disease, and a thorough history and physical examination are negative, only simple diagnostic studies should be performed. Complex and invasive studies rarely influence the outcome.** In special instances, gastrointestinal barium studies, cholecystography, ultrasonography, intravenous pyelography, endoscopy, colonoscopy, and small-bowel biopsy may be helpful. Although sonography is often the initial test in children, CT scans are currently being used more frequently to evaluate abdominal pain. For diagnosing appendicitis, the average sensitivity and specificity of ultrasound have been reported to be around 87% and 89%, respectively, whereas for CT scanning, they are 91% and 94%, respectively. Laparoscopy has been helpful in instances of recurrent pain when the diagnosis is not apparent despite multiple studies. Laparoscopy is particularly helpful in children with recurrent RLQ pain and premenarchal girls with undiagnosed recurrent abdominal pain.

LESS COMMON DIAGNOSTIC CONSIDERATIONS

Congenital intestinal obstruction, Hirschsprung's disease, duodenal atresia, midgut volvulus, and necrotizing enterocolitis may occur in the neonate. Abdominal distention, food refusal, and vomiting are typically present in all these conditions. Likewise, radiographs are usually diagnostic. Neonates with Hirschsprung's disease fail to pass meconium. Many with duodenal atresia or midgut volvulus demonstrate visible gastric peristalsis.

A twisted ovarian cyst should be considered in cases of acute lower abdominal pain in girls. A mass is usually palpable, but a thorough rectal examination may be difficult unless it is performed with the patient under general anesthesia. Ultrasonography may help detect an ovarian cyst. A history of mittelschmerz also suggests that the pain may be due to an ovarian cyst. In older girls, salpingitis and pelvic inflammatory disease must be considered whenever a fever is observed in association with lower abdominal pain. The fever is usually higher than that observed with appendicitis, and a vaginal discharge is usually present. If a Gram stain preparation of the vaginal secretion reveals gonococci, the diagnosis is clear.

Complete or incomplete intestinal obstruction resulting from adhesions should be considered as a cause of abdominal pain in any patient with an abdominal scar. This pain is usually cramping and is typically accompanied by bilious vomiting. Physical examination may reveal abdominal distention, and distended loops of bowel may occasionally be identified clinically or radiographically. In the early phase, high-pitched, tinkling bowel sounds may occur in rushes. If the obstruction continues, peristalsis becomes lower in pitch and less frequent.

Peptic ulceration and occasional perforation may develop in children experiencing major stress as the result of serious physical trauma (e.g., burns, severe head injuries). Unfortunately, diagnosis is frequently delayed because of the severity of the other associated problems. Peptic ulceration and perforation should be considered whenever children with abdominal symptoms have undergone major stress. Upright or decubitus radiographs may demonstrate free air in the peritoneal cavity.

Gallstones are rare in children and are most likely to occur in those with hemolytic anemias. Abdominal pain may be the presenting complaint in children with lower lobe pneumonias. Children with migraine headaches may also complain of abdominal pain.

Lactose intolerance can cause recurrent abdominal pain in children and should be considered if the onset of pain coincides with heavy lactose ingestion. Before invasive procedures are performed or a psychogenic origin is assumed, a lactose-restricted diet should be attempted. Functional abdominal pain, occasionally associated with nausea but without headache, may be due to abdominal migraine (migraine sans migraine). In rare cases, when abdominal pain, nausea, and vomiting are associated with orthostatic hypotension, they are relieved by the treatment of the hypotension. Blunt, nonpenetrating abdominal trauma can cause rupture of the spleen, liver, intestines, or kidneys and can result in abdominal pain. Crohn's disease should be considered in adolescents who have abdominal pain associated with weight loss, anemia, rectal bleeding, diarrhea, or passage of mucus from the rectum.

Acute pancreatitis, though rare in children, can be caused by trauma, viral infection (especially mumps), prolonged steroid therapy, or obstruction of the common bile duct due to a stone or an inflammatory process. Patients with this condition usually have marked nausea; vomiting; low-grade fever; and severe, constant upper abdominal pain radiating to the back.

Allergies to foods and drugs occasionally cause abdominal pain. Lead poisoning should be suspected if the child has paroxysms of diffuse abdominal pain alternating with constipation. A history of pica may or may not be obtained from the parents or patient.

Urinary tract infections, kidney stones, and ureteropelvic junction obstruction may cause abdominal pain. Children with ureteropelvic junction obstruction often have recurrent unilateral pain that commonly occurs at night after ingestion of large quantities of fluids.

Other, less common causes are lead poisoning (diffuse, crampy abdominal pain and mild anemia) and hereditary angioedema (family history of paroxysmal dyspnea, cutaneous swelling, and attacks of abdominal pain).

Differential Diagnosis of Abdominal Pain in Children

CONDITION	NATURE OF PATIENT	NATURE OF PAIN	LOCATION OF PAIN	ASSOCIATED SYMPTOMS	PRECIPITATING AND AGGRAVATING FACTORS	PHYSICAL FINDINGS	DIAGNOSTIC STUDIES
Gastroenteritis	All ages	Crampy	Diffuse	Diarrhea Vomiting Nausea	Viral infection	Hyperperistalsis Low-grade fever	
Intussusception	Younger than 5 yr; peak incidence 6 mo	Severe, crampy				Rushes of high-pitched peristalsis "Currant jelly" stools Walnut-size mass, palpated abdominally or rectally	Barium enema Abdominal radiographs
Constipation	Any age; peak incidence 5-12 yr	Recurrent, crampy (especially after meals)	Often RLQ		Eating	Feces in rectum Feces may be palpable in colon	Enema yields large amount of feces and relieves pain
Psychosomatic cause	Frequently 5-12 yr High-strung, perfectionist History of colic	Recurrent (3 or more episodes of central, nonradiating pain in 3 mo)		Headaches No vomiting or diarrhea Poor appetite	Psychological stresses	Absence of systemic signs	Laboratory and radiographic findings within normal limits

Appendicitis	Uncommon in young children Peak incidence 5-15 yr	Atypical in children Precedes anorexia and vomiting Worse with movement	Begins gradually in epigastrium or periumbilical area Progresses to constant RLQ pain			Serial examinations useful Fever Guarding persists when pain is not present Rebound in RLQ Decreased peristalsis	Leukocytosis Abdominal radiographs Ultrasonography CT scan
Mesenteric adenitis	As in appendicitis	As in appendicitis	RLQ	Symptoms of recent upper respiratory infection Good appetite	Viral infection Recent upper respiratory infection	No guarding when pain is not present Fever Similar to those in appendicitis Lymphocytosis	Complete blood count with differential Upper and lower gastrointestinal radiographs
Inflammatory bowel disease	Adolescence			Diarrhea		Growth failure Diffuse abdominal tenderness, often without rebound	Elevated erythrocyte sedimentation rate
Inguinal hernia			Lower quadrant	Undescended testicle Abdominal distention		Bulge in inguinal area	

CT, Computed tomography; *RLQ,* right lower quadrant.

Selected References

American Academy of Pediatrics North American Society for Pediatric Gastroenterology: Hepatology, and Nutrition: Chronic abdominal pain in children, *Pediatrics* 115:e370-381, 2005.

Baber KF, Anderson J, Puzanovovna M, Walker L: Rome II versus Rome III classification of functional gastrointestinal disorder, *J Pediatr Gastroenterol Nutr* 47:299-302, 2008.

Brown RT, Hewitt GD: Chronic pelvic pain and recurrent abdominal pain in female adolescents, *Endocr Dev* 7:213-224, 2004.

Gryskiewicz JM, Huseby TL: The pediatric abdominal examination, *Postgrad Med* 67:126-138, 1980.

Jones PF: The acute abdomen in infancy and childhood, *Practitioner* 222:473-478, 1979.

Klein MD: Clinical approach to a child with abdominal pain who might have appendicitis, *Pediatr Radiol* 37:11-14, 2007.

Kohli R, Li BK: Differential diagnosis of recurrent abdominal pain: new considerations, *Pediatr Ann* 33:113-122, 2004.

Kolts RL, Nelson RS, Park R, et al: Exploratory laparoscopy for recurrent right lower quadrant pain in a pediatric population, *Pediatr Surg Int* 22:247-249, 2006.

Lake AM: Chronic abdominal pain in childhood: diagnosis and management, *Am Fam Physician* 59:1823-1830, 1999.

Leung AC, Sigalet DL: Acute abdominal pain in children, *Am Fam Physician* 67:2321-2326, 2003.

Macarthur C, Saunders N, Feldman W: *Helicobacter pylori*, gastroduodenal disease, and recurrent abdominal pain in children, *JAMA* 273:729-734, 1995.

Mason JD: The evaluation of acute abdominal pain in children, *Emerg Med Clin North Am* 14:629-643, 1996.

McCollough M, Sharieff GQ: Abdominal pain in children, *Pediatr Clin North Am* 53:107-137, 2006.

McOmber ME, Shulman RJ: Recurrent abdominal pain and irritable bowel syndrome in children, *Curr Opin Pediatr* 19:581-585, 2007.

Noe JD, Li BU: Navigating recurrent abdominal pain through clinical clues, red flags, and initial testing, *Pediatr Ann* 38:259-266, 2009.

Riddell A, Carr SB: Recurrent abdominal pain in childhood, *Practitioner* 244:346-350, 2000.

Roberts DM, Ostapchuk M, O'Brien JG: Infantile colic, *Am Fam Physician* 70:735-742, 2004.

Rowland M, Bourke B, Drumm B: Do the Rome criteria help the doctor or the patient? *J Pediatr Gastroenterol Nutr* 41(Suppl 1):S32-S33, 2005.

Russell G, Abu-Arafeh I, Symon DN: Abdominal migraine: evidence for existence and treatment options, *Paediatr Drugs* 4:1-8, 2002.

Stevenson RJ: Abdominal pain unrelated to trauma, *Surg Clin North Am* 65:1181-1215, 1985.

Strouse PJ: Imaging and the child with abdominal pain, *Singapore Med J* 44:312-322, 2003.

Yacob D, DiLorenzo C: Functional abdominal pain: all roads lead to Rome (criteria), *Pediatr Ann* 38:253-258, 2009.

Zeiter DK, Hyams JS: Recurrent abdominal pain in children, *Pediatr Clin North Am* 49:53-71, 2002.

Backache

3

Low back pain causes countless visits to physicians, including 5% of all visits to family physicians. Two percent of the population consults a physician each year because of back pain. More than 80% of adults have had at least one episode of back pain, and many have had recurrent episodes since adolescence. It is the most common cause of disability in patients younger than age 45 years, and by age 50 years, 80% to 90% show evidence of degenerative disc disease at autopsy.

Despite the frequency of low back syndrome, it is poorly understood, physical examination is often unrewarding, and diagnostic test results are often negative or falsely positive. **Some patients have local or radicular signs but no evidence of morphologic abnormalities, even after testing with all available diagnostic technologies.** On the other hand, 50% to 60% of asymptomatic individuals have degenerative changes, and 20% have disc herniation without symptoms. To complicate matters even more, patients may change from one low back syndrome to another (e.g., from sciatica to chronic low back pain). **Therefore, low back pain should be considered a symptom that is rarely attributable to a specific disease or pathologic lesion.**

Low back pain most often has a mechanical origin. Mechanical causes include *acute lumbosacral strain, postural backache,* and *degenerative lumbosacral arthritis,* all of which may be caused by problems with muscles, tendons, ligaments, and discs. Other common causes are *sciatica* (often associated with a *herniated disc*), *lumbar spinal stenosis,* and *chronic low back pain.* Social and psychological factors are more pronounced in patients with *chronic low back pain,* and the severity of their symptoms does not match documented abnormalities.

NATURE OF PATIENT

Backaches in patients younger than 20 years old or older than 50 years suggest a serious *(red flag)* problem, as does back pain lasting longer than 6 weeks.

Backaches in children are relatively uncommon., Backache represents serious disease more often in young children than in adults, although the most common cause of backache in children is lumbosacral sprain. This type of sprain usually results from participation in sports. A sprained back is occasionally caused by *trauma* (e.g., injuries sustained during a motor vehicle accident or during participation in gymnastics). Thoracic back pain and structural kyphosis in adolescents are usually caused by Scheuermann's disease, a condition related to repetitive trauma in which the nucleus pulposus migrates through the cartilaginous layer between the vertebral body and the ring apophysis, resulting in its avulsion. The pain is located in the midscapular region.

Because low back pain may represent serious illness in children, a thorough history and physical examination should be performed. *Infection* should be a strong diagnostic consideration, especially in suspected intravenous (IV) drug users. *Spondylolisthesis* is a deficit in the pars interarticularis, which is the weakest part of the vertebra. It sometimes results in the anterior translocation of the affected vertebra, which is called *spondylolysis*. *Spondylolisthesis* and *spondylolysis* occur more often in teenagers than in younger patients. Pain usually develops after strenuous athletic activity, and the cause can be detected best with single-photon emission computed tomography (SPECT), because plain radiographs may not detect an early stress fracture.

Regardless of the cause, backache is most common in patients between 20 and 50 years of age. It occurs more often in people such as industrial workers and farmers, who do heavy manual labor. In young adults who complain of persistent backache, *nonbacterial inflammatory disease,* such as *Reiter's syndrome* and *ankylosing spondylitis,* should be considered. It is particularly important for the examiner to ask these patients about other inflammatory changes that may be associated with Reiter's syndrome (e.g., iritis, pharyngitis, urethritis, arthritis). Even if the patient has spondylolisthesis, the physician must rule out inflammatory causes of backache. *Postural backaches* are more common in multigravida patients and individuals who are obese or otherwise in poor physical condition. *Herniated discs* occur in young adults but are relatively uncommon.

The number of backaches caused by *disc disease* rises as age increases from 25 to 50 years. Disc syndromes are more common in men, particularly older ones. In older patients, backache is a common symptom but not a common chief complaint. When it is the chief complaint in patients older than 50 years, serious illness such as *lumbar spinal stenosis* with or without *cauda equina syndrome* must be considered, although the most common cause is *lumbosacral osteoarthritis.* Everyone probably experiences some degenerative joint disease in the low back, but as a rule, clinical problems arise only when this degeneration reaches a moderate degree. It is then usually preceded by some traumatic incident, possibly minor, that precipitates the onset of symptoms. **In patients older than 50 years who present with backache without a significant history of prior backaches, serious conditions such as cancer and multiple myeloma must be considered.**

NATURE OF SYMPTOMS AND LOCATION OF PAIN

To determine the cause of backache, the physician must consider important historical factors, such as age, location of pain (Table 3-1) possible radiation of pain, effects of back or leg motion, and previous trauma.

TABLE 3-1.   Differential Features of Common Causes of Pelvic Girdle Pain

CAUSES	SITE OF PAIN	AGGRAVATING AND RELIEVING FACTORS	PHYSICAL FINDINGS	OTHER FINDINGS
Degenerative disc disease with tender facet impingement	Buttock, posterior thigh	Worse with spinal extension; relieved by rest in fetal position	Restricted spinal movement, spinal segment	
Degenerative disc disease with nuclear prolapse dysfunction	Buttock, posterior thigh	Worse with spinal extension; relieved by rest in fetal position	Restricted spinal movement, tender spinal segment, nerve root	Radiographic findings abnormal
Sacroiliitis	Buttock, posterior thigh	Worse at rest; relieved with activity	Restricted spinal movement	Radiographic findings abnormal
Osteoarthritis of hip	Groin, occasionally buttock or knee	Worse with activity: relieved with rest	Restricted hip movement	Radiographic findings abnormal
Meralgia paresthetica anterosuperior	Lateral thigh paresthesia	Worse at night; relieved by local infiltration of anesthetic and steroids	Tenderness just below iliac spice	
Trochanteric bursitis	Lateral thigh	Worse at night with activity; relieved by local infiltration of aesthetic and steroids	Tenderness over greater trochanter	

From Little H: Trochanteric bursitis. Can Med J 120:456-458, 1979.

The pain of *acute lumbosacral strain* is characterized by a sudden onset often related to turning, lifting, twisting, or unusual physical activity. It is usually well localized at the lumbosacral region.

The pain of a *musculoskeletal strain* and a *postural backache* is often described as dull and persistent and associated with stiffness. Patients have difficulty locating a precise point of maximum pain, although the pain is usually centered in the lower lumbar region. After trauma, this pain may have an immediate or delayed onset. Patients may state that they felt something "give way." The pain typically radiates across the lower back and occasionally into the buttocks but rarely into the lower extremity. **Radiation of pain does not always indicate nerve root compression.**

The low back pain of *degenerative lumbosacral arthritis* has a gradual onset, is not usually precipitated by physical activity, and is usually associated with a history of morning stiffness. Many patients with this condition complain that their lumbosacral motion is limited by pain and stiffness that is often worse in the morning but improves an hour or so after they arise. Radiation of pain to the knee, calf, or lower leg is uncommon.

Many patients with *herniated disc syndrome* have a history of previous, less severe episodes. The pain usually has a sudden onset and often radiates into the buttock, down the posterolateral aspect of the leg, and sometimes to the foot. The pain of a disc syndrome has been compared with a toothache—sharp, lancinating, radiating pain that may be associated with paresthesias and muscle weakness (caused by nerve root pressure). Remitting pain usually indicates a posterolateral disc protrusion, but an intermittent backache can also be caused by a disc that does not produce significant root irritation. More than 90% of lumbar disc herniations occur at L4-L5 or L5-S1. If root irritation is present, neurologic findings (sensory loss, motor weakness, or hyporeflexia) are diagnostic. The patient may also have tenderness on palpation in the sciatic notch.

The qualitative characteristics of low back pain can be of considerable practical diagnostic importance. Variable, diffuse, and intense sensations of pressure often occur in patients without demonstrable organic disease. When the pain is described consistently and specifically, it is easier for the physician to demonstrate organic disease. Inflammatory disease (e.g., ankylosing spondylitis) and infectious processes (e.g., tuberculosis) are *not* likely if pain is related to posture, trauma, or overly strenuous activities, is episodic and intermittent, is aggravated by action, and is relieved by rest and recumbency.

Back pain in *sacroiliac syndromes* tends to be localized over the posterosuperior iliac spine. In *sacroiliitis* (inflammatory arthritis of the sacroiliac joints) the pain may alternate from side to side, although it is usually felt in the low back and buttocks and may radiate into the posterior thigh. **The pain of sacroiliitis does not have a radicular distribution.**

Occasionally, low back pain may be a manifestation of *irritable bowel syndrome*. In these cases, there is often associated midback pain, abdominal pain, and a history characteristic of an irritable colon. This pain does not radiate into the leg. The low back pain from *prostatitis* is usually a vague ache that is not affected by movement or coughing and is not associated with muscle spasm or limited mobility.

On rare occasions, the acute pain of *renal colic* manifests as excruciating pain in the back rather than in the flank or groin. The patient shows a gradual shift in the location of pain to the flank, with radiation into the groin. With renal colic the straight-leg raising test result is usually negative, and urinalysis generally shows hematuria.

Some patients with *depression* may experience chronic low back pain. It is often described as diffuse, accompanied by a sensation of severe pressure. When somatic pain is a manifestation of depression, the severity of the pain varies with the mental state: pain increases with anxiety and depression and often decreases with extreme fear. If an elderly patient describes a burning or aching back pain, particularly if it is superficial and unilateral, *herpes zoster* should be suspected, because this pain often precedes the herpetic skin lesions.

ASSOCIATED SYMPTOMS

With *lumbar osteoarthritis,* patients often have pain in other joints. Patients with *herniated disc syndrome* usually have neurologic symptoms such as sciatica, paresthesias, dysesthesias, hypesthesias, anesthesias, paresis, sphincter problems, and impotence. **Pressure on the unmyelinated fibers may cause *cauda equina syndrome,* a rare surgical emergency whose signs include central back pain associated with weakness of the leg muscles, impotence, urinary frequency, urinary retention (sometimes with overflow), incontinence, saddle anesthesia, and loss of sphincter tone.**

Low back pain associated with vaginal discharge suggests a *gynecologic* cause. In men, back pain associated with burning on urination, difficulty in urination, or fever suggests *prostatitis.* If herpes zoster is associated with back pain, underlying *cancer* should be strongly considered.

The physician should be aware of the *red flags* of serious disease. Cancer or infection is suggested by unexplained weight loss, immunosuppression, urinary infection, IV drug use, prolonged use of corticosteroids, patient age more than 50 years, and back pain not improved with rest. Spinal fracture is suggested by a history of trauma, even minor trauma in osteoporotic elderly patients, or prolonged steroid usage. Cauda equina syndrome or some other severe neurologic compromise is suggested by acute urinary retention, overflow incontinence, loss of sphincter tone, saddle anesthesia, or progressive motor weakness in the lower limbs.

PRECIPITATING AND AGGRAVATING FACTORS

Spondylolysis in adolescents is often precipitated by athletic activity. It often manifests as low back pain that is aggravated by activity and leads to an erroneous diagnosis of lumbosacral strain.

Acute lumbosacral strain is usually precipitated by lifting, twisting, unusual physical activity or position, or trauma. Many patients are older and overweight and have not been physically active. When acute lumbosacral strain occurs in athletes, it may be caused by poor equipment, inadequate coaching, insufficient warm-up or conditioning, or any body position that unnecessarily exaggerates lordosis. Acute lumbosacral strain in adolescent athletes may be precipitated or aggravated during periods of rapid growth, since the soft tissues, ligaments, and musculotendinous units do not keep up with bone growth. Patients with acute lumbosacral strain experience pain with motion but not with coughing and straining. *Postural backaches* worsen as the day progresses.

In patients with *herniated disc syndrome,* pain can be precipitated by trauma or certain types of movement, particularly twisting in the bent-back position, as when starting a lawn mower or outboard engine. Aging also facilitates the development of this syndrome; herniation of the nucleus pulposus is the result of degenerative changes that occur with aging of the disc. The pain of a disc syndrome may be exacerbated by coughing, laughing, straining at stool, sneezing, sitting, and lateral bending; in acute cases it may be aggravated by almost any activity that results in the movement of the lower back, particularly hyperextension. The pain caused by *degenerative lumbosacral arthritis* may also be increased by lateral bending and extension of the lumbar spine. The polyradicular pain of *spinal stenosis* worsens with lumbar extension; thus many older patients with this condition report relief when leaning forward on a shopping cart. Backaches that worsen during or just after menstruation suggest a *gynecologic* cause. Back pain that is aggravated by recumbence or infection or that wakens the patient at night suggest malignancy.

AMELIORATING FACTORS

Inflammatory back pain often improves with exercise, whereas mechanical pain worsens. Many patients with an *acute lumbosacral strain* state that lying prone and motionless relieves the pain. Most acute back pain relieved by rest is of a mechanical origin. This fact can be a significant point in differential diagnosis in that it rules out the malingerer, the somaticizing patient, or a patient with strong secondary gain. Many patients with low back pain from *osteoarthritis* state that their pain diminishes when they lie on the floor or on a firm mattress. Likewise, some patients with disc syndrome are relieved by lying down. This variable is therefore not helpful in the differential diagnosis of low back pain. Some patients with *disc syndrome* inform the physician that they feel better when walking or lying on their sides with their knees flexed (fetal position). This latter finding strongly suggests that the pain is caused by disc disease. Patients with inflammatory, infectious, or tumorous spinal disease usually have constant pain in all positions.

The back discomfort from *irritable bowel syndrome* may be relieved by defecation. The pain of *spinal stenosis* improves with lumbar flexion.

PHYSICAL FINDINGS

The investigation of low back pain should include a general medical, personal, sociologic, occupational, and sexual history. Special attention should be paid to previous backaches and factors that precipitate, aggravate, or ameliorate the pain as well as to a history of trauma or heavy physical activity. This section outlines a satisfactory examination of a patient with low back pain. **Physical examination should include rectal and pelvic evaluations, especially in patients older than 40 years and in those without a history or physical findings characteristic of the common causes of backache.** Particular attention should be devoted to observations made during examination of the breast, prostate, thyroid, lymph nodes, and peripheral pulses. Any evidence of systemic inflammatory disease, such as iritis, urethritis, or arthritis, should be noted. Examination of the spine should include determination of range of motion anteriorly, posteriorly, and laterally as well as inspection for pelvic tilt.

Examination of the back should also include observation of the patient in the anatomic position, determination of range of motion of both the trunk and the lumbar spine, cervical flexion with and without trunk flexion, and gait. With the patient sitting, knee and ankle reflexes should be checked, as should extension of each leg. In teenagers with low back pain, a *one-legged hyperextension test* should be performed because the result may suggest a pars stress fracture or spondylolysis. In this test, the patient stands on the leg of the same side in which there is pain and gently leans back. If the pain is reproduced, this may indicate spondylolysis. The examiner should also determine the strength of dorsiflexion of the toes and ankles, sensation to touch and pinprick in the lower extremity, and integrity of proprioception (Figs. 3-1 to 3-4) while the patient is in this position.

With the patient supine, five tests should be performed: straight-leg raising, Lasègue's compression (Fig. 3-5), bowstring, knee compression, and pelvic pressure. The range of motion of hip joints must be established, and painful areas of extremities must be palpated. With the patient prone, the spine should be palpated, as should the sacroiliac joints; the hips should be hyperextended and the knees flexed.

Physical findings in the patient with *acute lumbosacral strain* are usually limited to the lower back, which demonstrates some limitation of motion. The patient may have local swelling and tenderness on palpation as well as spasm of the paraspinal muscles. Neurologic findings are normal, unlike with a herniated disc, which is often associated with spasm of the hamstring muscles and neurologic findings in the lower leg. Palpation over the sciatic notch may reveal pain or tenderness with some radiation to the knee or upper calf, but sensory and motor examination of the lower extremities is intact. The lumbar lordotic curve often increases and may change minimally with bending. The patient frequently has limited range of motion of the lower back, particularly anteriorly and posteriorly but not as much laterally. Although a straight-leg raising test may cause back pain, it does not induce pain with a sciatic distribution.

When *osteoarthritis* causes low back pain, the patient may have symmetrical restriction of movement, unlike that with a *herniated disc,* which usually causes

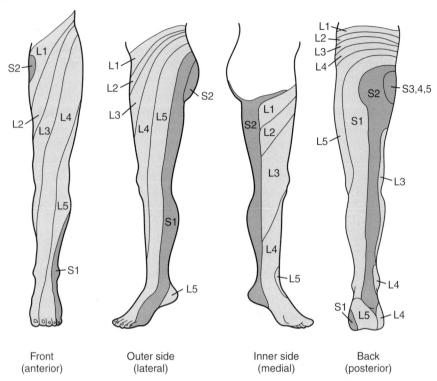

| | Front
(anterior) | Outer side
(lateral) | Inner side
(medial) | Back
(posterior) |

Figure 3-1. Dermatomes of skin. (From Lane F, ed: Medical Trial Technique Quarterly, 1980 annual issue, pp 456-466.)

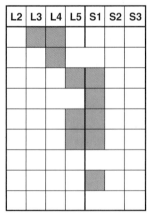

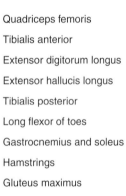

	L2	L3	L4	L5	S1	S2	S3
Quadriceps femoris		■	■				
Tibialis anterior			■				
Extensor digitorum longus				■			
Extensor hallucis longus				■			
Tibialis posterior			■	■			
Long flexor of toes					■		
Gastrocnemius and soleus					■	■	
Hamstrings				■	■		
Gluteus maximus				■	■		

Figure 3-2. Nerve supply of various muscles (main nerve roots are shaded). (From Lane F, ed: Medical Trial Technique Quarterly, 1980 annual issue, pp 456-466.)

asymmetrical limitation of motion. The patient may also have tenderness on palpation in the lumbosacral region or at L4, L5, or S1.

When low back pain results from *disc syndrome*, the physical findings often differ from those in a lumbosacral strain or osteoarthritis. Instead of increasing the lumbar lordotic curve, a disc syndrome usually reverses it, often with forward or lateral tilt or both. As with osteoarthritis and lumbosacral strain,

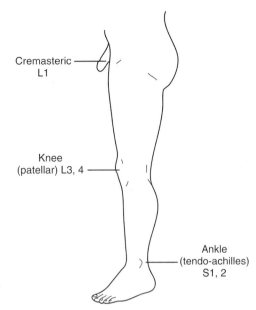

Figure 3-3. Root origin of reflexes.
(From Lane F, ed: Medical Trial Technique
Quarterly, 1980 annual issue, pp 456-466.)

spinal movement is limited with disc syndrome. The distinguishing features disc syndrome of are the production of sciatic pain after hyperextension or lateral tilt and diminution or absence of knee jerks. As with other causes of low back pain, the patient may have spasm of the paraspinal muscles and tenderness on palpation in the sciatic notch.

Restricted straight-leg raising implies root irritation and is suggestive but not diagnostic of a herniated disc. Positive results of crossed, straight-leg raising usually indicate a massive or central herniated disc or a mass lesion. The location of pain elicited by straight-leg raising often suggests the area of nerve root irritation. Pain in the back or lumbosacral region suggests a higher lesion than that for pain in the calf or along the distribution of the sciatic nerve. Another clue to a ruptured disc may be asymmetrical hamstring tightness.

Most patients with sciatic nerve root irritation, regardless of its cause, experience pain in the calf on straight-leg raising. They usually demonstrate Lasègue's sign as well.

Patients with herniated disc syndrome seldom represent a surgical emergency. Three basic factors influence the outcome of pressure on a nerve root: the amount of pressure on the nerve root, the duration of pressure, and the amount of myelin surrounding the nerve axon. Mild pressure with local edema and inflammation causes nerve root irritation, with some pain and paresthesias. Stretching of the root, which occurs with the straight-leg raising or Lasègue's test, aggravates the pain. With increased pressure the patient has impaired conduction, motor weakness, reflex diminution, and some sensory loss in addition to pain. Severe pressure produces marked motor paralysis, loss of reflexes, and anesthesia. Mild to moderate pressure for short periods is tolerated fairly well by myelinated fibers. However, prolonged pressure is poorly tolerated, particularly

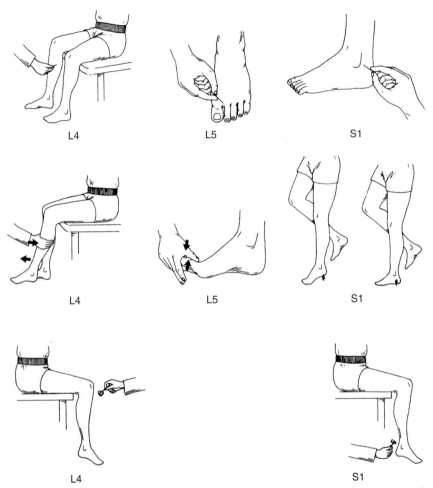

Figure 3-4. Neurologic screening examination of lower extremity in patients with low back pain. (From Birnbaum JS: The Musculoskeletal Manual, 2nd ed. Philadelphia, WB Saunders Co, 1986, p 124.)

by minimally myelinated nerves. If paralysis after compression of myelinated fibers persists for 24 hours, it may be irreversible. Myelin protects nerves from compression; however, the central parasympathetic nerve fibers to sphincters are unmyelinated. Therefore, loss of sphincter tone or urinary retention is a surgical emergency. If pressure on these unmyelinated fibers is not relieved immediately, permanent damage may ensue.

DIAGNOSTIC STUDIES

In patients with osteoarthritis or a mechanical cause of their low back pain, the erythrocyte sedimentation rate (ESR) and alkaline phosphatase (ALP) value are within normal limits. The ESR is elevated in *multiple myeloma, infectious spinal*

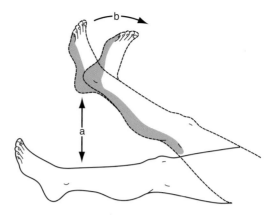

Figure 3-5. Sciatic nerve stretch test. Examiner uses Lasègue's test *(a)* to invoke pain down leg by raising limb with knee extended. If this fails to induce pain, compression of posterior tibial nerve in lateral popliteal space is painful if there is nerve root involvement, or pain may be invoked by sharp dorsiflexion of foot (Bragard's test) *(b)*. (From Jacobs B: American Family Physician, October 1978, p 13 [monograph].)

disease, and *ankylosing spondylitis.* The alkaline phosphatase value is elevated in patients with *Paget's disease.*

Plain radiography is most helpful in children and adolescents, although it is seldom indicated in otherwise healthy patients ages 20 to 50 years who present with acute low back pain. For patients with nonspecific low back pain, current guidelines recommend against routine imaging. Structures such as muscles, ligaments, and discs are often responsible for back pain but are not visualized on plain films. Radiographic examination has normal findings or may show increased lumbar lordosis in patients with acute lumbosacral or low back strain. When osteoarthritis causes low back pain, radiography frequently shows narrowing of the lumbar spaces, with spurring and often sclerosis of the vertebrae. Radiography may assist in the diagnosis of compression fractures, cancer, Paget's disease, and multiple myeloma.

Magnetic resonance imaging (MRI) is the most sensitive test for herniated discs and the most comprehensive way of evaluating degenerative changes and detecting tumors, fibrosis, cysts, and arachnoiditis. Computed tomography (CT) scans (with or without contrast media) are helpful in locating herniated discs and spinal tumors; however, current guidelines prefer MRI over computed tomography unless MRI is contraindicated or unavailable. **Imaging studies should be used not to make a diagnosis but to confirm one made by history and physical examination.** These studies should be performed after 7 weeks of conservative management in patients with low back pain unless evidence of a motor, sensory, reflex, sphincter, or autonomic deficit is present or if major trauma, infection, or neoplasia is suspected. Selective nerve root injections may also be helpful as a diagnostic tool in evaluating spinal pain with radicular features.

LESS COMMON DIAGNOSTIC CONSIDERATIONS

Although most backaches are caused by lumbosacral strain, disc disease, osteoarthritis, or postural backache, innumerable less common causes exist. Backaches can result from disease of almost any system and have been classified as viscerogenic, vascular, neurogenic, psychogenic, spondylogenic, genitourinary, musculoskeletal, and secondary to metastatic or primary tumors of bone or soft tissue. They also may be caused by functional-mechanical derangement in the musculoskeletal system resulting from poor posture or obesity. Back pain in children is a rare complaint and may have a serious organic cause. In older patients in whom back pain is a major complaint, particularly if it is the first attack, the physician must consider serious diseases such as metabolic disorders (osteoporosis, osteomalacia, chondrocalcinosis, Paget's disease); compression fractures; infections; and metastatic cancer from the breast, lung, or prostate. Infection and cancer are the most common diseases that cause back pain.

Ankylosing spondylitis most often occurs in young to middle-aged males. It has an insidious onset and lasts at least 3 months. Classically, it is associated with marked morning stiffness. In contrast to more common causes of backache, ankylosing spondylitis is associated with a significantly elevated ESR and, rarely, with fever. There may be a family history of the same illness. Other joints may be involved, and the pain is frequently worse at night. The HLA-B27 test result is seldom positive. Fifty percent of patients with ankylosing spondylitis experience transient arthritis of larger peripheral joints; sometimes they have conjunctivitis or urethritis.

Vertebral fractures, or *compression fractures,* may occur with severe trauma or more often with osteoporosis of the vertebrae in elderly patients. In these patients, vertebral fractures may occur after minor trauma. They also can occur after prolonged immobilization or steroid use. The back pain is usually at the level of the fracture and radiates locally across the back and around the trunk but seldom into the lower extremities. Vertebral fractures occur more frequently in the middle and lower dorsal spine. Radiography is useful in confirming the diagnosis.

Infectious diseases of the spine, more common in children and IV drug users, also cause backaches. Many patients with such infections have an elevated ESR and may be febrile. An infectious cause of backache should be considered in cachectic individuals or patients undergoing prolonged steroid or immunosuppressive therapy. Uncommon causes of disc space infection include actinomycosis, tuberculosis, brucellosis, and fungal infections.

Neoplastic disease can cause backache, particularly in elderly patients. Although primary neoplasms are rare, myeloma and metastatic disease are more common. In a patient with known cancer, the onset of back pain should suggest spinal metastasis. Metastatic carcinoma is more common in older patients and should be particularly suspected if they have a history of cancer. Often, after an insidious onset, waist-level or midback pain becomes progressively more severe and more persistent. The pain is usually not relieved by lying down and frequently worsens at night. Unexplained weight loss with severe back pain aggravated by rest should suggest metastatic carcinoma in the spine. Multiple myeloma can cause severe, unremitting backaches; these are present at rest and may worsen with recumbency. This diagnosis can be confirmed by radiographic findings in the spine, pelvis, or skull; elevated ESR; and abnormal serum protein electrophoretic patterns.

Differential Diagnosis of Backache

CONDITION	NATURE OF PATIENT	NATURE OF SYMPTOMS AND LOCATION OF PAIN	ASSOCIATED SYMPTOMS	PRECIPITATING AND AGGRAVATING FACTORS	AMELIORATING FACTORS	PHYSICAL FINDINGS	DIAGNOSTIC STUDIES
Acute lumbosacral strain	Adults (ages 20-50 yr): especially those who do strenuous work Children: often caused by trauma or sports	Sudden onset Pain usually localized to lumbosacral region		Precipitated by lifting, twisting, and unusual physical activity Aggravated by motion but not by coughing or straining	Lying prone and motionless	Neurologic findings negative Paraspinal muscle spasm and pain Straight leg raising causes back but not leg pain Limitation of motion in lumbosacral region anteriorly and posteriorly Increased lumbar lordosis	Usually not indicated
Postural backache (low back strain)	Obese, physically unfit adults	Vague low back pain Difficult to locate point of maximum pain Occasional radiation into buttocks		Worsens as day progresses		Neurologic findings negative Limitation of motion anteriorly and posteriorly Increased lumbar lordosis Straight-leg raising causes back pain, not leg pain	
Degenerative lumbosacral arthritis	Older than 50 yr	Gradual onset, not precipitated by physical activity Lumbosacral spine motion limited Pain worse in morning Pain radiation into leg uncommon	Often arthritis in other joints	Aggravated by lateral bending and extension of lumbar spine	Lying on back on floor Better 2 hr after arising	Neurologic findings negative Symmetrical restriction of movement	Radiograph shows disc space narrowing and spurring

Continued

Differential Diagnosis of Backache—cont'd

CONDITION	NATURE OF PATIENT	NATURE OF SYMPTOMS AND LOCATION OF PAIN	ASSOCIATED SYMPTOMS	PRECIPITATING AND AGGRAVATING FACTORS	AMELIORATING FACTORS	PHYSICAL FINDINGS	DIAGNOSTIC STUDIES
Lumbar disc disease	More common in males age 40 yr or older Rare in children	Sudden onset, previous episodes less severe Pain often radiates down posterolateral aspect of leg Buttock pain or paresthesia pain, possibly lancinating or resembling pain of severe toothache	Hypesthesia Dysesthesia Weakness of some leg muscles	Coughing Sneezing Hyperextension of lumbar spine	Lying on side with knees flexed	Neurologic signs in lower leg Asymmetrical limitation of motion Hamstring spasm Tender on palpation in sciatic notch Reversal of lumbar lordotic curve Forward or lateral tilt Pain of sciatic distribution after hyperextension of lateral tilt Restricted straight-leg raising	MRI CT scan
Chronic low back pain	All ages	Pain lasts longer than 6 mo Symptoms and disability dissociated from physical findings	Psychological and social dysfunction	Trauma of sciatica may be initial event	Few	Few	Findings usually negative Abnormalities demonstrated may not represent cause of pain
Spinal stenosis	More common in elderly males	Gradual onset Often mimics intermittent claudication, except pain usually in buttocks or thighs Often bilateral		Pain worse with spinal extension Exercise Not precipitated by exercise with spine flexed (e.g., bicycling)	Spinal flexion Pain slowly improves with cessation of walking	Polyradiculopathy Good pedal pulses	MRI CT scan

Differential Diagnosis of Backache—cont'd

CONDITION	NATURE OF PATIENT	NATURE OF SYMPTOMS AND LOCATION OF PAIN	ASSOCIATED SYMPTOMS	PRECIPITATING AND AGGRAVAT-ING FACTORS	AMELIO-RATING FACTORS	PHYSICAL FINDINGS	DIAGNOSTIC STUDIES
Gynecologic disorders			Vaginal discharge	Worse around menstruation or ovulation	Lying supine with knees flexed	Abnormal pelvic examination	
Prostatitis	Older men	Constant low back pain	Urinary hesitancy	Change in sexual frequency		Prostate tender on palpation No limitation of back motion No muscle spasm	White blood cells in prostatic secretion
Irritable bowel	Young women Stressed individuals	Pain occurs in midback	Mucus in stools Abdominal pain	Stress	Defecation	Colon tender on palpation	
Depression	Adults	Severity of pain varies with mental state Diffuse pressure-like pain	Early-morning wakefulness Fatigue Constipation Anorexia	Some "loss" or other event		Depressed affect	
Neoplasm (usually backache caused by metastases)	History of cancer, especially of breast and prostate First episode of backache occurs after age 50 yr	Gradual onset of pain, weight loss	Weight loss	May be worse lying down	Not relieved by recumbency	Rectal, pelvic, or breast examination may reveal primary tumor	Radiographs CT scan MRI
Herpes zoster	Elderly patients	Superficial burning pain	Herpetic lesions appear after onset of pain			Herpetic vesicles	

Continued

Differential Diagnosis of Backache—cont'd

CONDITION	NATURE OF PATIENT	NATURE OF SYMPTOMS AND LOCATION OF PAIN	ASSOCIATED SYMPTOMS	PRECIPITATING AND AGGRAVATING FACTORS	AMELIO-RATING FACTORS	PHYSICAL FINDINGS	DIAGNOSTIC STUDIES
Fracture	Older patients Osteoporosis	Usually sudden onset Pain at level of fracture		Trauma; minor trauma in osteoporotic patients and patients receiving long-term corticosteroids		May have palpable swelling at site of vertebral fracture	Radiographs

CT, Computed tomography; *MRI,* magnetic resonance imaging.

The back pain of *acute pancreatitis* is invariably associated with marked gastrointestinal symptoms. However, chronic low-grade pancreatitis may cause vague back pain without noticeable abdominal symptoms. Patients with posterior penetrating *ulcers* may have pain in the high midback as their chief complaint. This pain is usually not in the lumbar area and is occasionally relieved by antacids. Frequently, the patient has tenderness on epigastric palpation. Pain can be referred to the back from the urinary tract, uterus, prostate, and retroperitoneal structures.

Spinal stenosis can cause central low back pain that may radiate into one or both legs. The pain has the character of intermittent claudication: the patient is forced to rest after walking one or two blocks. An important diagnostic feature is that the pain is also relieved by flexion of the spine. It may occur at night, and the patient may find relief by walking, especially in a stooped position.

Spondylolisthesis and *spondylolysis* occur infrequently in the general population but are common causes of back pain in growing individuals. These conditions are caused by repetitive flexion and extension forces, particularly in congenitally predisposed individuals, and are more common in gymnasts and football linemen. The pain is severe, worse with activity, and relieved by rest. Diagnosis is confirmed by appropriate radiographic studies.

Selected References

American College of Radiology: *ACR Appropriateness Criteria*, :Available at http://www.acr.org/SecondaryMainMenuCategories/quality_safety/app_criteria.aspx/.

Bernstein RM, Cozen H: Evaluation of back pain in children and adolescents, *Am Fam Physician* 76:1669-1676, 2007.

Bhangle SD, Sapru S, Panush RS: Back pain made simple: an approach based on principles and evidence, *Cleve Clin J Med* 76:393-399, 2009.

Broder J, Snarski JT: "Back pain in the elderly.", *Clin Geriatr Med* 23:271-289, 2007.

Bueff HU, Van Der Reis W: Low back pain, *Prim Care* 23:345-364, 1996.

Chou R, Qaseem A, Snow V, et al: Diagnosis and treatment of low back pain: a joint clinical practice guideline from the American College of Physicians and the American Pain Society. [Erratum appears in Ann Intern Med. 5;148:247–8, 2008.]

Datta S, Everett CR, Trescot AM, et al: An updated systematic review of the diagnostic utility of selective nerve root blocks, *Pain Physician* 10:113-128, 2007.

Glancy GL: Diagnoses and treatment of back pain in children and adolescents: an update, *Adv Pediatr* 53:22-240, 2006.

MacDonald J, D'Hemecourt P: Back pain in the adolescent athlete, *Pediatr Ann* 36:703-712, 2007.

Rosomoff HL, Rosomoff RS: Low back pain: evaluation and management in the primary care setting, *Med Clin North Am* 83:643-663, 1999.

Siemionow K, McLain RF: When back pain is not benign: a concise guide to differential diagnosis, *Postgrad Med* 119:62-69, 2007.

Siemionow K, Steinmetz M, Bell G, et al: Identifying serious causes of back pain: cancer, infection, fracture, *Cleve Clin J Med* 75:557-566, 2008.

Sieper J, van der Heijde D, Landewé R, et al: New criteria for inflammatory back pain in patients with chronic back pain: a real patient exercise by experts from the Assessment of SpondyloArthritis international Society (ASAS), *Ann Rheum Dis* 68:784-788, 2009.

Swenson R: Differential diagnosis: a reasonable clinical approach, *Neurol Clin North Am* 17:43-63, 1999.

Winters ME, Kluetz P, Zilberstein J: Back pain emergencies, *Med Clin North Am* 90:505-523, 2006.

Belching, Bloating, and Flatulence

4

In this chapter, *belching* is defined as the eructation of gas through the mouth; *bloating* is gaseous abdominal distention; and *flatulence* is the passage of intestinal gas through the rectum.

BELCHING

Belching is not a symptom of organic disease. The only cause of belching is the swallowing of air *(aerophagia)*. Air is swallowed or, more accurately, sucked into the stomach and released in the form of a belch. Air swallowing may occur with eating or drinking; more air is swallowed with liquids than with solids. Aerophagia also occurs as a conscious or, more often, an unconscious nervous habit unassociated with food ingestion. It can also be associated with mouth breathing, gum chewing, orthodontic appliances, and poorly fitting dentures. Chronic, repetitive, *unintentional* belching is usually caused by repetitive inhalation of air and its regurgitation from the stomach or esophagus in the form of a belch. Some patients who demonstrate these findings consciously or unconsciously relax the upper esophageal sphincter during inspiration. Belching occurs in patients with dyspepsia and may be an uncommon sign of gastroesophageal reflux. It cannot be used to differentiate between them.

Nature of Patient
Excessive belchers tend to be nervous, anxious, and tense. Belching is often normal in infants, although excessive belching may be the result of excessive air swallowing during feeding. If the seal of the infant's lips is inadequate around the real or artificial nipple, air may be ingested during nursing. This may be exaggerated if during feeding the child is held in a position that is too horizontal.

Some patients with gastric or biliary disorders develop a habit of trying to relieve abdominal discomfort by swallowing (sometimes unconsciously) air and belching it up again; they believe that this provides some relief from their abdominal discomfort.

If associated pathology can be confidently ruled out, patients must be reassured that nothing serious is wrong. It may help to describe how a patient with a laryngectomy can be trained to swallow air; accordingly, a patient with a belching problem can be *un*trained. Simply instructing some patients not to belch when they feel the urge to do so may gradually stop their habit of swallowing air and belching it back. Antifoaming agents have not been particularly helpful. Instead, patients should be instructed to avoid chewing gum, eating quickly, smoking, and drinking carbonated beverages.

Associated Symptoms

The most common associated symptom is abdominal distention, representing gas in the stomach. Most swallowed air that is not belched up is reabsorbed in the small intestine. Usually, intestinal gas is derived by fermentation of intestinal contents. Some patients who swallow large amounts of air may experience or perceive abdominal discomfort until they belch. An urge to belch accompanied by chest pain on belching is a rare finding that may indicate an inferior wall myocardial infarction.

Precipitating and Aggravating Factors

The most common precipitating factor is air swallowing and subsequent relaxation of the esophageal sphincter to produce a belch. Nervous concern about belching can initiate a vicious circle of unconscious air swallowing and more belching. For some individuals, a supine position prevents swallowed gastric air from escaping into the esophagus, and an upright position facilitates belching. *Emotional stress* increases the likelihood of air swallowing. Ingestion of carbonated beverages, gum chewing, and poorly fitting dentures may also aggravate belching.

Diagnostic Studies

Although belching is invariably caused by swallowing air, this fact does not rule out coexisting unrelated pathology. If other symptoms warrant further tests, cholecystography, upper gastrointestinal (GI) studies, and chest radiography should be considered.

Less Common Diagnostic Considerations

Oral eructation of intestinal gas rarely occurs. In patients with this condition, the odor is offensive, resembling that of methane or hydrogen sulfide. It suggests fermentation in stagnating gastric contents secondary to gastroparesis, vagotomy, or pyloric obstruction from an ulcer or tumor.

BLOATING AND FLATULENCE

Bloating and flatulence are two common complaints reported to physicians. The problem has been recognized since the time of Hippocrates, who taught that "passing gas is necessary to well-being." In the days of early Rome, it was noted that "all Roman citizens shall be allowed to pass gas whenever necessary." Because swallowed air is reabsorbed in the small bowel, most of the gas in the distal small bowel and colon is produced within the bowel by fermentation. Small-bowel bacterial overgrowth can lead to malabsorption syndrome characterized by flatulence, diarrhea, chronic abdominal pain, and bloating; symptoms are often seen in patients with irritable bowel syndrome. In most instances, flatulence is not of any clinical significance, but because various pathologic conditions may be associated with it, their presence should be investigated if the flatulence is excessive.

Bloating may be caused by gaseous distention of the stomach, small bowel, or colon. This condition occurs more frequently in patients with *gastroparesis, malabsorption* of various sugars and fat, and *colonic bacterial fermentation* of unabsorbed foods. In some patients, disturbed visceral motility and increased sensitivity to normal luminal distention may cause the sensation of bloating.

Flatulence is usually caused by excessive production of gas (in the large bowel and less frequently in the small bowel) in an otherwise normal individual or increased discomfort from normal amounts of abdominal gas in healthy individuals. If bloating and flatulence have persisted for several years without the development of signs of serious organic pathology (e.g., weight loss, ascites, jaundice), the patient can be reassured that the flatulence is not of great clinical significance. However, it must always be remembered that some patients with *gallbladder disease, colon carcinoma, irritable bowel syndrome, diverticulitis,* and *diverticulosis* may present with a chief complaint of abdominal discomfort, bloating, and, occasionally, flatulence. Patients with colon carcinoma may present with vague abdominal discomfort or distention.

Nature of Patient

Flatulence is particularly common in infants up to age 3 months. This condition, referred to as *3-month colic,* is caused by immature nervous control of the gut, which permits gas to become trapped in bowel loops.

Malabsorption may lead to excessive fermentation of unabsorbed nutrients; this may produce an increase in flatulence. It can occur in patients with pancreatic insufficiency, pancreatic carcinoma, biliary disease, celiac disease, or bacterial overgrowth in the small intestine.

Native Americans and other patients, particularly of African or Mediterranean descent, who complain of excessive bloating or flatulence may have malabsorption and subsequent fermentation due to *lactose intolerance.* Lactose intolerance does not usually occur in infants or preschool children unless a lactase deficiency develops secondary to other disorders, such as bacterial or viral infections of the small bowel, giardiasis, or sensitivity to cow's milk or gluten (celiac disease). This diagnosis is confirmed if diarrhea develops or if the bloating or flatulence is exacerbated after ingestion of a lactose load (found in milk, ice cream, and other dairy products).

Flatulence may also be seen in patients with *diverticulitis* or *diverticulosis*. Flatulence is common in patients on a diet high in fiber or legumes, often recommended for hypercholesterolemia.

Nature of Symptoms

Most gas that passes from the rectum has an unpleasant, foul odor. The gases that cause this odor are produced by intestinal bacteria. Because of their odor, these gases are detectable in minute quantities. Lactose malabsorption and lactase deficiency can cause abdominal pain; distention; flatulence; and loose, watery stools—symptoms similar to those of irritable bowel syndrome. **Although irritable bowel syndrome is more common, lactose intolerance must always be considered because its management is simple and effective.**

Associated Symptoms

Flatulence of no clinical significance may be associated with abdominal distention, bloating, borborygmi, abdominal discomfort, and cramping pain. When flatulence or bloating occurs, moderate abdominal pain may be involved, even in the absence of organic disease. Patients may be unable to obtain relief by passing flatus. In some individuals, this state is caused by disordered motility of the gut; it cannot propel the gas forward through the bowel. This is not caused by an increased volume of gas but rather by the patient's inability to propel the gut gas forward. Some individuals have an exaggerated pain response to bowel distention despite a normal volume of intestinal gas.

Diverticulitis should be suspected if flatulence is accompanied by lower abdominal pain, constipation, or diarrhea. *Giardiasis* should be suspected as the cause of flatulence, particularly if it is accompanied by foul-smelling, watery, or semisolid stools or abdominal distention.

Precipitating and Aggravating Factors

The symptoms of bloating and flatulence are exacerbated by the ingestion of nonabsorbable or incompletely absorbable carbohydrates, including sorbitol, a sugar used as a noncaloric sweetener for candy and other dietetic foods. These carbohydrates provide a substrate for the intestinal bacterial production of carbon dioxide and hydrogen.

Flatulogenic foods include milk, ice cream, and other dairy products; onions; dry beans; celery; carrots; raisins; bananas; apricots; prune juice; apple juice; many vegetables; pretzels; bagels; wheat germ; Brussels sprouts; and fiber. Bloating and flatulence may develop in patients with a lactase deficiency from ingestion of many dairy products. The flatulogenic properties of these foods vary greatly among individuals.

Constipation may also aggravate the symptoms of abdominal distention. This process can be explained by the increased smooth muscle spasm in the colon around the gas bubbles. **Although constipation may aggravate abdominal bloating, diarrhea does not usually relieve such distention.**

Many patients with *gas entrapment syndromes* experience a worsening of the pain when bending over to tie their shoes or when wearing tight garments. Occasionally, this pain is exacerbated by flexion of the leg on the abdomen.

Ameliorating Factors

Factors that may be associated with decreasing symptoms are diets low in indigestible carbohydrates or lactose, avoidance of reclining after meals, exercise, and ingestion of buttermilk or broad-spectrum antibiotics. Passage of flatus often relieves the sensation of abdominal bloating, at least temporarily. Any abdominal pain syndrome that is greatly relieved by passage of flatus should suggest gas entrapment.

Physical Findings

When gas is trapped in the splenic flexure, palpation of the left upper quadrant (LUQ) can cause abdominal pain or pain in the chest (pseudoangina). With gas entrapment in the hepatic flexure, the pain is most frequently in the right upper quadrant (RUQ) and may simulate gallbladder discomfort.

Diagnostic Studies

The physician should consider the following studies when appropriate: upper and lower gastrointestinal radiographic examination, colonoscopy, cholecystography, and stool analysis for fat and occult blood. If these tests do not reveal organic disease, the patient should be reassured, and dietary modification recommended. Likewise, a diagnostic trial of a lactose load can be used to determine presumptively whether a lactase deficiency is present. If the load exacerbates bloating, flatulence, or diarrhea, the patient should avoid foods with lactose. Analysis of breath hydrogen before and after a lactose load is a more specific test for lactase insufficiency. Hydrogen breath tests may also be used to diagnose intestinal bacterial overgrowth. In patients in whom celiac disease is suspected, endomysial antibodies, tissue transglutaminase and total IgA should be measured.

More complicated tests can be performed, such as D-xylose absorption, mucosal biopsy, and the analysis of flatus for the volume and composition of the various intestinal gases. Large quantities of carbon dioxide or hydrogen suggest malabsorption and fermentation of nonabsorbable carbohydrates, such as fruits and beans. Lactase deficiency can also lead to excessive quantities of hydrogen in the flatus.

Less Common Diagnostic Considerations

Incomplete or intermittent bowel obstruction, malabsorption syndromes, small-bowel diverticula, maldigestion due to pancreatic or biliary disease, and short-bowel syndrome may cause bloating or flatulence.

Differential Diagnosis of Belching, Bloating, and Flatulence

CONDITION	NATURE OF PATIENT	NATURE OF SYMPTOMS	ASSOCIATED SYMPTOMS	PRECIPITATING AND AGGRAVATING FACTORS	AMELIORATING FACTORS	PHYSICAL FINDINGS	DIAGNOSTIC STUDIES
Belching							
Aerophagia	Nursing infants Nervous, anxious, and tense children and adults	Occurs with eating or drinking Conscious or unconscious nervous habit	Abdominal distention	Infants: nursing while in horizontal position Mouth breathing Gum chewing Orthodontic appliances Emotional stress Poorly fitting dentures Supine position Gastric or biliary disorders	Behavior modification: avoidance of gum chewing, eating quickly, smoking, and drinking carbonated beverages Upright position	Those of gas in stomach	
Bloating and Flatulence							
Excessive intestinal bacterial fermentation causing increased gas	Most common cause at any age, especially in elderly adults	Flatulence Bloating	Abdominal discomfort or pain	Ingestion of non-absorbable carbohydrates, onions, bananas, ice cream	Avoidance of all carbohydrates, particularly non-absorbable ones Passage of flatus		hydrogen breath test
Increased awareness of normal amount of gas							
Malabsorption	Pancreatic insufficiency Pancreatic carcinoma Biliary disease Celiac disease Bacterial overgrowth in small intestine	Increased flatulence	Diarrhea	Nonabsorbable carbohydrates		Greasy, foul-smelling stools	Stool analysis GI radiographs / ultrasound/ CT scan, endomysial abs/tissue trans gluta-minase/IgA

Continued

Differential Diagnosis of Belching, Bloating, and Flatulence—cont'd

CONDITION	NATURE OF PATIENT	NATURE OF SYMPTOMS	ASSOCIATED SYMPTOMS	PRECIPITATING AND AGGRAVATING FACTORS	AMELIORATING FACTORS	PHYSICAL FINDINGS	DIAGNOSTIC STUDIES
Lactase deficiency	Common in patients of African or Mediterranean descent and Native Americans	Bloating Excess flatulence	Diarrhea Occasional abdominal pain	Lactose load (from dairy products)	Avoidance of lactose Lactase supplement	Abdominal distention	Mucosal biopsy Lactose load Hydrogen breath test
Giardiasis	Campers and hikers at higher risk	Increased flatulence	Abdominal distention Watery diarrhea, often foul-smelling	Drinking water infested with *Giardia*			Stool analysis for *Giardia* Duodenal aspirate for *Giardia*
Gas entrapment:							
Splenic flexure			Pseudoangina	Abdominal pain worsened by bending or wearing tight garments	Passage of flatus	LUQ pain on palpation Pain worsened by flexion of left leg on abdomen	Fluoroscopy for trapped gas
Hepatic flexure			Pain resembling gallbladder discomfort		Passage of flatus	RUQ pain on palpation Pain worsened by flexion of right leg on abdomen	

GI, Gastrointestinal; *LUQ,* left upper quadrant; *RUQ,* right upper quadrant.

Selected References

Agrawal A, Whorwell PJ: Review article: abdominal bloating and distension in functional gastrointestinal disorders: epidemiology and exploration of possible mechanisms, *Aliment Pharmacol Ther Jan 1* 27:2-10, 2008.

Antao B, Lavin V, Shawis R: Repetitive eructation (belching in children): is it pathological? *Int J Adolesc Med Health* 18:649-651, 2006.

Bouchier IAD: Flatulence, *Practitioner* 224:373-377, 1980.

Clearfield HR: Clinical intestinal gas syndromes, *Prim Care* 23:621-628, 1996.

Gasbarrini A, Lauritano EC, Gabrielli M, et al: Small intestinal bacterial overgrowth: diagnosis and treatment, *Dig Dis* 25:237-240, 2007.

Levitt MD, Bond JH: Flatulence, *Annu Rev Med* 31:127-137, 1980.

Rao SSC: Belching, bloating and flatulence, *Postgrad Med* 101:263-278, 1997.

Raskin JB: Intestinal gas, *Geriatrics* 38:77-93, 1983.

Shaw AD, Davies GJ: Lactose intolerance: problems in diagnosis and treatment, *J Clin Gastroenterol* 28:208-216, 1999.

Suarez F, Levitt MD: Abdominal symptoms and lactose: the discrepancy between patients' claims and the results of blinded trials, *Am J Clin Nutr* 64:251-252, 1996.

Van Ness MM, Cattau EL: Flatulence: pathophysiology and treatment, *Am Fam Physician* 31:198-208, 1985.

Breast Lumps

5

Over their lifetimes, most women detect a lump in the breast. Approximately 80% of breast masses are discovered by the patient before mammography or physician examination. Most of these lumps are benign cysts. A woman's estimated lifetime risk for development of breast cancer is 12%. Five-year relative survival is 98% for localized disease, 84% for regional disease, and 23% for distant-stage disease. In 2008, 40,480 breast cancer deaths occurred in the United States. Therefore, it is crucial to be able to separate benign from malignant lesions promptly. The main cause of delayed diagnosis is inappropriate reassurance that a mass is benign without the performance of a biopsy.

Benign breast disease is a continuum of entities, from fibroadenoma and cysts with atypia to cystic changes with marked atypia. The most common breast lesions are *fibrocystic breasts, fibroadenomas, breast cancer, mastitis* (especially in lactating women), *fat necrosis,* and *gynecomastia,* which by definition occurs only in males. Breast lumps occur in as many as 50% of premenopausal women. Most of these lumps are benign, but because breast cancer is part of the differential diagnosis, this is a problem of great concern.

Breast lumps are masses in the breast noted on physical examination and may be either benign or malignant. *Benign breast disease* is a pathologic diagnosis and usually applies to masses that have undergone tissue sampling. It includes fibrocystic disease; fibroadenoma; and uncommon conditions such as mastitis, lipoma, traumatic fat necrosis, and galactocele. At biopsy, 90% to 95% of all benign breast disease is found to be fibrocystic or fibroadenoma. *Fibrocystic disease* is a poorly defined group of pathologic breast lesions that includes cysts, fibrosis, adenosis, ductal ectasia, hyperplasia, and papilloma.

NATURE OF PATIENT

Breast masses are rare in children and are seen more often in adolescents, but malignancy is rare in both groups. Benign breast disease is common in women younger than 30 years. Of women with benign breast disease, 45% have fibrocystic disease, whereas about 45% have fibroadenomas. In those with benign breast disease after age 30 years, 85% have fibrocystic breasts, and 10% have

58

fibroadenomas. In other words, fibroadenomas become less common with increasing age. Breast cysts are uncommon in elderly patients, but 50% of the patients in whom they occur are using estrogen supplements.

Menstrual status, previous history of breast-feeding, parity, family medical history, and drug use are also important in assessing the risk of breast cancer. Users of oral contraceptives have a lower incidence of breast cancer. Factors that increase the risk for breast cancer include a mother or sister who had breast cancer, early menarche, late menopause, and nulliparity. There is twice the risk of breast cancer in a patient whose mother or sister had breast cancer and three times the risk if both the mother and sister had breast cancer. Also, a rare genetic type of familial breast cancer appears to be inherited as an autosomal dominant trait. Other factors that increase the risk for breast cancer are age greater than 50 years, first pregnancy after age 35, obesity, and benign proliferative breast disease (ductal and lobular hyperplasia or atypia).

Gynecomastia is normal in the neonatal period, during puberty, and in older men. It also occurs in certain familial syndromes and various pathologic states (cirrhosis, prolactinoma, ulcerative colitis, prostatic and testicular carcinoma, orchitis, cryptorchidism) and among users of many drugs (angiotensin-converting enzyme [ACE] inhibitors, lansoprazole, spironolactone, H_2 antagonists, and anabolic steroids). Gynecomastia in neonates is probably related to the high levels of estrogen in the placental and fetal circulation. In neonatal gynecomastia, involvement is usually bilateral, and fluid may occasionally be expressed from the nipple. Gynecomastia develops in 40% of pubertal boys (ages 13-14 years). When bilateral and mild, it may be diagnosed by the physician, but the patient and family do not recognize it unless it is marked. Unilateral gynecomastia is a more frequent patient complaint. Generally, gynecomastia can be diagnosed by physical examination. If physical findings are not certain, then men should be referred for diagnostic mammography. Breast cancer in men accounts for 1% of all breast cancers. At presentation, more than 40% of men with breast malignancy have stage III or IV disease; therefore, any mass suspicious for malignancy in men should be referred directly for tissue sampling.

Prevalence of breast cancer in pregnancy is approximately 3 in 10,000 pregnancies, accounting for approximately 3% of all breast cancers. Therefore, imaging of a breast lump should not be postponed in pregnancy.

NATURE OF SYMPTOMS

The most common breast complaints are nipple discharge, breast pain, and a lump in the breast. Nipple discharge, usually bilateral, can be caused by drugs such as oral contraceptives and phenothiazines. Discharges that are unilateral, pink or bloody, nonmilky, or associated with a mass are suggestive of cancer.

Fibroadenoma is the most common breast lump that occurs during adolescence, but because it is asymptomatic, it is usually detected on physical examination by the patient or physician. These lumps are usually single, unilateral, and located in the upper outer quadrant, although they may be multiple or bilateral in 25% of patients. Fibroadenomas do not vary in size with the menstrual cycle, whereas the lumps of fibrocystic breast disease often enlarge premenstrually.

ASSOCIATED SYMPTOMS

Pain in the breast *(mastodynia)* in young women suggests fibrocystic disease, especially if the pain is bilateral and increases premenstrually. **Pain in one breast in postmenopausal women is highly suggestive of a malignant process.** Cyclic breast pain that increases premenstrually suggests a benign condition, especially fibrocystic breast disease. Mastodynia may also be caused by papillomas, sclerosing adenosis, ductal ectasia, sporadic puerperal mastitis, breast lipomas, traumatic fat necrosis, and galactoceles. Other causes of chest wall pain include pectoral or intercostal muscle sprain, mastitis, costochondral separation, and costochondritis.

If the lump is fixed to the skin or if nipple discharge or axillary adenopathy is present, cancer is probable. Although nipple discharge, particularly if it is bloody, suggests cancer, it occasionally occurs with fibrocystic disease and in males with adrenogenital syndrome.

If lactation is associated with a breast lump, *prolactinoma* or pregnancy should be suspected.

PRECIPITATING AND AGGRAVATING FACTORS

Risk factors for breast cancer have been discussed earlier in this chapter. The pain and tenderness of fibrocystic breasts often worsen during the premenstrual period. Gynecomastia is exacerbated by several drugs, including marijuana, spironolactone, methyldopa, phenytoin, cimetidine, finasteride, diazepam, tricyclic antidepressants, phenothiazines, histamine H_2-receptor blockers, and digitalis. Fat necrosis may be precipitated by external trauma as well as surgical trauma.

AMELIORATING FACTORS

Cyst size is reduced and pain decreases in patients with fibrocystic breast disease when they become menopausal. Oral contraceptives, pregnancy, and reduction in the ingestion of methylxanthines contained in coffee, tea, cola, and chocolate also often alleviate the symptoms of fibrocystic disease.

PHYSICAL FINDINGS

Typically cancers are firm, have indistinct borders, and have attachments to the skin or deep fascia with dimpling or nipple retraction. Benign lesions are typically discrete with well-defined margins. They are usually mobile. Unfortunately, cysts cannot be reliably differentiated from solid masses on physical examination.

Fibroadenomas are usually unilateral and occur in the upper outer quadrant. They usually manifest as smooth, oval, occasionally irregular 3- to 4-cm firm to elastic lumps that are freely movable. Fibrocystic disease is usually bilateral and symmetrical, with multiple tender, soft, or cystic round lumps that have regular borders. They are occasionally single or unilateral. In contrast, malignant breast lumps are typically hard; irregular; fixed; and associated with a nipple lesion or discharge, adenopathy, and occasionally pain.

Clinical breast examination as a screening tool has a sensitivity of 40% to 69% and a specificity of 88% to 99%. The sensitivity range of breast self-examination is reported as only 12% to 41%. Therefore, all suspicious lesions must undergo biopsy to enable a histologic diagnosis, even if mammography results are negative and not all the typical findings of cancer are present.

Gynecomastia is usually unilateral but may be bilateral. In contrast to breast tissue from gynecomastia, cancerous lesions are not usually palpable under the male nipple. The lumps of fat necrosis are usually firm, solitary, and irregular and may be attached to the overlying skin.

DIAGNOSTIC STUDIES

Though most professional organizations (including the American Cancer Society) recommend annual mammography screening beginning at age 40 years for women of average risk, the U.S. Preventive Services Task Force has now recommended mammography every 2 years for women between the ages of 50 and 74 years (recommending that consideration of mammography for women 40 to 49 years be made on an individual basis).

It is important to differentiate *screening* mammography, which is usually done with two views, from *diagnostic* mammography, done in multiple views. For evaluation of a palpable mass, the physician needs to order a *diagnostic* mammogram. Mammographic signs of cancer are as follows:

- Irregularity of the mass
- Mass appearing smaller on mammogram than on physical examination
- Nipple retraction
- Increased stromal density on sequential examinations
- Calcification appearing on the mammogram

Biopsy should be performed on all suspicious lesions so a histologic diagnosis may be obtained. The sensitivity of screening mammography is 77% to 95% with a specificity of 94% to 97%. Digital mammography may be more sensitive than plain film mammography in women younger than 50 years, premenopausal women, and women with dense breasts. **Because mammograms can miss some lesions, biopsy should be performed on any suspicious mass that is palpable on physical examination.**

Ultrasound is useful in differentiating between cystic and solid lumps, especially in young women with dense breasts. Ultrasound is the preferred first radiologic test in evaluating a breast lump in women younger than 30 years. When the ultrasound findings are suggestive of malignancy or equivocal, the procedure is followed by mammography in this population. When both mammography and ultrasound findings are negative or benign, the negative predictive value is very high (>97%). Although fine-needle aspiration is useful in evaluating cystic lesions, it has largely been replaced by image-guided core needle biopsy for evaluation of masses and abnormalities on mammography. Stereotactic core needle biopsies have reduced the need for open surgical biopsy. Biopsy is indicated when the mammogram suggests cancer or a suspicious lesion is palpable on physical examination.

Magnetic resonance imaging (MRI) of the breast is generally reserved for staging of newly diagnosed breast cancer and for postoperative evaluation of breast cancer patients. It is also recommended as a screening tool for women at very high risk for the disease.

LESS COMMON DIAGNOSTIC CONSIDERATIONS

Less common causes of benign breast lumps include papillomas, sclerosing adenosis, duct ectasia, lobular neoplasia, and apocrine metaplasia. A solitary *papilloma* is the most common benign cause of nipple discharge and bleeding. It is usually unilateral and located in the subareolar region. It most often occurs in perimenopausal women and does not increase the risk of cancer. In contrast, multiple papillomas increase cancer risk fourfold and most often occur in premenopausal women. With multiple papillomas, nipple discharge is rare. The lesions are bilateral in 25% of patients and occur distal to the nipple. See Table 5-1.

Ductal ectasia results from ductal dilatation and stasis of ductal contents, with a subsequent inflammatory reaction. It is often associated with nipple discharge and occasionally with ductal calcification. In women older than 55 years, nipple discharge is most often caused by ectasia, although one third of patients with nipple discharge have ductal papilloma.

Mondor's disease is superficial thrombophlebitis of the anterolateral portion of the breast and chest wall. It may occur spontaneously or secondary to injury or surgery. The skin may be retracted along the course of the thrombosed vein.

Sporadic puerperal mastitis, which seldom occurs in lactating mothers, may result in a breast abscess manifesting as a lump. Fever, chills, and tenderness are usually present.

TABLE 5-1. Screening for Breast Cancer using Film Mammography Clinical Summary of U.S. Preventive Services Task Force Recommendation

POPULATION	WOMEN AGED 40-49 YEARS	WOMEN AGED 50-74 YEARS	WOMEN AGED ≥75 YEARS
Recommendation	Do not screen routinely. Individualize decision to begin biennial screening according to the patient's context and values. Grade: C	Screen every 2 years. Grade: B	No recommendation. Grade: I (insufficient evidence)
Risk Assessment	This recommendation applies to women aged ≥40 years who are not at increased risk by virtue of a known genetic mutation or history of chest radiation. Increasing age is the most important risk factor for most women.		
Screening Tests	Standardization of film mammography has led to improved quality. Refer patients to facilities certified under the Mammography Quality Standards Act (MQSA), listed at www.fda.gov/cdrh/mammmography/certified.html.		
Timing of Screening	Evidence indicates that biennial screening is optimal. A biennial schedule preserves most of the benefit of annual screening and cuts the harms nearly in half. A longer interval may reduce the benefit.		
Balance of Harms and Benefits	There is convincing evidence that screening with film mammography reduces breast cancer mortality, with a greater absolute reduction for women aged 50 to 74 years than for younger women. Harms of screening include psychological harms, additional medical visits, imaging, and biopsies in women without cancer, inconvenience due to false-positive screening results, harms of unnecessary treatment, and radiation exposure. Harms seem moderate for each age group. False-positive results are a greater concern for younger women; treatment of cancer that would not become clinically apparent during a woman's life (overdiagnosis) is an increasing problem as women age.		
Rationale for No Recommendation (I Statement)			Among women 75 years or older, evidence of benefit is lacking.
Relevant USPSTF Recommendations	USPSTF recommendations on screening for genetic susceptibility for breast cancer and chemoprevention of breast cancer are available at www.preventiveservies.ahrq.gov.		

For a summary of the evidence systematically reviewed in making these recommendations, the full recommendation statement, and supporting documents, please go to http://www.preventiveservices.ahrq.gov.

Differential Diagnosis of Breast Lumps

CONDITION	NATURE OF PATIENT	NATURE OF SYMPTOMS	ASSOCIATED SYMPTOMS	PRECIPITATING AND AGGRAVATING FACTORS	AMELIORATING FACTORS	PHYSICAL FINDINGS	DIAGNOSTIC STUDIES
Fibroadenoma	Usually age 20–40 yr Rare in postmenopausal women unless they are estrogen	Usually asymptomatic	May enlarge, especially during adolescence and pregnancy			Usually solitary Multiple or bilateral in 15%–25% of cases Firm, mobile, smooth, rubbery	Mammography Fine-needle biopsy
Fibrocystic breasts	Frequency increases with age; incidence peaks especially around menopause, and then declines	Cyclic breast pain, especially around menstruation Usually bilateral	Rare nipple discharge, usually not bloody	Pain and tenderness worsen premenstrually	Menopause Reduction in ingestion of methylxanthines in tea, coffee, cola, and chocolate Oral contraceptives	Multiple tender breast lumps Usually bilateral and in upper outer quadrants Occasionally single or unilateral	Mammography Ultrasonography
Cancer	Usually older than 40 yr Chapter 1 in 10 women	Usually none until late in disease	Occasional pain in one breast in postmenopausal patient Bloody nipple discharge Axillary adenopathy	Increased incidence if mother and/or sister had breast cancer Early menarche Late menopause Over age 50 Nulliparous	Decreased incidence in users of oral contraceptives	Hard, irregular, fixed lump	Mammography Biopsy Fine-needle aspiration biopsy Ductal endoscopy MRI in selected cases

Fat necrosis	Older women More common in large, pendulous breasts	Painful, tender on palpation		Trauma; surgical trauma	Firm, solitary, irregular lump May be attached to skin
Gynecomastia	Males, especially pubertal and elderly Alcoholics	Breast enlargement Unilateral or bilateral, often tender	Adrenogenital syndrome	Drugs: oral and topical estrogens, marijuana, spironolactone, methyldopa, phenytoin, cimetidine, digitalis, finasteride, lansoprazole, ACE inhibitors	Increased breast tissue under nipple

ACE, Angiotensin-converting enzyme; MRI, magnetic resonance imaging.

Selected References

Brennan M, Houssami N, French J: Management of benign breast conditions. Part 2: breast lumps and lesions, *Austral Fam Physician* 34:253-255, 2005.

Daniels IR, Layer GT: How should gynaecomastia be managed? *ANZ J Surg* 73:213-216, 2003.

Goodson WH, Moore DH: Causes of physician delay in the diagnosis of breast cancer, *Arch Intern Med* 162:1343-1348, 2002.

Gunham-Bilgen I, Bozkaya H, Ustun EE, et al: Male breast disease: clinical, mammographic, and ultrasonographic features, *Eur J Radiol* 43:246-255, 2002.

Hamed H, Fentiman IS: Benign breast disease, *Int J Clin Pract* 55:458-460, 2001.

Hazard HW, Hansen NM: Image-guided procedures for breast masses, *Adv Surg* 41:257-272, 2007.

Hines SL, Tan W, Larson JM: A practical approach to guide clinicians in the evaluation of male patients with breast masses, *Geriatrics* 63:19-24, 2008.

Kerlikowske K, Smith-Bindman R, Ljung B-M, et al: Evaluation of abnormal mammography results and palpable breast abnormalities, *Ann Intern Med* 139:274-284, 2003.

Kriege M, Brekelmans CT, Boetes C, et al: Efficacy of MRI and mammography for breast cancer detection with a familial or genetic predisposition, *N Engl J Med* 351:427-437, 2004.

Kuhl CK: Current status of breast MR imaging. Part 2: Clinical applications, *Radiology* 244:672-691, 2007.

Liang Z, Du X, Liu J, et al: Comparison of diagnostic accuracy of breast masses using digitized images versus screen-film mammography, *Acta Radiol* 49:618-622, 2008.

Parikh JR: ACR Appropriateness Criteria on palpable breast masses, *J Am Coll Radiol* 4:285-288, 2007.

Park YM, Kim EK, Lee JH, et al: Palpable breast masses with probably benign morphology at sonography: can biopsy be deferred? *Acta Radiol* 49:1104-1111, 2008.

Rim A, Chellman-Jeffers M: Trends in breast cancer screening and diagnosis, *Cleve Clin J Med* 75(Suppl 1):S2-S9, 2008.

Saslow D, Boetes C, Bruke W, et al: American Cancer Society guidelines for breast screening with MRI as an adjunct to mammography.[Erratum appears in CA Cancer J Clin57:185, 2007.], *CA Cancer J Clin* 57:75-89, 2007.

Silverstein MJ, Recht A, Lagios MD, et al: Special report: Consensus conference III. Image-detected breast cancer: state-of-the-art diagnosis and treatment, *J Am Coll Surg* 209:504-520, 2009.

Singletary SE, Cristofanilli M: Defining the clinical diagnosis of inflammatory breast cancer, *Semin Oncol* 35:7-10, 2008.

Smith RA, Saslow D, Sawyer KA, et al: American Cancer Society guidelines for breast cancer screening: update 2003, *CA Cancer J Clin* 53:141-169, 2003.

Stein L, Chellman-Jeffers M: The radiologic workup of a palpable breast mass, *Cleve Clin J Med* 76:175-180, 2009.

U.S. Preventive Services Task Force: Screening for breast cancer: U.S. Preventive Services Task Force recommendation statement, *Ann Intern Med* 151:716-726, W-236, 2009.

Chest Pain

6

Chest pain is one of the most common complaints of adult patients. Whether the patients admit it or not, they are usually concerned that this pain is caused by some type of cardiac disease. Therefore, the physician must be thoroughly familiar with the differential diagnosis of chest pain. Catastrophic events such as acute coronary syndrome, aortic dissection, pulmonary embolism, pericarditis, and esophageal rupture must be considered. Although the physician must realize that it is in the patient's interest not to overlook any acute cardiac illness, it is just as essential that cardiac disease not be incorrectly diagnosed or inferred because such misdiagnosis may cause some patients to inappropriately fear they have a cardiac condition.

Common causes of chest pain are angina pectoris; myocardial infarction; musculoskeletal chest wall conditions (especially in children), including costochondritis, benign overuse myalgia, fibrositis, and referred pain; trauma; cervicodorsal arthritis; psychoneurosis; esophageal reflux; esophageal spasm; pleuritis; and mitral valve prolapse (Table 6-1). **The most common cause of noncardiac chest pain is gastroesophageal reflux.** Less common causes of chest pain include precordial catch syndrome in children, microvascular dysfunction in women, lung tumors, gas entrapment syndromes, pulmonary hypertension, pulmonary embolus, pericarditis, and panic disorder. Cocaine is implicated as the cause of nontraumatic chest pain in 14% to 25% of patients in urban centers. Patients with biliary disease, including cholelithiasis, cholecystitis, and common duct stones, may also present with pain in the chest. A patient complaining of burning chest pain in a dermatomal distribution should be examined for the lesions of herpes zoster (though pain may be experienced prior to appearance of the lesions).

NATURE OF PATIENT

Chest pain due to *coronary artery disease* (CAD) or other serious organic pathology is rare in young people. In children, chest pain most likely results from the *musculoskeletal system* (e.g., strain, trauma, overuse, precordial catch, costochondritis), an *inflammatory process* (e.g., pleurisy or Tietze's syndrome/costochondritis), or a *psychiatric problem* (e.g., anxiety, conversion disorder, depression). When pain similar in quality to angina pectoris occurs in a child or adolescent, *reflux*

TABLE 6-1.   Noncardiac Causes of Chest Pain

Resemble angina slightly	anxiety* Pulmonary hypertension* Esophagitis, esophagospasm* Radiculitis Cervicodorsal arthritis Bursitis Shoulder disease Pericarditis Pneumonia Aneurysm Gastrointestinal distention with gaseous entrapment* Peptic ulcer Gallbladder disease* Diaphragmatic or paraesophageal hernia*
Not typical of angina	anxiety* Costochondritis Nonspecific myositis

*Relieved by nitroglycerin.
From Seller RH: Cardiology. In Rakel RE, Conn HF, eds: Family Practice, 2nd ed. Philadelphia, WB Saunders, 1978.

esophagitis, mitral valve prolapse, or *cocaine abuse* should be suspected. Although they are uncommon, myocarditis and pericarditis may cause cardiac chest pain in children. Rarely, children with congenital anomalies of the coronary arteries may have ischemic pain. Although *pulmonary embolism* is uncommon in children, it should be suspected in any postoperative, immobilized, or bedridden patient.

Women are at increased risk for pulmonary embolism if they are taking oral contraceptives. They are more likely than men to have atypical symptoms rather than chest pain as manifestations of cardiac ischemia. These atypical symptoms include back pain, nausea, vomiting, dyspnea, and severe fatigue. Women with typical chest pain and no evidence of obstructive coronary artery disease are likely to have coronary microvascular dysfunction.

In adults, any cause of chest pain may occur. Some patients experience chest wall pain after *aortocoronary bypass* in which internal mammary artery grafts are used. In older patients, *CAD, cervicodorsal arthritis, tumors, esophagitis,* and *pulmonary embolism* are the most common causes.

In athletes chest pain may originate from the heart, lung, or esophagus, but musculoskeletal causes, such as costochondritis, intercostal muscle strain, and stress fractures, must be strongly considered. The musculoskeletal cause may originate in myofascial structures, articular surfaces, the ribs, or the sternum. The pain may be induced by direct trauma, overuse, or gastroesophageal reflux disease (GERD), and asthma may also be induced by exercise.

NATURE OF PAIN

Although the physician must differentiate chest pain of cardiac origin from other types of pain, it is not sufficient to establish whether or not the pain is of cardiac origin. Patients with pain of cardiac origin should receive varying forms of therapy and have different prognoses, depending on whether their pain is caused by *angina pectoris, Prinzmetal's angina, hypertrophic cardiomyopathy (HCM), mitral valve prolapse,* or *pericarditis.* An accurate diagnosis can usually be made from a precise history. In eliciting the history of chest pain, the examiner should note the following five specific characteristics of the discomfort: location of pain, quality of pain, duration of pain, factors that precipitate or exacerbate the pain, and ameliorating factors.

The distinctive clinical characteristics of *angina pectoris* are that the pain is paroxysmal (lasting 30 seconds to a few minutes), dull, pressing, squeezing, or aching; it is located substernally; and it may radiate to the precordium, upper extremities, neck, or jaw. The term *anginal salute* refers to the way patients hold a clenched fist over the sternum to describe the pain. Some patients experience no chest pain and only neck, arm, or jaw discomfort. The location of pain in patients with angina pectoris may vary greatly from person to person, but it differs little with recurrent episodes in the same patient. Thus, if the patient complains of chest pain in different locations during separate episodes, the pain is probably not caused by angina pectoris. Pain of biliary tract or esophageal origin is likely to be substernal, whereas the pain of pericarditis is likely to be precordial.

Patients with angina pectoris describe their pain as tightness, pressure, or heaviness and infrequently as a burning sensation. Burning is relatively uncommon and suggests the possibility of *peptic esophagitis,* the most frequent imitator of CAD. **Rarely if ever is anginal pain described as knifelike, sharp, or sticking. Although some patients describe the pain as "sharp," they usually mean that it is severe in intensity rather than knifelike in quality.** The pain of *pulmonary hypertension,* which often occurs in patients with mitral stenosis or primary pulmonary disease, may be indistinguishable from the pain of angina pectoris. The pain of pulmonary hypertension is usually described as a dull, pressing, substernal pain. It is precipitated by exertion and relieved by rest or administration of nitroglycerin. Although this pain may radiate to either arm, it radiates more often to the right arm. Patients with pulmonary hypertension and CAD may experience chest pain as a result of pulmonary hypertension, CAD, or both.

The most frequent cause of noncardiac angina-like chest pain is esophageal dysfunction. This pain is usually due to gastroesophageal reflux, although esophageal dysmotility may be less frequently etiologic. Dull, achy, or burning chest pain may also be experienced by patients with *pulmonary hypertension, cervicodorsal arthritis, gallbladder disease, diaphragmatic or paraesophageal hernias,* and *mitral valve prolapse.* The associated exacerbating or ameliorating factors are most helpful in establishing the diagnosis.

Sharp, sticking pains, especially if they last only a few seconds, are more characteristic of *anxiety, costochondritis, cervicodorsal arthritis, mitral valve prolapse, chest wall syndrome, pericarditis,* and *pleuritic processes.* The location of the pain is usually not helpful in differentiating the cause of the chest pain in these conditions, with a few exceptions. Pain on the side of the chest, particularly if it is exacerbated by respiration, is more likely to be pleuritic. Pain localized to the costochondral junction or specific intercostal spaces is most likely caused by *costochondritis* or *intercostal myositis.* The pain of chest wall syndrome may

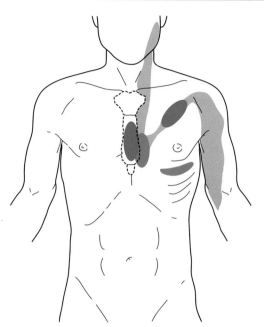

Figure 6-1. Regions of anterior chest where spontaneous pain is most often experienced and where tenderness may be elicited are shown in shades of blue. The *light blue areas* represent radiation of pain. (Modified from Epstein SE, Gerber LH, Borer JS: Chest wall syndrome: a common cause of unexplained cardiac pain. JAMA 241:2793-2797, 1979.)

occur during exercise or at rest; occasionally, it is nocturnal. The pain may be described as "sticking" but also as "dull" and "pressing." The most critical finding in the diagnosis of chest wall syndrome is detection of chest wall tenderness on physical examination. It is more common in athletes. It is frequently located substernally, at the left parasternal region, near the shoulder, and in the fourth or fifth left intercostal space (Fig. 6-1). Pain that is positional, pleuritic, sharp, or reproduced by palpation portends a much lower probability of ischemic heart disease.

The presence of cervicodorsal arthritis or reflux esophagitis does not rule out the possibility that chest pain is caused by coronary disease. Patients may have two conditions, each of which contributes to the chest pain. For example, a patient may have pain from esophagitis as well as pain from angina pectoris. When two conditions coexist, the patient may be able to distinguish between the two types of chest pain. For example, if questioned carefully, a patient may describe a dull substernal pain often induced by exercise and relieved by nitroglycerin but not antacids as well as another dull substernal pain radiating to the neck and arms that is not as thoroughly relieved by nitroglycerin but is occasionally ameliorated by antacids. When this patient is investigated further, s/he may have both CAD and reflux esophagitis.

ASSOCIATED SYMPTOMS

Fatigue is the most common presenting symptom in elderly patients with acute coronary syndrome. The pain of *mitral valve prolapse* may occasionally be indistinguishable from that of CAD in that it may occur with exertion and can occasionally be relieved by nitroglycerin. More often the chest pain of mitral valve prolapse has features not typical of angina that should alert the physician that the pain is not of coronary origin. The chest pain of mitral valve prolapse usually occurs during rest. Although it may last for a few minutes, it may also last for several hours. It is often described as "sticking" and is not substernally located. It is frequently alleviated by lying down; the pain of *angina pectoris* is often worsened by recumbency, as is the pain of *reflux esophagitis*. **If atypical chest pain is associated with arrhythmias (particularly tachyarrhythmias) and lightheadedness or syncope, mitral valve prolapse should be suspected.**

Patients with *pneumonia* or *pulmonary embolism* may have chest pain but usually also have fever, cough, or hemoptysis. Patients who have protracted or vigorous coughing may experience chest pain resulting from intercostal muscle or periosteal trauma. Local chest wall tenderness is usually present.

Patients with *HCM* may have typical angina pectoris, but their chest pain is not necessarily caused by CAD. **In patients with HCM the most common symptom is dyspnea (often precipitated by exercise), which usually precedes the development of chest pain.** In any patient with angina pectoris who has coexisting or antecedent dyspnea, a careful search for HCM should be made.

Dyspnea may be the only symptom associated with anginal pain in patients with effort-induced cardiac ischemia.

Although the pain from *esophagitis* is often similar to that from anginal pain, the associated symptoms are helpful in establishing the differential diagnosis. The pain of esophagitis is usually not related to exertion but is related to overeating and recumbency. The pain typically wakens the patient at night. This symptom is rare in patients with angina pectoris unless they have angina decubitus. Patients with angina decubitus usually have congestive heart failure, and their pain is often precipitated by minimal exertion.

Burning, indigestion-like chest or epigastric pain has been shown to occur frequently in patients with cardiac ischemia who presented with undifferentiated chest pain.

Cervicodorsal arthritis may produce chest pain. This pain is seldom similar to that of angina pectoris. More often it is sharp and piercing but may occasionally be described as a deep, boring, dull discomfort. The major characteristics of *nerve root pain* are:

- Pain with body movement
- Pain on coughing and sneezing
- Pain after prolonged recumbency

The pains may occur in any part of the chest or shoulder girdle, may radiate down the arms, and may be bilateral or unilateral. Chest pain may be precipitated by bending or hyperextension of the upper spine or neck. The pain is usually not related to exercise, is fleeting, and thus is not truly relieved by rest.

The chest pain associated with *pericarditis* may be pleuritic or heavy and steady.

PRECIPITATING AND AGGRAVATING FACTORS

Anginal pain is often precipitated by physical exertion, emotional stress, sexual activity, exposure to cold, and occasionally eating (Table 6-2). *Prinzmetal's angina* occurs at rest. Chest pain due to pulmonary hypertension is also induced by exertion.

Chest pain from *reflux esophagitis* is often precipitated by overeating and recumbency. It frequently awakens the patient at night. Chest pain from *esophageal spasm* can be precipitated by swallowing certain substances, particularly cold liquids and anything that stimulates the production of endogenous gastrin. Thus, chest pain that follows ingestion of alcohol should suggest esophageal spasm. Chest pain during exercise such as jogging may be caused by esophageal reflux rather than angina pectoris. The former is relieved by antacids.

If the pain is exacerbated or reproduced when pressure is applied over the painful area, *costochondritis, Tietze's syndrome, rib fractures, chest wall syndrome,* and *nonspecific myositis* are more likely. Reproduction or exacerbation of pain with chest wall pressure does not usually occur in patients with ischemic cardiac pain.

Although a few patients with chest pain due to HCM obtain relief with nitrates, the pain is usually exacerbated and the murmur intensified by nitroglycerin. Just as chest pain associated with dyspnea should alert the physician to the possibility of HCM, chest pain exacerbated by nitrates should suggest HCM, as should the associated lightheadedness, dizziness, or syncope.

In instances of recurrent chest pain, especially in young adults, cocaine should be suspected.

AMELIORATING FACTORS

Nitroglycerin usually relieves *angina pectoris* within 2 to 4 minutes; rest alone usually brings relief in less than 10 minutes. Unfortunately, a positive response to nitroglycerin does not confirm CAD as the cause of pain. Nitroglycerin works primarily by relaxing smooth muscle. **Nitroglycerin also may relieve chest pain due to peptic esophagitis and esophageal spasm, biliary dyskinesia and cholelithiasis, gas entrapment syndrome, pulmonary hypertension, mitral valve prolapse, and, occasionally, psychoneurotic chest pain** (see Table 6-1).

Pain can be caused by CAD and yet not be relieved by nitroglycerin. The pain may be too severe, or the nitroglycerin may be outdated or administered improperly. If the symptoms suggest CAD and sublingual nitroglycerin does not provide relief, the physician should determine whether the patient is taking the medication properly. A helpful method is to take a tiny piece of paper, crumple it into the size of a nitroglycerin tablet, and have the patient place it under the tongue. The patient should be instructed to:

1. Let the nitroglycerin dissolve and remain under the tongue unswallowed.
2. Expect a warm, flushing feeling.
3. Keep the saliva under the tongue until the pain is relieved. At this point the patient may either swallow the saliva or expectorate it.

TABLE 6-2. Diagnosis of Chest Pain

CONDITION	TYPICAL	ATYPICAL	DIZZINESS, VERTIGO, SYNCOPE	NITRATES	CARDIAC AUSCULTATION	QRS COMPLEX	ST SEGMENT–T WAVE CHANGES	STRESS ECG FINDINGS	SYMPTOMS REPRODUCED AT BEDSIDE
Coronary heart disease	+++	+	Rare	++++	– to +++	Common	Common	+++	–
Angina with normal coronary arteries	++	++	Rare	++	–	Occasional	Common	+++	–
Hypertrophic cardiomyopathy	+++	+	++	+	– to +++ Variable	Common	Common	+++	Rare
Mitral valve prolapse	+	+++	++	+	– to +++ Variable	Rare	Common	++	Rare
Hyperventilation syndrome	+ Rare	++	++	–	–	–	Rare	+	+
Esophageal disease	+ (?)	+++	–	+	–	–	–	–	–
Radicular syndromes	+	+++	+	+ (?)	–	–	–	–	+++
Chest wall syndromes	–	+++	–	–	–	–	–	–	+++

ECG, Electrocardiogram.
From Levine HJ: Difficult problems in the diagnosis of chest pain. Am Heart J 100:108-117, 1980.

Valsalva's maneuver may also give prompt relief from angina pectoris, but it does not usually relieve the chest pain of obstructive HCM. Occasionally, patients with HCM obtain relief from chest pain by squatting, which decreases outflow obstruction. Relief of a patient's chest pain by an antacid strongly suggests that the discomfort is caused by *reflux esophagitis*. Relief of chest pain by recumbency suggests *mitral valve prolapse*. Relief of chest pain by passage of flatus suggests *gas entrapment* in the hepatic or splenic flexure.

PHYSICAL FINDINGS

Few physical findings are diagnostic of *angina pectoris*. Sinus tachycardia or bradycardia may coincide with anginal pain. Signs of *congestive heart failure* in patients with chest pain suggest that the pain is probably caused by myocardial ischemia. If a careful examination performed during an episode of ischemic heart pain reveals a palpable systolic bulge near the apex, a paradoxical splitting of the second sound, a diastolic filling sound (S_3 or S_4), or a transient mitral regurgitant murmur, ischemic heart disease is strongly suggested as the cause of chest pain. Likewise, *hypertension, diabetic retinopathy*, or the presence of cutaneous manifestations of atherosclerosis such as *xanthomas* increases the probability of CAD as the cause of chest pain.

Squatting decreases outflow tract obstruction and thus diminishes the characteristic midsystolic murmur of *HCM*. The systolic murmur of HCM is increased with the patient in the upright position and during Valsalva's maneuver. Atrial and ventricular arrhythmias (dysrhythmias) are common in HCM and may occasionally be the earliest manifestation. Chest wall tenderness on palpation or auscultation of pericardial or pleural friction suggests a musculoskeletal pericardial or pleural problem, respectively. Likewise, epigastric tenderness on palpation suggests a GI etiology, especially in children and adolescents presenting with chest pain.

Tenderness in the region of spontaneous pain, especially if the quality of pain can be reproduced by pressure on the area, strongly suggests *chest wall syndrome*. Certain maneuvers (e.g., horizontal arm flexion, *crowing rooster* maneuver) may also cause the pain of chest wall syndrome. *Mitral valve prolapse* is suggested by auscultation of a midsystolic *click*, late systolic murmur, or both. Patients may have mitral valve prolapse with absent or transient auscultatory findings.

DIAGNOSTIC STUDIES

The findings of a resting electrocardiogram (ECG) may be normal in 50% of patients with angiographically confirmed CAD. An abnormal ECG and elevated troponin values obtained during a bout of chest pain are more likely to be abnormal. Troponin values usually rise within 2-3 hours of an acute myocardial infarction (MI), and remain elevated for around 10-14 days, allowing for late diagnosis of MI. Approximately 80% of patients with an acute MI will exhibit elevated troponin values within 2-3 hours of the event. The MB isoenyzme of creatinine kinase (CK-MB) may also be used in the diagnosis of acute MI. This typically rises within 4-6 hours of the event, but make take as long as 12 hours in some patients. Values typically return to normal within 36-48 hours. This means that CK-MB cannot be used for late diagnosis of MI (as can troponin), however, it can be used to diagnose reinfarction, or extention of infarction. Because of its increased specificity and rapid elevation, troponin is preferred over CK-MB for the diagnosis of actue MI.

Stress echocardiography and stress myocardial perfusion scanning using single-photon emission computed tomography (SPECT), have greatly enhanced the ability to diagnose CAD with noninvasive tests. Both have similar sensitivities for detecting coronary artery disease. Stress echocardiography may be slightly more specific, but interpretation is more subjective than perfusion imaging. SPECT myocardial perfusion imaging is somewhat better at localizing the perfusion defect. Whereas coronary angiography has a role in treating an acute ST-elevation MI, in patients with chronic-stable chest pain, it should be reserved for patients in whom angina is not adequately controlled with medications, and in whom left main stenosis or multi-vessel disease is suggested by stress testing. Ambulatory 24-hour esophageal pH monitoring is useful in diagnosing reflux esophagitis, although a 14-day course of a proton-pump inhibitor, is more sensitive, more specific, and cheaper.

The ECG in *mitral valve prolapse* may show changes similar to those in CAD. ECG changes, if present, usually include ST-segment depression and T-wave inversion or abnormalities in leads II, III, and AVF and occasionally in the precordial leads.

ECG findings are usually abnormal in patients with *obstructive HCM*, although a normal ECG may be obtained. The most common ECG abnormalities are those indicative of left ventricular hypertrophy and intraventricular conduction defects, and nonspecific ST-segment–T-wave changes. The ECG findings (P-wave abnormalities) most helpful in the diagnosis of HCM are those not generally seen in patients with CAD. These P-wave abnormalities suggestive of atrial enlargement are common in patients with HCM and uncommon in patients with CAD. An ECG picture of transmural infarction (Q waves in the anteroseptal or inferior leads) may also be seen in some patients with HCM.

The echocardiogram is the preferred study for the diagnosis of both mitral valve prolapse and obstructive HCM. Helical CT of the chest is the preferred study to diagnosis pulmonary embolism.

Because women often have atypical symptoms of CAD, a higher index of suspicion is required, and those with intermediate risk should be evaluated with noninvasive studies such as nuclear scan and stress echocardiogram. Microvascular disease is suggested (especially in women) by a positive stress test result coupled with a negative coronary angiogram findings.

A short course of a proton pump inhibitor and esophagoscopy are most useful in the diagnosis of GERD.

LESS COMMON DIAGNOSTIC CONSIDERATIONS

The pain of *costochondritis* and *costochondrodynia* is usually localized to the costochondral junction. The pain may be constant or exacerbated by movement of the chest wall, including respiratory motion. The physician may confirm the diagnosis by applying pressure over the painful area, thus replicating the pain.

Differential Diagnosis of Chest Pain

CONDITION	NATURE OF PATIENT	NATURE OF PAIN	ASSOCIATED SYMPTOMS	PRECIPITATING AND AGGRA- VATING FACTORS	AMELIORAT- ING FACTORS	PHYSICAL FINDINGS	DIAGNOSTIC STUDIES
Angina pectoris	Adult	Achy, dull, tight, severe, pressing Not usually sharp or sticking Substernal	Women are more likely to have atypical symptoms such as back pain, nausea, and fatigue	Exertion Cold exposure Emotional stress	Nitroglycerin Rest Valsalva's maneuver	Sinus tachycardia, bradycardia, or apical systolic bulge coincident with pain Xanthomas Signs of heart failure	Exercise ECG Coronary arteriography Radionuclide tests Stress echocardiography
Variant angina (Prinzmetal's angina)	Adult	Achy, dull, tight, severe, pressing Not usually sharp or sticking Substernal		Often occurs at rest or at night	Nitroglycerin Rest		ECG during attack Coronary arteriography
Gastroesopha- geal reflux disease	Any age	Burning Tightness May be identical to that of angina	Water brash "Heartburn"	Overeating Recumbency (may awaken from sleep) Occasionally precipitated by exertion	Antacids Proton pump inhibitors		Esophagoscopy Ambulatory monitoring of esophageal pH Short course of high-dose proton pump inhibitors
Esophageal spasm	Especially obese adults	May be identical in quality to angina		Often induced by ingestion of alcohol or cold liquids	Occasionally relieved by nitroglycerin		Esophageal manometry

Condition	Age	Character of Pain	Associated Symptoms	Precipitating/Aggravating Factors	Relieving Factors	Physical Findings	Diagnostic Tests
Mitral valve prolapse	Any age	Not usually substernal Often has sticking quality May last several hours Not typical of angina	Palpitations Arrhythmias Often occurs at rest Syncope		Beta blockers Recumbency	Click/late systolic murmur	Echocardiogram Phonocardiogram
Hypertrophic cardiomyopathy	Any age	Pain may be similar to that of angina	Dyspnea Arrhythmias Lightheadedness	Pain may be aggravated by nitroglycerin	Beta blockers Squatting	Murmur intensified by nitroglycerin and Valsalva's maneuver Decreased by squatting	Echocardiogram
Intercostal myositis	Any age but more common in children and athletes	May have sticking quality		May intensify with inspiration		Localized tenderness on palpation No pleural friction	
Costochondritis				Severe coughing	"Splinting" of tender area		
Cervicodorsal arthritis	Adult	May be sharp or sticking Duration only a few seconds		May be precipitated by certain movements (e.g., neck exercises and twisting) Not related to stress			Radiographs of cervicodorsal spine
Pulmonary embolus	Usually adult	Sharp, severe, often pleuritic	Tachypnea Hemoptysis	Prolonged immobilization Oral contraceptives, especially in smokers		Deep vein thrombosis Tachypnea Minimal cyanosis	Spiral CT D-dimer assay $\dot{V}/\dot{Q}$ scan Pulmonary angiography

Continued

Differential Diagnosis of Chest Pain—cont'd

CONDITION	NATURE OF PATIENT	NATURE OF PAIN	ASSOCIATED SYMPTOMS	PRECIPITATING AND AGGRAVATING FACTORS	AMELIORATING FACTORS	PHYSICAL FINDINGS	DIAGNOSTIC STUDIES
Pneumonia			Fever Cough			Egophony Dullness on percussion	
Chest wall syndrome	Adult More common in athletes	Often sharp and sticking Fleeting		May be aggravated by recumbency and certain positions		Local tenderness on palpation "Crowing rooster" maneuver may precipitate pain	
Pericarditis	Any age	Sharp or dull Protracted duration	Fever Recent viral infection			Pericardial friction	ECG Echocardiogram CBC
Myocardial infarction	Adult	Severe Crushing Precordial Protracted duration	Sweating Fatigue Nausea		Not relieved by nitroglycerin		Cardiac troponins ECG Serial CK-MB levels Radionuclide studies
Gas entrapment syndrome	Any age Often obese	Dull, achy	Flatulence	Aggravated by bending and tight garments	Passage of flatus Nitroglycerin	Flexing thigh and palpation of colon may elicit pain	Gas in hepatic or splenic flexure on radiographs

CBC, Complete blood count; CK-MB, creatine kinase, muscle-brain subunits (CK2, found primarily in cardiac muscle); CT, computed tomography; ECG, electrocardiogram; V̇/Q̇ ventilation/perfusion.

Cervical angina, also called *pseudoangina,* is a rare cause of chest pain and is similar to that of angina pectoris in quality, location, and radiation. The pain is not brought on by exertion but is often precipitated by cervical motion, sneezing, or coughing and aggravated by lateral tilting of the head. The diagnosis is confirmed by finding cervical disc disease on magnetic resonance imaging.

Gas entrapment syndrome (gas trapped in the hepatic or splenic flexure) is suggested by a history of chest pain when the patient bends at the waist or wears a tight garment. The pain may be exacerbated by bending, flexing the thigh on the chest, or palpating the colon. The pain may be relieved by passage of flatus or ingestion of sublingual nitroglycerin.

The pain of *pulmonary hypertension* may be indistinguishable from that of angina pectoris and other causes of exercise-induced chest wall pain. It can also be relieved by sublingual nitroglycerin. It should be suspected in patients with mitral stenosis or other causes of pulmonary hypertension, pulmonary disease, an accentuated second pulmonary sound, or ECG signs of right atrial disease (peaked P waves) or right ventricular overload. The pain of a pulmonary embolus in the acute phase may be caused by pulmonary hypertension. Subsequently, the pain is related to pulmonary infarction with associated pleurisy. The pain is usually not related to exercise and tends to become more constant (often with a pleuritic component) in the later stages.

Pericarditis should be suspected in the patient with continual chest pain associated with diffuse ECG changes. This pain tends to be aggravated by changes in position. A pericardial friction rub confirms the diagnosis.

Lung and mediastinal tumors often manifest as chest pain, which tends to be constant, especially in the later stages. **Whenever the diagnosis of chest pain is not clear, particularly in adult patients, the examiner should obtain a chest radiograph to look for possible tumors.**

Selected References

ACC/AHA Guidelines for the Clinical Application of Echocardiography: executive summary, *J Am Coll Cardiol* 29:862-868, 1997.

Bhardwaj R: Chest pain, dynamic ECG changes, and coronary artery disease, *J Assoc Physicians India* 55:556-559, 2007.

Chambers J, Bass C: Atypical chest pain: looking beyond the heart, *Q J Med* 91:239-244, 1998.

Eden BM: Chest pain in women: what's the difference? *Nurse Pract* 33:24-34, 2008:quiz 35.

Epstein SE, Gerber LH, Borer JS: Chest wall syndrome: a common cause of unexplained cardiac pain, *JAMA* 241:2793-2797, 1979.

Fass R: Evaluation and diagnosis of noncardiac chest pain, *Dis Mon* 54:627-641, 2008.

Fraker T Jr, Fihn S, et al: 2007 chronic angina focused update of the ACC/AHA 2002 guidelines for the management of patients with chronic stable angina: a report of the American College of Cardiology/American Heart Association Task Force on Practice Guidelines Writing Group to develop the focused update of the 2002 guidelines for the management of patients with chronic stable angina, *J Am Coll Cardiol* 50:2262-2672, 2007.

Gumbiner CH: Precordial catch syndrome, *Southern Med J* 96:38-41, 2003.

Hayden GE, Brady WJ, Perron AD, et al: Electrocardiographic T-wave inversion: differential diagnosis in the chest patient, *Am J Emerg Med* 20:252-262, 2002.

Hendel R, Berman D, Di Carli M, et al: ACCF/ASNC/ACR/AHA/ASE/SCCT/SCMR/SNM 2009 appropriate use criteria for cardiac radionuclide imaging: a report of the American College of Cardiology Foundation Appropriate Use Criteria Task Force, the American Society of Nuclear Cardiology, the American College of Radiology, the American Heart Association, the American Society of Echocardiography, the Society of Cardiovascular Computed Tomography, the Society for Cardiovascular Magnetic Resonance, and the Society of Nuclear Medicine, *Circulation* 119:e561-87, 2009.

Jones JH, Weir WB: Cocaine-induced chest pain, *Clin Lab Med* 26:127-146, 2006.

Katz PO: Approach to the patient with unexplained chest pain, *Semin GI Dis* 12:38-45, 2001.

Lauer M: What is the best test for a patient with classic angina? *Cleveland Clinic Journal of medicine* 74:123-126, 2007.

Limacher M, Handberg E: Evaluating women with chest pain for the diagnosis of coronary artery disease, *Dis Mon* 48:647-658, 2002.

Earls J, White R, Woodard P, et al: Expert Panel on Cardiac Imaging. ACR Appropriateness Criteria: chronic chest pain–high probability of coronary artery disease. [online publication], Reston (VA), 2010, American College of Radiology.

Owens TR: Chest pain in the adolescent: state of the art reviews, *Adolesc Med* 12:95-105, 2001.

Pandak WM, Arezo S, Evett S, et al: Short course of omeprazole: a better first approach to noncardiac chest pain than endoscopy, manometry, or 24-hour esophageal pH monitoring, *J Clin Gastroenterol* 35:307-317, 2002.

Rashford S: Acute pleuritic chest pain, *Australian Fam Phys* 30:841-846, 2001.

Ringstrom E, Freedman J: Approach to undifferentiated chest pain in the emergency department: a review of recent medical literature and published practice guidelines, *Mt Sinai J Med* 73:499-505, 2006.

Sharkey AM, Clark BJ: Common complaints with cardiac implications in children, *Pediatr Clin North Am* 38:657-666, 1991.

Sik EC, Batt ME, Heslop LM: Atypical chest pain in athletes, *Curr Sports Med Rep* 8:52-58, 2009.

Winters ME, Katzen SM: Identifying chest pain emergencies in the primary care setting, *Prim Care* 33:625-642, 2006.

Colds, Flu, and Stuffy Nose

The differential diagnosis of colds, flu, and stuffy nose might appear unimportant, because most of these conditions have no specific cures. However, because upper respiratory infections (URIs) are the most common affliction of adults and children, the sheer case volume requires the physician to be particularly expert in the diagnosis and symptomatic treatment of these conditions.

Many different *viruses* are responsible for causing colds, URIs, and flu. The physician must be able to differentiate these viral infections from *allergic rhinitis* (both perennial and seasonal), *chronic rhinitis,* and the common complications of these viral infections, which include *sinusitis, otitis media, bronchitis,* and *pneumonia.* These last four complications are usually secondary to superimposed bacterial infections, which will respond to appropriate antibiotic therapy. The constitutional complaints often associated with URI may also represent the prodrome of other viral infections, such as *infectious mononucleosis, measles,* and *mumps.*

NATURE OF PATIENT

Children typically experience more severe constitutional symptoms with URIs or colds than adults do. After a *common cold,* adults with a history of bronchitis, allergies, asthma, heavy cigarette smoking, or immune incompetence and children with a history of recurrent bronchitis, allergies, or cystic fibrosis develop lower respiratory tract infections more frequently than other people. Pregnancy is occasionally the cause of rhinitis.

Influenza tends to be milder in neonates and children; severity increases with age. Many elderly patients develop superimposed *bacterial pneumonia.* More than 70% of deaths recorded during known influenza epidemics have occurred in patients over age 65. Other high-risk groups include patients with acquired immunodeficiency syndrome (AIDS), chronic cardiorespiratory disease, chronic renal disease, diabetes, and third-trimester pregnancies. *Rhinitis medicamentosa* should be suspected in patients who frequently use nasal drops, sprays, or inhalers.

The physician must be especially alert for the development of complications of common URIs. *Sinusitis* is more likely to occur in a patient with a history of recurrent sinusitis. *Otitis media* is more common in young children, *bronchitis* in smokers and patients with underlying *pulmonary disease*, and *pneumonia* in older and diabetic patients.

NATURE OF SYMPTOMS AND ASSOCIATED SYMPTOMS

Symptoms of common *viral URIs* are well known. These symptoms largely depend on the particular infective viral agent, the patient's age, and the underlying medical conditions. The incubation period is 1 to 3 days. Patients usually have profuse nasal discharge and congestion and complain of stuffy nose, sneezing, postnasal drip, cough, and sore throat. They may also complain of headache, fever, malaise, and hoarseness and may note pharyngeal exudates, oropharyngeal vesicles, and lymphadenopathy. It is notable that colds in adults are rarely associated with a substantial fever. Acute bacterial rhinosinusitis is characterized by purulent rhinorrhea, facial pain or pressure, nasal obstruction, and often a worsening of symptoms after an initial improvement. Children may experience vomiting, diarrhea, abdominal pain, and wheezing.

Although a URI is the most frequent cause of nasal airway obstruction, other causes must be considered, including polyps, foreign bodies, herpes simplex, furuncles (folliculitis of nasal vibrissae), and less common infections. In neonates, unilateral nasal obstruction may be caused by a congenital abnormality (e.g., choanal atresia). In a child with unilateral nasal obstruction as the presenting symptom, the physician should consider a foreign body.

Although the symptoms of influenza and common URI may be similar, *influenza viral infections* can often be differentiated from the symptoms of a common cold by the sudden onset of typical signs of flu: shivering, chills, malaise, insomnia, marked aching of the limb and back muscles, dry cough, retrosternal pain, loss of appetite, and especially the coexistence of cough and fever greater than 37.8° C within 48 hours of the onset of symptoms. The sudden onset of fever and cough is highly predictive of influenza. A patient with *type A influenza* may not have coryza (profuse nasal discharge).

In addition to acute stuffy nose, chronic stuffy nose is a common complaint. *Chronic rhinitis* is most frequently caused by *allergy* (both seasonal and perennial), *nonallergic rhinitis with eosinophilia* (NARES), drugs (topical and systemic), and *vasomotor rhinitis* (nonallergic rhinitis). Chronic rhinitis is characterized by nasal congestion, postnasal drip, rhinorrhea, sneezing, and nasal itchiness. It is difficult to determine the specific cause on the basis of the symptoms alone.

The physician must especially recognize *allergic rhinitis* and *chronic rhinitis* as causes of nasal stuffiness. The two types of allergic rhinitis are perennial and seasonal. Patients with *perennial rhinitis* usually complain of nasal airway blockage with a persistent watery mucoid drainage. Their nasal turbinates are pale and boggy. Patients with *seasonal rhinitis* usually complain of sneezing, itchy eyes, lacrimation, and a watery nasal discharge. Their symptoms have a seasonal variation, unlike those of patients with the perennial type.

Chronic, or idiopathic, rhinitis is not known to have a specific cause. Most patients have persistent engorgement of the nasal turbinates, which leads to nasal obstruction and profuse watery rhinorrhea. They often complain of persistent nasal obstruction that may alternate from side to side. Sneezing is not as common as it is in allergic rhinitis.

When symptoms of a cold and cough persist longer than the patient's fever, the URI may have subsided, and the persistent symptoms may be caused by bacterial rhinosinusitis. Bacterial rhinosinusitis should be suspected if the symptoms last more than 7 days and are associated with maxillary pain or tenderness, unilateral facial or dental pain, and bloody/purulent nasal secretions.

PRECIPITATING AND AGGRAVATING FACTORS

Nasal sprays, antihypertensive drugs, hormones, and psychotropic agents often cause chronic nasal congestion. The more frequent offenders are methyldopa, prazosin, beta blockers, diuretics, antireflux agents, estrogens, oral contraceptives, thioridazine, chlordiazepoxide, amitriptyline, and perphenazine. Aspirin and nonsteroidal anti-inflammatory drugs (NSAIDs) can cause nasal stuffiness, rhinorrhea, asthma, and nasal polyposis.

Symptoms of chronic rhinitis are exacerbated by allergy, stress, hormonal changes (e.g., those associated with menstruation and menopause), marked temperature variations, and chemical irritants.

AMELIORATING FACTORS

Ameliorating factors are not particularly helpful in differential diagnosis.

PHYSICAL FINDINGS

The physical examination is most helpful in the detection of complications such as otitis media, sinusitis, pneumonia, and other bacterial infections. The physician should suspect something more serious than a simple URI if the temperature is greater than 102° F (38.8° C). If the patient has severe sore throat, exudative pharyngitis, earache, severe head or neck pain, or wheezing, the physician must exclude complications such as *streptococcal pharyngitis, otitis media, sinusitis, meningitis,* and *bacterial pneumonia,* because these conditions respond well to appropriate antibiotic therapy.

Patients with *acute sinusitis* often have pain over the involved sinuses that is usually unilateral and dull in the early stages but may become bilateral and more severe later. Coughing, sneezing, and percussion over the involved sinuses often exacerbate the pain. Percussion of the teeth may produce pain when the maxillary sinuses are infected. Some patients may even have a toothache as an early manifestation of sinusitis. Patients with ethmoid sinusitis often experience retro-orbital pain on coughing or sneezing. They may also demonstrate chemosis,

Differential Diagnosis of Colds, Flu, and Stuffy Nose

CONDITION	NATURE OF PATIENT	NATURE OF SYMPTOMS AND ASSOCIATED SYMPTOMS	COMPLICATIONS	PRECIPITATING AND AGGRAVATING FACTORS	PHYSICAL FINDINGS	DIAGNOSTIC STUDIES
Common cold/viral upper respiratory tract infections	Anyone	Constitutional symptoms worse in children Incubation period 1-3 days Profuse nasal drainage Nasal congestion Sneezing Postnasal drip Cough Sore throat Headache Fever (>102° F) Hoarseness General malaise	Lower RTI, especially in adults with history of bronchitis, allergies, asthma, heavy cigarette smoking, immune incompetence Sinusitis, especially in patients with history of recurrent sinusitis Bronchitis in smokers and patients with pulmonary disease Pneumonia in elderly and diabetic patients Nasal airway obstruction Streptococcal pharyngitis Meningitis		Mucopurulent nasal discharge Nasopharyngeal mucosal infection and swelling Temperature usually >102° F Pharyngeal exudates less frequent than with bacterial infections Lymphadenopathy	Throat culture (to rule out streptococcal infection and pharyngitis) Monospot test (to rule out infectious mononucleosis)
	Children	Vomiting Diarrhea Abdominal pain Wheezing	Lower RTI in children with history of recurrent bronchitis, allergies, cystic fibrosis Otitis media Pneumonia		Fever, may be >102°F Wheezing when bronchiolitis is associated	
Influenza viral infection	Any age; patients who are immunocompromised or elderly or have chronic lung disease or diabetes are at greater risk		Elderly frequently have bacterial pneumonia		Fever >37.8° C, cough within 48 hr of onset of symptoms	Rapid test for influenza virus and culture if anthrax is suspected

	History/Onset	Clinical features	Complications	Precipitating factors	Physical findings	Diagnostic studies
Allergic rhinitis						
Perennial	Onset before age 20 yr Family history of allergic disease	Nasal airway blockage Persistent watery nasal discharge No seasonal variation			Pale, boggy nasal turbinates Watery nasal discharge	Nasal smear: eosinophils
Seasonal		Sneezing Itchy eyes Lacrimation Watery nasal discharge Seasonal variation		Allergens Dust Pollen Spores	Pale, boggy nasal turbinates	
Chronic (idiopathic) rhinitis		Persistent nasal obstruction May alternate sides Profuse watery rhinorrhea Sneezing not common		Allergy Stress Hormonal changes Marked temperature changes Chemical irritants	Swollen nasal turbinates	
Sinusitis	Prior history of sinusitis	Often recurrent pain over sinuses Early: unilateral dull Later: bilateral severe		Coughing Sneezing Percussion of involved sinuses		Sinus CT scan Transillumination of sinuses
Maxillary		May manifest as toothache			Pain with percussion of teeth	
Ethmoid		Retro-orbital pain Mucopurulent nasal discharge (may be bloody)	Visual loss Cavernous sinus thrombosis Brain abscess	Coughing and sneezing may cause retro-orbital pain	Chemosis Proptosis Extraocular muscle palsy Orbital fixation	

Continued

Differential Diagnosis of Colds, Flu, and Stuffy Nose—cont'd

CONDITION	NATURE OF PATIENT	NATURE OF SYMPTOMS AND ASSOCIATED SYMPTOMS	COMPLICATIONS	PRECIPITATING AND AGGRA-VATING FACTORS	PHYSICAL FINDINGS	DIAGNOSTIC STUDIES
Rhinitis medica-mentosa	Frequent users of nasal drips, sprays, or inhalants Hypertensive patients taking certain anti-hypertensive drugs	Nasal congestion Nasal stuffiness		Nasal medications Reserpine Beta blockers Clonidine Hydralazine Methyldopa Prazosin Estrogens Oral contraceptives Chlordiaz-epoxide Amitriptyline	Mucosa injected	Nasal smear: no eosinophils

CT, Computed tomography; RTI, respiratory tract infection.

proptosis, extraocular muscle palsy, or orbital fixation. A mucopurulent nasal discharge, with or without blood, is frequently present.

Examination should include not only palpation and percussion over the sinuses but also careful observation of the pharynx, cranial nerves, eyes (including evaluation of visual acuity), ears, nose, and mouth. Visual loss, cavernous sinus thrombosis, and brain abscesses are serious potential sequelae. When correctly performed, transillumination may be helpful in the diagnosis of frontal and maxillary sinusitis.

DIAGNOSTIC STUDIES

Rapid "strep" tests may be useful in diagnosing streptococcal pharyngitis. The monospot test is helpful in the diagnosis of infectious mononucleosis. Nasal smears allow detection of eosinophils in allergic rhinitis. Computed tomography (CT) permits visualization of the sinuses, deviated septa, and intracranial lesions. A rapid test for influenza virus, such as *Z Stat Flu* (ZymeTx, Inc., Oklahoma City, OK) and blood cultures for anthrax should be performed if anthrax infection is suspected, however, with recent influenza outbreaks in the US, recommendations have been to treat influenza empirically based on clinical impression as opposed to testing the general population. Allergy skin testing should be performed in patients with rhinitis and when the diagnosis is not clear. White blood cells counts greater than 15,000/mm^3 suggest a bacterial origin of acute URIs in children. White blood cell counts greater than 8000/mm^3 make influenza less likely. A positive *Z stat Flu* test result and the absence of leukocytosis strongly suggest influenza. Nucleic acid amplification tests and DNA microarrays are being used more frequently in the early diagnosis of respiratory viral infections. These tests are proving to be cost-effective.

LESS COMMON DIAGNOSTIC CONSIDERATIONS

Frequent respiratory infections should alert the physician to the possibility of an anatomic abnormality, immune incompetence, or cystic fibrosis. Less common causes of nasal blockage are nasal polyps, sick building syndrome, occupational rhinitis (both allergic and irritant), tumors, foreign bodies, collagen vascular disorders, congenital malformations in neonates, and medications and atrophic rhinitis, especially in the elderly. Lyme disease may manifest as flulike symptoms.

The advent of bioterrorism requires that we add anthrax infection to the differential diagnosis of influenza-like illnesses.

Selected References

Benninger M, Segreti J: Is it bacterial or viral? Criteria for distinguishing bacterial and viral infections, *Suppl J Fam Pract* 57(Suppl):S5-S11, 2008.

Bush A: Recurrent respiratory infections, *Pediatr Clin North Am* 56:67-100, 2009.

Chan EM, Kuhn FA: An update on the classifications, diagnosis, and treatment of rhinosinusitis, *Curr Opin Otolaryngol Head Neck Surg* 17:204-208, 2009.

Drake-Lee A, Ruckley R, Parker A: Occupational rhinitis: a poorly diagnosed condition, *J Laryngol Otol* 116:580-585, 2002.

Fine AM, Wong JB, Fraser HS, et al: Is it influenza or anthrax? A decision analytic approach to the treatment of patients with influenza-like illnesses, *Ann Emerg Med* 43:318-328, 2004.

Georgitis JW: Prevalence and differential of chronic rhinitis, *Curr Allergy Asthma Rep* 1:202-206, 2001.

Henrickson KJ: Cost-effective use of rapid diagnostic techniques in the treatment and prevention of viral respiratory infections, *Pediatr Ann* 34:24-31, 2005.

Hulson TD, Mold JW, Scheid D, et al: Diagnosing influenza: the value of clinical clues and laboratory tests, *J Fam Pract* 50:1051-1056, 2001.

Knight A: The differential diagnosis of rhinorrhea, *J Allergy Clin Immunol* 95:1080-1083, 1995.

Le BM, Presti R: The current state of viral diagnostics for respiratory infections, *Mo Med* 106:283-286, 2009.

Mahr TA, Sheth K: Update on allergic rhinitis, *Pediatr Rev* 26:278-283, 2005.

Monto A, Gravenstein S: Clinical signs and symptoms predicting influenza infection, *Arch Intern Med* 160:3243-3247, 2000.

Solomon WR: Newer approaches to the diagnosis of rhinitis, *Ear Nose Throat* 65:42-46, 1986.

Constipation

8

Constipation is common in Western society. The frequency of constipation diagnoses depends on both the patient's and the physician's definitions of the problem. One bowel movement each day is what most patients consider normal. However, many physicians may accept two or three hard and dry stools a week as normal if this pattern is usual for the individual. Some experts believe that anyone who strains to defecate or does not effortlessly pass at least one soft stool daily is constipated. By this definition, constipation is very common.

Constipation may also be defined as a change in the person's normal bowel pattern to less frequent or more difficult defecation. In this chapter, *constipation* is defined as straining with bowel movements or bowel movements that occur fewer than three times per week. The American College of Gastroenterology defines constipation as "unsatisfactory defecation characterized by infrequent stools, difficult stool passage, or both." The Rome III criteria are generally used to define chronic functional constipation in adults, infants, and young children. They define chronic as the presence of these symptoms for at least 3 months. Constipation has been attributed to the deficiency of dietary fiber in the customary Western diet, which has replaced fiber with excessive ingestion of refined carbohydrates.

Constipation is usually not caused by a serious disease. In most patients it can be corrected by decreasing the amount of refined carbohydrates and increasing the amount of fiber ingested. It is particularly important for the examiner to ask whether the constipation is of recent onset and constitutes a change in previous bowel habits, since such findings may indicate serious disease.

The most common causes of constipation are laxative habit, diets high in refined carbohydrates and low in fiber, change in daily habits or environment, drug use, irritable bowel syndrome (IBS), and painful defecation due to a local anorectal problem. In many instances, it is important to differentiate IBS from chronic constipation. Pain or abdominal discomfort must be present to diagnose IBS. In many cases, multiple factors contribute to the patient's constipation. Less common causes include bowel tumors, fecal impaction, pregnancy, and metabolic disorders (e.g., hypothyroidism, diabetes, hypercalcemia).

The common causes of constipation can be divided into three categories: simple constipation, disordered motility, and secondary constipation. *Simple constipation* usually results from a diet that contains excessive refined carbohydrates and is deficient in fiber. It may be influenced by environmental factors. *Disordered motility*, the next most common category, is seen with idiopathic slow transit (most common in elderly persons), idiopathic megacolon and megarectum (more common in children), irritable bowel syndrome, and uncomplicated diverticular disease. *Secondary constipation* can be a response to drugs (especially codeine, opiates, and calcium channel blockers); chronic use of laxatives; prolonged immobilization; and organic disease of the anus, rectum, or colon (anal fissures, strictures, and carcinoma).

NATURE OF PATIENT

Constipation is uncommon in neonates and is usually caused by *anal fissures* or *feeding problems*. It rarely results from congenital problems such as *Hirschsprung's disease*. Cow's milk occasionally causes constipation. In children the most common cause of constipation is a change in daily habits or environment. The earlier that constipation begins in childhood, the greater the likelihood of an organic cause.

Disorders of defecation in children are common, difficult to manage, and negatively perceived by the family. Approximately 85% to 95% of constipation in children is functional. In children ages 6 months to 3 years, it frequently results from some *psychological cause*. Early diagnosis of psychological causes of constipation in children facilitates treatment. For example, toilet training may have occurred recently, or constipation may have developed because the child had a condition, such as a rectal fissure, that caused painful defecation. Fearing painful defecation, the child suppressed the urge to defecate, perpetuating the production of hard, dry stools, which continued to irritate the rectal fissure.

In adults, most constipation is caused by *dietary fiber deficiency* or *laxative habit*. Laxative use is more common in women than men. Constipation is a common complaint in elderly persons, although 80% to 90% of patients older than 60 years have one or more bowel movements per day. Despite this fact, 50% of patients older than 60 years use laxatives. This apparent discrepancy may be a result of older persons' greater preoccupation with bowel function in comparison with younger people. Constipation in elderly patients most often is caused by inappropriate diet, decreased activity, poor dentition, use of constipating medications, and impaired motility. Constipation ranks with joint pain, dizziness, forgetfulness, depression, and bladder problems as one of the major causes of misery in older patients.

Irritable bowel syndrome occurs more frequently in patients with chronic fatigue syndrome, fibromyalgia, and temporomandibular joint (TMJ) syndrome.

Obstipation (regular passage of hard stools at 3- to 5-day intervals) and *fecal impaction* are most common in elderly patients. Some patients with fecal impaction have continuous soiling (liquid passing around hard stools), which they describe as diarrhea. Elderly patients who are confined to bed, drink small amounts of fluid, or take constipating drugs are particularly vulnerable to fecal impaction. Although fecal impaction is more common in elderly persons, the physician must be aware that it can occur in any patient subjected to sudden immobility, bed rest, or a marked change in diet or fluid consumption.

Tumors of the bowel are uncommon in children and young adults, but their frequency increases after age 40 years. **In any patient older than 40 years who presents with recent constipation or a marked change in bowel habits, the physician must rule out carcinoma of the colon and rectum.**

NATURE OF SYMPTOMS

The most important factor in determining whether constipation should be investigated for a serious cause or treated symptomatically and by dietary modification is whether it is chronic or of recent onset. The second most important factor is the presence of *alarm symptoms*. Patients who have long-standing constipation and those whose constipation developed with a recent depressive illness, change in diet, recent debility, or ingestion of constipating medicine can be treated symptomatically. Their clinical status should be reassessed after a few weeks of appropriate therapy. **Patients with unexplained constipation of recent onset or a sudden aggravation of existing constipation associated with abdominal pain, unexplained weight loss, passing of blood or mucus, a progressive decrease in the number of bowel movements per day, or a substantial increase in laxative requirements should be investigated even in the absence of abnormal physical findings. These patients should undergo colonoscopy. Constipation occurs in less than one third of patients with carcinoma of the colon and is less common than diarrhea in these patients.**

Ribbon-like stools suggest a motility disorder. They can also be caused by an organic narrowing of the distal or sigmoid colon. A progressive decrease in the caliber of the stools suggests an organic lesion. If the patient complains of stools that have a toothpaste-like caliber, fecal impaction should be suspected.

Tumors of the descending colon are more common in older adults with right-sided lesions, increasing in frequency as the patient grows older. One third of colon cancers in patients older than 80 years are right sided, and fewer than half of these patients have altered bowel habits. They usually present late with an anemia or a palpable mass on the right side of the colon.

ASSOCIATED SYMPTOMS

In children, simple constipation is often associated with abdominal distention, decreased appetite, irritability, reduced activity, and soiling. Obstipated children (i.e., those who pass hard, dry stools every 3 to 5 days) may also have overflow soiling. If soiling persists after the constipation or obstipation has improved, the physician should search for some *psychological disturbance;* fecal impaction is relatively rare in children. When children have abdominal distention associated with constipation, the problem is usually caused by improper diet or decreased motility; intestinal obstruction is a rare cause of constipation in children. Acting out, school problems, and difficulties with interpersonal relationships should suggest that the constipation has a psychological cause.

If constipation is associated with steatorrhea and greenish yellow stools, a *small-bowel* or *pancreatic lesion* should be suspected. Constipation with early-morning rushes, hypogastric cramps, tenesmus, and passage of blood suggests that the constipation is of colonic origin.

In adults, colicky pain; abdominal distention; anemia; decreased effectiveness of laxatives; weight loss; anorexia; and blood, pus, or mucus in the stool should suggest a *colonic tumor*. Weight loss, anorexia, and anemia are usually observed only in the late phases of colonic tumors. Rectal discomfort, leakage of stool, bleeding, urgency, tenesmus, diarrhea alternating with constipation, and rectal prolapse all suggest a *rectosigmoid tumor*. In contrast, abdominal distention and sudden onset of obstipation suggest a more proximal colon lesion.

If constipation alternates with diarrhea or is accompanied by passage of hard scybala or intermittent left- or right-sided iliac pain that occasionally radiates through the torso to the back, constipation is probably caused by *irritable bowel syndrome*. A change in stool frequency or consistency associated with abdominal pain also suggests an irritable colon, as do abdominal distention and mucus in the stools.

Fecal incontinence, which some patients actually describe as diarrhea, should suggest *fecal impaction*. Most patients with this condition must strain during defecation, do not have normally formed stools, often have a toothpaste-like stool, and often have continuous soiling. Rectal examination usually reveals large quantities of hard feces in the rectal ampulla.

Constipation that develops after painful *hemorrhoids* suggests that the constipation is secondary to suppression of defecation because it induces pain. Patients with this condition, as well as others with local anorectal problems, often report blood in the bowel movements. When questioned, they usually recognize that the blood is on the surface of the stool, on the toilet paper, or in the toilet bowl rather than mixed in with the stool.

PRECIPITATING AND AGGRAVATING FACTORS

Patients and their family members should be questioned about stressful problems such as divorce, death of a spouse, and loss of a job. Twenty percent of children have moderate constipation when they begin to become effectively toilet trained. Functional constipation may be precipitated by hospital admission, traveling, suppression of the urge to defecate, uncomfortable lavatory environment (e.g., latrine), and/or immobilization. Reduction in laxative dose or change in brand of laxative occasionally precipitates constipation.

In elderly patients, constipation can be aggravated by limited variety in meals, decreased fluid or fiber intake, poor dentition, increased costs of fresh high-fiber foods (e.g., fruits, vegetables), impaired motility, debilitating illnesses, confinement to bed, and frequent ingestion of constipating drugs.

Certain drugs typically cause constipation. These include antacids that contain aluminum hydroxide or calcium, anticholinergics, antiparkinsonian drugs, diuretics, tricyclic antidepressants, opiates (in analgesics or cough medicine), phenytoin, cough medications calcium channel blockers, iron-containing compounds, and certain antihypertensive and antiseizure drugs. The patient may be taking one of these constipating agents but may experience symptoms only when a second drug is added.

AMELIORATING FACTORS

A diet high in fiber (e.g., whole-grain cereals, bran, vegetable fiber) and low in refined sugar often alleviates constipation. Many patients find that weight reduction diets that are low in carbohydrates and high in fiber relieve constipation. Increased fluid intake, particularly in patients who do not drink enough fluids or take diuretics, is often helpful. Relief of painful anorectal problems frequently alleviates constipation. If a change in daily routine has caused constipation, instructing the patient to readjust daily activities to permit bowel movements at the time of the urge to defecate is often effective.

PHYSICAL FINDINGS

A rectal examination should be performed in all patients with a significant complaint of constipation. This examination allows the physician to determine whether the rectum is full or empty, whether an anorectal problem exists (e.g., fissure, hemorrhoids), and whether a rectal mass is present. A stool specimen should be obtained to check for occult blood.

The physician should also conduct an abdominal examination, with special attention to the colon, to detect palpable masses (fecal or otherwise) or abdominal tenderness. Normally, the colon is neither palpable nor tender. If the colon can be palpated and it is tender, particularly over the descending or ascending regions, an irritable bowel syndrome is probable. Stigmata of myxedema and abdominal distention should suggest that the constipation is secondary to hypothyroidism. Anemia, manifested by tachycardia and conjunctival pallor, should suggest a right-sided colonic lesion. Abnormal bowel sounds, abdominal distention, or surgical scars suggest a specific cause for the constipation.

DIAGNOSTIC STUDIES

In most instances of chronic constipation, a trial of dietary changes, including increased fiber and fluids and decreased refined carbohydrates, will alleviate the constipation and the need for additional tests. A stool diary (date, frequency, time, symptoms of constipation [straining, bloating, incomplete evacuation], and medication) may be helpful. Examination of stools for occult blood and measurement of the hematocrit or hemoglobin and the erythrocyte sedimentation rate are appropriate, inexpensive, and noninvasive tests to evaluate constipation. In instances of alarm symptoms, colonoscopy and barium enema study are also helpful.

Newer studies, considered cost-effective in specific instances, are a colonic transit study with radiopaque markers, anorectal manometry, and balloon expulsion tests.

LESS COMMON DIAGNOSTIC CONSIDERATIONS

In neonates, *Hirschsprung's disease* (aganglionic megacolon) is the most prevalent of the less common causes of constipation. Early diagnosis is important. To differentiate between Hirschsprung's disease and chronic constipation, the physician should be aware that each condition is associated with characteristic symptoms. In Hirschsprung's disease, symptoms usually date from birth, soiling is absent, and the rectum is empty. With chronic constipation, onset may occur from ages 6 months to 3 years, soiling is common, and the rectum is usually full of feces.

Other less common causes of constipation in children include anorectal stenosis, chronic lead poisoning, hypothyroidism, hyperparathyroidism, medication, anal fissures, allergy to cow's milk, and neurologic abnormalities such as spina bifida.

If constipation is associated with nausea, polyuria, fatigue, and sometimes a history of kidney stones, *hypercalcemia,* though uncommon, may be the cause. Other metabolic and endocrinologic causes of constipation are diabetes, pregnancy, and hypothyroidism. Constipation may be the presenting symptom in patients with classic *myxedema.* Myxedematous patients frequently have an adynamic bowel with moderate abdominal distention. An adynamic bowel also occurs with senility, scleroderma, autonomic neuropathy, and spinal cord injuries and diseases. Idiopathic megacolon and megarectum can also produce severe constipation.

Psychiatric causes of constipation include depressive illness and anorexia nervosa. Occasionally, constipation is induced in depressed patients as the result of the anticholinergic effect of antidepressant drugs.

Marked prostatic enlargement may contribute to constipation. Disease or weakness of the abdominal muscles, neurologic diseases, diverticular diseases, occult rectal prolapse, pancreatic carcinoma, and lead poisoning are all rare causes of constipation.

Differential Diagnosis of Constipation

CONDITION	NATURE OF PATIENT	NATURE OF SYMPTOMS	ASSOCIATED SYMPTOMS	PRECIPITATING AND AGGRAVATING FACTORS	AMELIORATING FACTORS	PHYSICAL FINDINGS	DIAGNOSTIC STUDIES
Simple Constipation							
Low dietary fiber	Most common cause of constipation in adults	Dry, hard stools Stool frequency less than 5 times/wk Straining during stool	Children: may be associated with abdominal distention	Excessive intake of refined carbohydrates	Increased dietary fiber Decreased intake of refined carbohydrates	Ascending or descending colon tender to palpation Feces palpable in sigmoid colon	
Functional (environmental and daily-habit changes)	Most common cause of constipation in children Common cause in adults	Vague abdominal discomfort	Children: Abdominal distention Decreased appetite Irritability Decreased activity Soiling	Toilet training Traveling Uncomfortable lavatories Immobilization	Resume prior habits		
Disordered Motility							
Irritable bowel syndrome	Any age, especially young adults More frequent in patients with chronic fatigue syndrome, fibromyalgia, and TMJ syndrome	Change in stool frequency and consistency Constipation alternates with diarrhea Mucus in stools	Abdominal distention Abdominal pain	Stress	Increased dietary fiber Decreased environmental stress	Colon tender on palpation	

Continued

Differential Diagnosis of Constipation—cont'd

CONDITION	NATURE OF PATIENT	NATURE OF SYMPTOMS	ASSOCIATED SYMPTOMS	PRECIPITATING AND AGGRAVATING FACTORS	AMELIORATING FACTORS	PHYSICAL FINDINGS	DIAGNOSTIC STUDIES
Obstipation/fecal impaction	Most common in elderly and those subject to sudden immobility, bed rest, or decreased fluid consumption	Regular passage of hard stools at 3- to 5-day intervals; Patients describe continuous soiling as diarrhea; Toothpaste-caliber stools; Fecal incontinence; Straining during stool				Large quantities of hard feces in rectal ampulla	
Idiopathic slow transit	Most common in elderly people	Dry, hard stools; Decreased stool frequency		Decreased exercise; Decreased dietary fiber; Decreased fluid intake	Increased exercise; Increased dietary fiber; Increased fluids; Improved dentition	Rectum empty	Barium enema
Hirschsprung's disease (aganglionic megacolon)	Rare cause of constipation in children	Present from birth; Soiling absent					
Secondary Constipation							
Anal fissure	Affects any age	Patient suppresses painful defecation; Hard stools	Blood on surface of feces, on toilet paper, or in toilet			Anal fissure	Anoscopy
Hemorrhoids	Adults	Patient suppresses painful defecation	Blood on surface of feces, on toilet paper, or in toilet	Pregnancy; Prior hemorrhoid problems		Hemorrhoids	Anoscopy

Drug-induced constipation	Chronic laxative users Patients taking other medications Most common in elderly patients	Laxatives Codeine Morphine Analgesics NSAIDs Aluminum-containing antacids Antiparkinsonian drugs Cough mixtures Antidepressants Iron and calcium supplements Antihypertensives Calcium channel blockers			
Bowel tumors	Uncommon in children Frequency increases after age 40 yr	Constipation in less than one third of patients with colon cancer; diarrhea more common Early-morning rushes Decreased laxative effectiveness Blood, pus, or mucus in stool	Elderly patients with right-sided lesions may present late with anemia Weight loss Anorexia Colicky abdominal pain and distention	Possible palpable mass	Rectal examination Stool examination for occult blood Colonoscopy Barium enema
Rectosigmoid tumors		Rectal discomfort Stool leakage Urgency, tenesmus Progressive narrowing of stool caliber	Rectal bleeding Rectal prolapse		Sigmoidoscopy
Proximal colon tumors		Sudden onset Obstipation	Abdominal distention	Anemia	Colonoscopy Barium enema

NSAIDs, Nonsteroidal anti-inflammatory drugs; TMJ, temporomandibular joint.

Selected References

Arce DA, Ermocilla MD, Costa H: Evaluation of constipation, *Am Fam Physician* 65:2283-2290, 2002.

Bonapace ES, Fisher RS: Constipation and diarrhea in pregnancy, *Gastroenterol Clin North Am* 27:197-211, 1998.

De Lillo AR, Rose S: Functional bowel disorders in the geriatric patient: constipation, fecal impaction, and fecal incontinence, *Am J Gastroenterol* 95:901-905, 2000.

Drost J, Harris LA: Diagnosis and management of chronic constipation, *JAAPA* Nov 19:24-29, 2006.

Jacobs TQ, Pamies RJ: Adult constipation: a review and clinical guide, *J Nat Med Assoc* 93:22-30, 2001.

Keller J, Layer P: Intestinal and anorectal motility and functional disorders, *Best Pract Res Clin Gastroenterol* 23:407-423, 2009.

Malagelada JR: A symptom-based approach to making a positive diagnosis of irritable bowel syndrome with constipation, *Int J Clin Pract* 60:57-63, 2006.

Masi P, Miele E, Staiano A: Pediatric anorectal disorders, *Gastroenterol Clin North Am* 37:709-730, 2008.

Nowicki MJ, Bishop PR: Organic causes of constipation in infants and children, *Pediatr Ann* 28:293-299, 1999.

Remes-Troche JM, Rao SS: Diagnostic testing in patients with chronic constipation, *Curr Gastroenterol Rep* 8:416-424, 2006.

Solzi GF, DiLorenzo C: Are constipated children different from constipated adults? *Digest Dis* 17:308-315, 1999.

Stark ME: Challenging problems presenting as constipation, *Am J Gastroenterol* 94:567-574, 1999.

Talley NJ: Differentiating functional constipation from constipation-predominant irritable bowel syndrome: management implications, *Rev Gastroenterol Disord* 5:1-9, 2005.

Thompson WG, Heaton KW: Functional bowel disorders in apparently healthy people, *Gastroenterology* 79:283-288, 1980.

Cough

9

When evaluating patients with a cough, the physician should remember that:
1. Most healthy people seldom cough.
2. The main function of coughing is airway clearance.

The complaint of cough should be taken seriously, because it is one of the few ways by which abnormalities of the respiratory tree manifest themselves. Cough can be divided into three categories:

- Acute, lasting less than 3 weeks
- Subacute, lasting 3 to 8 weeks
- Chronic, lasting more than 8 weeks

Cough can be initiated by irritation of upper or lower airways. The most common causes of an acute cough are upper and lower respiratory *infections* (most often *viral upper respiratory tract infection), asthma, bronchitis, laryngitis,* and *allergies* (often seasonal), *pneumonia, exacerbation of chronic obstructive pulmonary disease (COPD),* and *heart failure.*

Common causes of a subacute cough include *postinfection state* and *cough-variant asthma.*

The most common causes of a chronic cough (duration more than 8 weeks) are *chronic bronchitis, postnasal drip (PND; currently called "upper airway cough syndrome") asthma, gastroesophageal reflux,* and medications such as angiotensin-converting enzyme *(ACE) inhibitors.* In many instances, chronic cough has multiple causes. Other common causes are *COPD, heart failure, tuberculosis, lung tumor,* and *habit* (Table 9-1).

The most common causes of recurrent cough in children are recurrent viral upper respiratory tract infections, reactive airway disease, asthma, viral bronchitis, and allergies.

NATURE OF PATIENT

Viral infections represent the most common cause of *acute* cough at all ages. This is particularly true of preschool children and even more likely if they are in close daily contact with many other children. In school-age children, *mycoplasmal pneumonias* are quite common. Because the incubation period is long

Table 9-1.   Causes of Chronic or Persistent Cough

Irritants	Cigarette smoking Dry air Dust Pollutants
Respiratory Tract Problems	Asthma Bronchiectasis Chronic obstructive pulmonary disease Chronic rhinitis Chronic sinusitis Disease of the external auditory canal Environmental and occupational factors Foreign body Heart failure Interstitial lung disease Pneumonitis Sick building syndrome Vocal cord dysfunction or polyps
Other	Angiotensin-converting enzyme inhibitor therapy Adenopathy Aortic aneurysm Malignancy Reflux esophagitis

Adapted from Ritz HJ: Pinning down the cause of a chronic cough. JAAPA 17:27-38, 2004; with permission from Haymarket Media, Inc. and American Academy of Physician Assistants.

(approximately 21 days), infection spreads slowly. *Bacterial pneumonias* also cause coughing and have their highest incidence in winter months. **Recurrent viral bronchitis is most prevalent in preschool and young school-age children and is the most common cause of a persistent cough in children of all ages.** There may be a genetically determined host susceptibility to frequently recurring bronchitis. Young patients with recurrent cough are often asthmatic. Physicians should be suspicious of underlying asthma contributing to a recurrent cough when there is a family history of allergies, atopy, or asthma.

A chronic cough in children (Table 9-2) is frequently caused by *allergic rhinitis, chronic sinusitis,* or *enlarged adenoids.* A chronic cough in children during the winter months is often due to bronchitis from dry air. Although it is rare, chronic cough in very young children (younger than age 12 months) should suggest congenital malformations or neonatal infections, including viral and chlamydial pneumonias. Other relatively uncommon causes of chronic cough in young infants include recurrent aspiration of milk, saliva, or gastric contents and cystic fibrosis. A chronic cough in children between ages 1 and 5 years should suggest bronchiectasis or cystic fibrosis after the more common causes have been ruled out. **In both children and adults, chronic cough may be the only manifestation of gastroesophageal reflux.**

Chronic cough in adults most often is caused by *chronic bronchitis* (especially in smokers), *gastroesophageal reflux disease* (GERD), *postnasal drip, asthma, environmental irritants, allergies,* and *habit.* Chronic cough resulted

TABLE 9-2.   Causes of Chronic Cough in Children According to Age

Infancy (age <1 yr)	Congenital malformations Congenital and neonatal infections: • Viral pneumonitis • Rubella • Cytomegalovirus • Aspiration • Milk • Gastric contents • Saliva Cystic fibrosis Asthma
Preschool (1 to 5 yr)	Inhaled foreign body Suppurative lung disease: • Chonic atelectasis • Bronchiectasis • Cystic fibrosis Bronchitis associated with chronic upper respiratory tract disease Asthma
School-age	Cigarette smoking *Mycoplasma pneumoniae* infections Nervous or psychogenic cough Cystic fibrosis
Common to all age groups	Recurrent viral bronchitis Asthma Pertussis Cystic fibrosis

Modified from Padiman R: The child with persistent cough. Del Med J 73:149-156, 2000.

from GERD, postnasal drip, or asthma in 99% of nonsmokers with a normal chest radiograph in one study. In older adults, any chronic cough without an obvious explanation should suggest *tumor* or *tuberculosis.*

NATURE OF SYMPTOMS

When the cough is of sudden onset and associated with fever or symptoms of an acute infection, a *viral* cause is most likely. The cough is noisy, produces minimal sputum, and is often worse at night. With *bacterial* and *mycoplasmal infections,* cough is often the most prominent symptom. Its onset may occur over hours or days, and the sputum produced is usually thick and yellowish. In mycoplasmal infections, the cough may be severe and persist for 1 to 4 months, although all other signs and symptoms abate within 7 to 10 days.

The cough caused by a viral upper respiratory infection (URI) or viral bronchitis usually lasts for 7 to 10 days. If the cough persists for longer than 14 days, a secondary bacterial infection may exist. If the cough is associated with shortness of breath and bilateral wheezing, asthma is likely. The cough of asthma is usually nonproductive or productive of minimal clear mucoid secretions.

An asthmatic cough is often worse in the late afternoon and at night; is associated with wheezing; is brought on by specific irritants; and is more common in patients with a family history of asthma, allergies, or atopy.

Patients with an acute or chronic cough secondary to upper airway cough syndrome (previously called *postnasal drip*) may not be aware of this condition. They should be questioned about swallowing mucus, frequent throat clearing, *hawking*, or cough that is worse in the morning. Examination may reveal mucoid secretions in the posterior pharynx, a cobblestone appearance of the mucosa, or signs of sinusitis. Although PND is usually caused by sinusitis, it may be caused by vasomotor or allergic rhinitis or nonallergic rhinitis with eosinophilia syndrome (NARES). It is important to differentiate these variant causes of rhinitis for effective treatment (Table 9-3).

A nocturnal cough associated with shortness of breath should suggest *paroxysmal nocturnal dyspnea* or *congestive heart failure*. A nocturnal cough without associated dyspnea indicates an *allergic origin*. On the other hand, a chronic cough that abates at night suggests a psychogenic or *habit cough*. A cough that recurs in the late afternoon or early evening is often due to asthma or allergy. This type of cough may occur in people who work in the city (where the pollen count is low) and then return in the late afternoon or evening to their suburban homes (where the pollen count is higher). A seasonal incidence of cough is highly suggestive of an allergic cause.

In smokers a chronic, minimally productive cough, often worse in the morning, is probably related to the irritating effect of inhaling tobacco smoke. Although it is more common in cigarette smokers, it also can occur in cigar and pipe smokers who inhale.

The evaluation of all patients whose chief complaint is cough should include a complete history, with particular attention to duration and character of the cough, smoking history, environmental and occupational experiences, antecedent allergies, asthma, sinusitis, symptoms of upper respiratory infection, heartburn, and shortness of breath or fainting while coughing *(tussive syncope)*. *Gastroesophageal reflux* should also be considered if cough is precipitated by chocolate, caffeine, or other foods (e.g., onions) that facilitate reflux. Exercise-induced cough may also be caused by reflux.

TABLE 9-3. Differentiating Vasomotor Rhinitis (VMR), Nonallergic Rhinitis With Eosinophilia Syndrome (NARES), and Allergic Rhinitis

FEATURE	VMR	NARES	ALLERGIC RHINITIS
Positive skin test results	No	No	Yes
Elevated serum immunoglobulin E levels	No	No	Yes
Eosinophils on nasal smear	No	Yes	Possible
Response to nasal corticosteroid	Yes	Yes	Yes
Triggered by odors	Yes	Yes	Possible

Modifed from Ritz HJ: Pinning down the cause of chronic cough. JAAPA 17:27-32, 2004.

ASSOCIATED SYMPTOMS

If a runny nose, a sore throat, or generalized aches and pains are present, the cough probably has an *infectious* cause. The presence of fever, chills, exudative or non-exudative pharyngitis, conjunctivitis, otitis, abdominal pain, headache, or pleuritic chest pain suggests the presence of *bacteria* or *mycoplasma*. Because PND (one cause of cough) may coexist with other conditions that produce chronic cough (e.g., bronchiectasis, heart failure, bronchogenic carcinoma, tuberculosis), the physician should not automatically assume that the PND is the only cause of the cough. If episodic wheezing or shortness of breath occurs in a patient complaining of cough, asthma is likely. When a cough is associated with heartburn or a sour taste in the mouth, gastroesophageal reflux is likely. **When chronic cough is caused by *silent* GERD, the chest radiograph findings are negative; the methacholine inhalation challenge result is negative; the patient is a nonsmoker and is not exposed to environmental irritants or ingesting an ACE inhibitor; there are no eosinophils in the sputum; and the cough does not improve after being treated for asthma or PND or with inhaled or systemic steroids.** It may, however, be improved by a trial of a proton-pump inhibitor. Stridor associated with cough suggests pathology, such as a foreign body or infection, in the larynx, upper trachea, or subglottic region.

An *allergic* cause of an otherwise unexplained cough is most likely if sneezing; a boggy, edematous nasal mucosa; conjunctivitis; tearing; itching of the roof of the mouth; or itching of the eyes is present.

Elderly patients, whose physical activity may be restricted by arthritis or other associated disease, may not present with the usual symptoms of dyspnea on exertion. The chief complaint instead may be a chronic unexplained cough that occurs only at night while the patient is recumbent or that worsens at night. **Therefore, any unexplained nocturnal cough in elderly patients should suggest congestive heart failure.**

PRECIPITATING AND AGGRAVATING FACTORS

In all cases of unexplained cough (particularly in children) precipitated by exercise, an asthmatic cause should be suspected, even with no typical wheezing. Some coughs are precipitated by exposure to very dry, superheated air, which frequently occurs in patients whose homes are heated with forced hot air. This cough may be exacerbated by sensitivity to spores in the dry, superheated air.

Chronic debilitating conditions such as alcoholism, malnutrition, diabetes, uremia, leukemia, and antitumor therapy may facilitate the development of infections that produce coughing. Long-term *cigarette smoking,* chronic exposure to *industrial irritants,* or *chronic respiratory disease* in childhood predisposes the patient to the development of lung disease and cough.

Patients with *allergic rhinitis* and *chronic sinusitis* are predisposed to PND and its resulting cough. This cough may be worse at night when the patient is recumbent because more mucus drips into the throat while the patient is in this position. Cough due to *gastroesophageal reflux* may also be worse when the patient is recumbent and may be precipitated by coffee, tea, caffeine, chocolate, alcohol, and/or exercise. Other coughs that worsen in the recumbent position or at night include those caused by allergies; paroxysmal nocturnal dyspnea; asthma; and breathing of dry, hot air.

Cough may be due to occupational or environmental factors, such as hypersensitivity, *pneumonitis*, indoor irritants (cigarette smoking, cooking fumes, dust mites) and *sick building syndrome*. Occupational and environmental factors must be considered in all patients.

AMELIORATING FACTORS

In patients with allergic rhinitis, antihistamine therapy and/or nasal steroids may ameliorate coughing by reducing secretions in the nose and paranasal sinuses. If cough, especially nocturnal cough, is relieved by inhaled steroids, asthma is likely. If smokers with chronic cough stop smoking, the cough usually abates. In one study, 77% of patients who ceased smoking lost their coughs, most after 1 month of not smoking. Coughing was greatly reduced in 13%. A cough relieved by the administration of a proton-pump inhibitor is probably due to GERD.

PHYSICAL FINDINGS

The ears, nose, mouth, throat (including indirect laryngoscopy), sinuses, neck, lungs, and cardiovascular system should be examined. **The patient should always be asked to cough so that the cough characteristics may be heard and the sputum examined.** A mucopurulent sputum suggests *infection,* although some *allergic* coughs are productive.

In patients with acute cough secondary to infection, the chest examination is often normal but the pharynx may be injected or pale, boggy, and swollen. The sinuses should be palpated, percussed, and transilluminated for evidence of *sinusitis.* When the mucosa of the nose or oropharynx has a cobblestone appearance (from chronic stimulation of submucosal lymphoid follicles), *PND* is probably causing the cough. If the lung fields are hyperresonant on percussion and auscultation reveals distant breath sounds, scattered rhonchi or wheezes, or prolonged expiration, *COPD* should be suspected. Bilateral expiratory wheezing suggests asthma, but unilateral wheezing suggests a foreign body or infection. Basilar rales suggest heart failure. Localized crackles suggest an infectious process.

Cough may be the earliest symptom of *heart failure,* particularly in patients with pulmonary hypertension or mitral stenosis. Cough may occur before the usual findings in chronic congestive heart failure (rales, edema, tachycardia, and gallop) are evident.

DIAGNOSTIC STUDIES

Tests used to determine the cause of cough include a complete blood count, an eosinophil count, sinus and chest radiographs, 24-hour monitoring of esophageal pH, and cytologic and microscopic sputum examination. If a large number of eosinophils are observed in a stained sputum specimen, an allergic cause is probable. Pulmonary function tests, bronchoscopy, and cardiovascular studies may help in some cases.

A chest radiograph should be performed in all patients with chronic cough. The chest radiograph findings may be negative in some patients with diffuse infiltrative lung disease. Approximately 5% of patients with sarcoidosis have normal chest films. Likewise, patients with cough due to a tracheobronchial lesion may have a normal chest radiograph.

If an asthmatic cough is suspected and wheezing is absent, pulmonary function tests that measure response to isoproterenol should be performed. In rare instances, bronchial provocation with methacholine may be performed, but only with extreme care. If these tests are positive, asthma is the most likely cause of the cough.

A simple outpatient diagnostic test for a cough due to congestive heart failure is the administration of a potent oral diuretic for 2 to 3 days. If the patient loses several pounds through diuresis and demonstrates marked improvement of the cough, the cough is probably caused by pulmonary congestion secondary to heart failure. Ultrasonography may also be used to estimate the ejection fraction.

LESS COMMON DIAGNOSTIC CONSIDERATIONS

Most people who complain of cough do not have *bronchogenic carcinoma*. However, 70% to 90% of patients with bronchogenic carcinoma experience a cough at some time during the course of the disease. Various studies have documented that cough is the presenting symptom for 21% to 87% of patients with bronchogenic carcinoma. The possibility of bronchogenic carcinoma is especially strong in chronic cigarette smokers who have a cough that lasts for months or who demonstrate a marked change in the character of the cough. Pulmonary tumors are often characterized by a change in the cough pattern, hemoptysis, chest pain, and enlarged supraclavicular nodes.

In patients with a *lung abscess*, cough is the dominant symptom more often than bloody sputum, pain, or dyspnea. The cough observed in patients with *bronchiectasis* is usually of long duration; productive of loose, moist, purulent sputum; and occasionally associated with hemoptysis. The cough of *tuberculosis* is often chronic (although it may be acute) and associated with hemoptysis, fever, night sweats, apical rales, and weight loss.

The physician should be particularly suspicious of disorders of the trachea or larynx in patients with inspiratory stridor or a dry, brassy, high-pitched, and unproductive cough. If the cough is associated with marked dyspnea, tachypnea, tachycardia, calf tenderness, prolonged immobility, atrial fibrillation, pleural friction, or hemoptysis, *pulmonary embolism* should be suspected.

Patients ranging in age from 3 months to 6 years may experience *croup* (laryngotracheobronchitis). This cough has a barking quality. Intercostal retraction with inspiration, inspiratory or expiratory wheezing, hoarseness, and difficulty with air movement all suggest this potentially critical condition. Hospitalization for intensive therapy may be necessary. In young children an inhaled foreign body must also be considered as the cause of coughing. Cough in very young infants suggests a congenital malformation such as tracheoesophageal fistulas or laryngeal clefts. Cough in the newborn may be due to interstitial pneumonia from congenital rubella or cytomegalic virus infections.

A rare and usually unrecognized cause of chronic cough is impaction of cerumen, a foreign body, or hair in the ear canal, which stimulates a cough through a reflex (ear-cough) mechanism. This cough is triggered by irritation of the external auditory canal or tympanic membrane.

Exposure to noxious gases, dusts, industrial pollutants, and smog can produce cough, particularly in people who have underlying lung disease.

ACE inhibitors and beta blockers, including β_2-blocker eyedrops, may cause a chronic nonproductive cough.

Reflux esophagitis does not usually present with cough, but patients with this condition may cough when they are recumbent. **It should be considered in all instances of unexplained chronic cough.**

Although it is rare, ornithosis should be considered in patients who have a dry, hacking, unproductive cough with fever and are in contact with fowl or pet birds. Physical findings in these patients are often normal except for fever and cough. Coccidioidomycosis should be suspected if cough develops after the patient has visited an endemic area such as the San Joaquin Valley. **Pertussis is reemerging and should be suspected in children of recent immigrants from countries where they may not have been vaccinated.** It may occur rarely in the adult immigrants.

When a complete history and thorough physical and laboratory examinations reveal no cause for a cough, a *subdiaphragmatic process* (abscess or tumor) should be considered. If no organic cause for a chronic cough is found, Tourette's syndrome or another *psychogenic cause* should be considered. Patients with such conditions do not cough at night and often can stop coughing if so instructed. This cough is seldom productive. In children it may be an attention-getting device; in adults it may be associated with other signs of anxiety.

A diagnosis of unexplained cough (previously called *idiopathic*) should be made only after a thorough search for and treatment of both common and uncommon causes of cough have been performed.

Differential Diagnosis of Cough

CONDITION	NATURE OF PATIENT	NATURE OF SYMPTOMS	ASSOCIATED SYMPTOMS	PRECIPITAT-ING AND AGGRAVAT-ING FACTORS	AMELIO-RATING FACTORS	PHYSICAL FINDINGS	DIAGNOSTIC STUDIES
Acute Cough							
Viral upper respiratory tract infec-tions	Most common cause of acute cough in all ages	Acute onset of noisy cough (over hours or days) Cough worse at night and may persist for 7-10 days Sputum thick and yellowish but minimal amount produced	Fever Runny nose Sore throat General aches and pains			Pharynx injected or pale, boggy, and swollen Coarse rhonchi	
Mycoplasmal bronchitis or pneumonia	Common cause of acute cough in school-age children Frequent cause of persistent cough in adults	Long incubation period (about 21 days) Severe cough may persist for 1-4 months Other symptoms (e.g., fever) abate within 10 days	Same as for bacterial pneumonia but not usually as severe			Scattered rales Signs of pneumonia	Chest radio-graph Cold aggluti-nins Complement fixation
Viral bron-chitis	Recurrent infections are most common cause of per-sistent cough in children, who are often asthmatic	Cough may persist for 7-10 days	Fever				

Continued

Differential Diagnosis of Cough —cont'd

CONDITION	NATURE OF PATIENT	NATURE OF SYMPTOMS	ASSOCIATED SYMPTOMS	PRECIPITATING AND AGGRAVATING FACTORS	AMELIORATING FACTORS	PHYSICAL FINDINGS	DIAGNOSTIC STUDIES
Allergies	History of allergy in family	Minimally productive May be nocturnal Recurrent cough without dyspnea May have seasonal incidence	Sneezing Conjunctivitis Tearing Itching of eyes and roof of mouth Postnasal drip		Antihistamines	Boggy, edematous nasal mucosa	Stained sputum smear for eosinophils
Bacterial pneumonia		Noisy cough Incidence highest in winter Acute onset Cough worse at night	Fever, chills Signs of acute infection Pharyngitis Conjunctivitis Otitis Abdominal pain Headache Pleuritic chest pain	Chronic debilitating conditions		Signs of pneumonia	Chest radiograph Sputum and blood cultures
Chronic or Recurrent Cough							
Postnasal drip	May not be aware of condition	Frequent throat clearing and hawking Cough worse in morning		Recumbency Chronic sinusitis Vasomotor rhinitis Allergic rhinitis Nonallergic rhinitis with eosinophilia		Mucoid secretions in posterior pharynx Palpation, percussion, and transillumination of sinuses reveal sinusitis Mucosa of nose/oropharynx: cobblestone appearance	

Asthma	May have family history of allergies, atopy, or asthma	Recurrent cough; Minimally or not productive (if productive, secretions clear and mucoid)	Shortness of breath	Exercise; May be worse during seasonal allergies		Bilateral wheezing	Pulmonary function tests; Response to isoproterenol and methacholine
Chronic obstructive pulmonary disease	Elderly patients		Shortness of breath			Lungs hyperresonant to percussion; Auscultation reveals distant breath sounds, scattered rhonchi, wheezes, or prolonged expiration	Pulmonary function tests
Chronic bronchitis	Most common cause of chronic cough in adults (especially smokers)	May be minimally productive; Often worse in morning			Smoking cessation	Scattered rhonchi	
Congestive heart failure	Elderly patients present differently; May have only chronic, unexplained cough	Cough often nocturnal	Dyspnea on exertion; Paroxysmal nocturnal dyspnea	Recumbency; Exercise	Diuresis	Rales; Pitting edema; Tachycardia; Gallop	Chest radiograph; Potent diuretic for 2-3 days should improve symptoms; Ejection fraction
Gastroesophageal reflux	Usually adults	Irritative, nonproductive cough	Heartburn, eructation	Recumbency; Ingestion of chocolate, caffeine, or alcohol; Exercise	Antireflux measures, including diet, drugs, and elevating head of bed	Usually none	Upper gastrointestinal radiograph; Esophagoscopy; Esophageal pH monitoring

Selected References

de Jongste JC, Shields MD: Chronic cough in children, *Thorax* 58:998-1003, 2003.

Dudha M, Lehrman SG, Aronow WS, et al: Evaluation and management of cough, *Compr Ther* 35:9-17, 2009.

Irwin RS, Baumann MH, Bolser DC, et al: Diagnosis and management of cough: ACCP evidence-based clinical practice guidelines, *Chest* 129(Suppl 1):1S-23S, 2006.

Mello CJ, Irwin RS, Curley FJ: Predictive values of the character, timing, and complications of chronic cough in diagnosing its cause, *Arch Intern Med* 156:997-1003, 1996.

Padman R: The child with persistent cough, *Del Med J* 73:149-156, 2000.

Patrick H, Patrick F: Chronic cough, *Med Clin North Am* 79:361-372, 1995.

Philp EB: Chronic cough, *Am Fam Physician* 56:1395-1402, 1997.

Pratter MR: Unexplained (idiopathic) cough: ACCP evidence-based clinical practice guidelines, *Chest Jan* 129:220S-221S, 2006.

Ramanuja S, Kelkar P: Habit cough, *Ann Allergy Asthma Immunol* 102:91-95, 2009.

Ritz HJ: Pinning down the cause of chronic cough, *JAAPA* 17:27-32, 2004.

Tarlo SM: Cough: occupational and environmental considerations: ACCP evidence-based clinical practice guidelines, *Chest* 129(Suppl 1):186S-196S, 2006.

Diarrhea

10

In this chapter, *diarrhea* is defined as an increase in frequency, fluidity, or volume of bowel movements relative to the usual habit for a person. Acute diarrhea is second in frequency only to acute respiratory tract disease in American families. Severe, acute diarrhea is more prevalent in vulnerable groups such as the elderly, travelers, those immunosuppressed from human immunodeficiency virus (HIV), those taking steroids, and those undergoing chemotherapy. **Diarrhea most frequently results from *acute gastroenteritis* caused by a virus or (less often) by bacteria or protozoa.**

Infectious diarrhea is more prevalent in patients with close living (including shipboard) or working conditions and who are exposed to contaminated food and water or inadequate sewage disposal. Other common causes of diarrhea are *irritable bowel syndrome* (IBS) (previously called irritable colon, mucous colitis, or functional diarrhea), diabetes, and ingestion of *antibiotics, anti-inflammatory agents, magnesium-containing substances, alcohol, lactose intolerance, and celiac disease* (gluten sensitivity). The diarrhea of IBS, diabetes, lactose intolerance, continuous drug ingestion, or alcoholism is usually chronic.

When evaluating a patient's complaint of diarrhea, the physician must inquire about the following matters:

1. The usual frequency and pattern of bowel movements
2. The current pattern of bowel movements
3. Nocturnal diarrhea
4. Blood or mucus in the stool
5. Travel within the United States or abroad
6. Recent dietary changes
7. Exacerbation of diarrhea by particular foods such as dairy products
8. Recent drug ingestion
9. Change in the nature of food intake
10. Any significant previous medical or surgical history

NATURE OF PATIENT

In all age groups, *viral gastroenteritis* is the most common cause of acute diar-rhea. This is usually a benign, self-limiting condition in adults but can result in severe dehydration in infants and children. In infants younger than 3 years, *rotavirus* is responsible for about 50% of wintertime nonbacterial gastroenteri-tis. This winter peak is even greater in temperate climates, such as that found in the United States. *Salmonella* as a cause of gastroenteritis is more common in children ages 1 to 4 years. Epidemics of *Shigella* have been noted in children ages 1 to 4 years and in people living in closed environments, particularly those with substandard sanitation (e.g., in prisons and custodial institutions).

In infants and toddlers, functional gastrointestinal (GI) disorders include functional diarrhea and constipation.

Giardiasis is not common in children, but infants are susceptible. Infants may be quite ill, in contrast to adults, who are often asymptomatic. However, acute or subacute diarrhea with marked symptomatology may also occur in some adults with giardiasis. Reports of symptomatic giardiasis have increased, primarily among hikers and campers, who are most likely to drink *Giardia*-infested water.

Whenever diarrhea in infants less than 1 year of age corresponds to increased ingestion of dairy products, *lactose intolerance* (lactase deficiency) should be suspected. This form of diarrhea is not limited to infants and young children. It occurs in 15% of persons of northern European descent, up to 80% of African Americans and Hispanics, and up to 100% of Native Americans and Asians. Although these people may not have previously demonstrated lactose intoler-ance, lactase production normally decreases with age. This decrease is more pro-nounced in some people, and diarrhea seems to follow acute or chronic ingestion of large quantities of lactose as found in milk, cheese, ice cream, and other dairy products. Transient lactase deficiency is common after infectious gastroenteritis.

Middle-aged women with chronic diarrhea are more likely to have functional diarrhea or *irritable bowel syndrome*. This condition seems to have a predilec-tion for young women who are raising children, especially if they have the added responsibility of a job outside the home. It affects other stressed people as well. Another form of diarrhea reported to be more frequent among middle-aged women is that due to the misuse or surreptitious use of purgatives. Patients who use laxatives surreptitiously often demonstrate other features of hysteri-cal behavior. The addition of sodium hydroxide to the stool provides a simple test for some forms of laxative abuse. The over-the-counter laxative products Ex-Lax, Feen-A-Mint, and Correctol contain phenolphthalein, which turns the stool red when alkali (sodium hydroxide) is added.

Patients with *diabetes* and associated neurologic dysfunction may also have chronic diarrhea. Some diabetic patients have gastric stasis and poor bowel motility, permitting bacterial overgrowth in the small bowel, which may pro-duce uncontrollable, explosive, postprandial diarrhea. Patients with this condi-tion may refrain from eating before leaving their homes to avoid uncontrollable diarrhea at an inconvenient time. A therapeutic trial of antibiotics may stop the diarrhea by combating the bacterial overgrowth.

Although acute diarrhea is usually benign and self-limiting, the following patients are particularly prone to serious complications from acute and chronic diarrhea: neonates, elderly people, patients with sickle cell disease, and those who are immunocompromised (by underlying disease or chemotherapy). Diarrhea due to enteric infections from protozoal, fungal, bacterial, and viral pathogens is common in patients with acquired immunodeficiency syndrome (AIDS).

NATURE OF SYMPTOMS

It is important to note the onset and duration of symptoms, weight loss, nocturnal diarrhea, and whether contacts are sick. A useful approach to the differential diagnosis of diarrhea is to separate *acute diarrhea* (which has an abrupt onset; lasts for less than 1 week; and may be associated with a viral prodrome, nausea, vomiting, or fever) from *chronic diarrhea* (in which the initial episode lasts longer than 2 weeks or symptoms recur over months or years). **The acute onset of diarrhea in a previously healthy patient without signs or symptoms of other organ system involvement suggests an infectious cause that most often is viral.** Norwalk virus has caused outbreaks of diarrhea among travelers on cruises. When vomiting and diarrhea begin suddenly and occur in many people at the same time, a preformed bacterial toxin (e.g., staphylococcal enterotoxin) is often the cause. Symptoms usually begin 2 to 8 hours after ingestion of contaminated food, most often in the summer months, when food may be inadequately refrigerated. With *Salmonella, Shigella,* or *Campylobacter,* symptoms are delayed for 24 to 72 hours while the organisms multiply in the body. With *Giardia* this delay may be 1 to 2 weeks.

Chronic diarrhea is most commonly caused by *IBS, medications, dietary factors, chronic inflammatory bowel disease,* and *colon cancer.* IBS may manifest as chronic or intermittent diarrhea (which classically alternates with constipation) or as flare-ups of diarrhea that occur during stressful periods. Stools are looser and more frequent with the onset of pain. A history of hard, often marble-like stools alternating with soft bowel movements, especially if associated with mucus in the toilet bowl or on the surface of the stool, suggests IBS. Although a patient suffers from chronic IBS, a superimposed case of viral gastroenteritis, salmonellosis, or giardiasis must still be considered. In such patients, a new cause of diarrhea should be sought if the usual diarrhea associated with the irritable colon changes or exacerbates.

Persistent diarrhea with frothy, foul-smelling stools that sometimes float suggests a *pancreatic* or *small-bowel* cause. Foul-smelling, watery, explosive diarrhea with mucus is often seen in *giardiasis*. The latency period may be 1 to 3 weeks. The onset of diarrhea due to giardiasis may be acute or gradual; it may persist for several weeks or months.

Functional diarrhea almost never occurs at night and seldom awakens the patient. It is typically present in the morning. Copious amounts of mucus may be present, but blood is seldom in the stool except that from hemorrhoidal bleeding. If questioned, the patient may admit to noticing undigested food in the stool and rectal urgency. Nocturnal diarrhea almost always has an organic cause.

ASSOCIATED SYMPTOMS

It is also diagnostically helpful to classify acute diarrhea into two types: *toxin-mediated diarrhea* (small-bowel diarrhea) and *infectious diarrhea* (colonic diarrhea) (Table 10-1). Patients with toxin-mediated diarrhea have an abrupt onset (often a few hours after eating potentially contaminated foods, especially unpasteurized dairy products and undercooked meat or fish) of large-volume, watery diarrhea associated with variable nausea, vomiting, increased salivation, crampy abdominal pain, and general malaise but little or no fever. The onset of neurologic symptoms in association with diarrhea suggests *Clostridium* toxin *(botulism)*.

Diarrhea of an infectious cause should be suspected with a history of prior good health, acute onset of diarrhea, and no signs or symptoms of involvement of systems other than the GI tract. This type of diarrhea is caused by *colonic mucosal invasion* and has also been referred to as *dysentery syndrome.* The presence of fever, vomiting, nausea, abdominal cramps, headache, general malaise, and myalgia along with watery diarrhea suggests *viral gastroenteritis* and *Salmonella* or *Campylobacter.* Infectious diarrhea, particularly that due to *Campylobacter,* often triggers an episode of postinfectious IBS (see Table 10-1).

Diarrhea of *colonic origin* should be suspected if fever, early-morning rushes, hypogastric cramps, tenesmus, blood in the stools, or soft stools mixed with copious mucus are associated with diarrhea. Patients with fever and symptoms of small-bowel or colonic diarrhea may have *shigellosis;* this is more common in the summer. Diarrhea caused by *Salmonella* may have an acute or subacute onset or may present as chronic diarrhea. When a patient known to have intermittent chronic diarrhea due to IBS has an increase in diarrhea, the cause may be additional stress or infectious diarrhea (e.g., *Salmonella*) superimposed on IBS. *Campylobacter jejuni* has been implicated in a large number of cases of food-borne diarrhea. It is usually associated with fever, bloody diarrhea, and abdominal pain.

When right lower quadrant pain is associated with diarrhea, *Yersinia* or *Campylobacter* infections may simulate *appendicitis.* The bacterial infections often cause diffuse abdominal tenderness and no rebound, thus militating against a diagnosis of appendicitis.

Blood on the surface of stools or on toilet paper suggests blood of anal origin, most often a bleeding hemorrhoid or small anal fissure, particularly if the bleeding occurs after hard stools are passed.

Alarm symptoms include onset of GI bleeding in patients older than 50 years, weight loss, nocturnal symptoms, and a family history of colorectal cancer. Constant abdominal pain associated with diarrhea in patients older than

Table 10-1. Infectious Diarrheas

ONSET	CHARACTERISTICS	DURATION	ETIOLOGY	SOURCE	LABORATORY TESTS	TREATMENT
1-6 hr	Nausea, vomiting, abdominal pain, diarrhea	24-48 hr	Staphylococcus aureus	Poorly refrigerated meats, egg or potato salad, cream pastries	Vomitus, stool for toxin	Supportive
9-48 hr	Diarrhea, fever, muscle aches	Variable	Listeria	Deli meats, hot dogs; unpasteurized milk; fresh, soft cheese	Not helpful	Ampicillin (TMP/SMZ)
	Cause of spontaneous abortions and stillbirths					
12-72 hr	Diarrhea, vomiting, blurred vision, diplopia	Variable	Clostridium botulinum	Home-canned/poorly canned food (low acid); honey	Stool for organism, toxin	Supportive, antitoxin
24-48 hr	Abdominal cramping, bloody diarrhea, mucus	4-7 days	Shigella	Feces-contaminated food or water	Routine stool culture	Quinolones, TMP/SMZ
	Vomiting, diarrhea, abdominal pain, fever	1-3 wk	Yersinia	Undercooked pork, unpasteurized milk	Organism-specific stool culture	Supportive Quinolones, TMP/SMZ
	Watery diarrhea, nausea, vomiting	24-60 hr	Norwalk virus	Undercooked shellfish, salads, fruits	Serum antibody titers	Supportive care Pepto-Bismol
24-72 hr	Bloody diarrhea, fever, abdominal pain	2-10 days	Campylobacter	Undercooked poultry, unpasteurized milk, contaminated water	Routine stool culture	Supportive care Consider quinolones, erythromycin
	Profuse, watery diarrhea; vomiting	3-7 days	Vibrio cholerae	Contaminated water, fish, shellfish	Organism-specific stool culture	Aggressive ORT Quinolones or doxycycline for adults; TMP/SMZ for children
1-3 days	Watery diarrhea, low-grade fever, vomiting	4-6 days	Rotavirus	Feces-contaminated foods	Stool test for rotavirus antigen	Supportive care
	Diarrhea, cramps, fever/chills, vomiting	4-7 days	Salmonella (not S. typhi)	Contaminated eggs, poultry, unpasteurized milk; juice; contaminated water	Routine stool culture	Supportive care Consider quinolones, azithromycin

Continued

TABLE 10-1.   Infectious Diarrheas—cont'd

ONSET	CHARACTERISTICS	DURATION	ETIOLOGY	SOURCE	LABORATORY TESTS	TREATMENT
1-8 days	Watery diarrhea, abdominal cramps, vomiting	3-7 days	Enterotoxigenic *Escherichia coli* (ETEC)	Contaminated water; food contaminated with feces; contact with farm animals, petting zoos	Organism-specific stool culture	Supportive care Consider TMP/SMZ or quinolones
	Bloody diarrhea, abdominal pain	5-10 days	Enterohemorrhagic *E. coli* (EHEC), including *E. coli* 0157 : H7	Undercooked beef; unpasteurized milk, juice	Organism-specific stool culture	Antibiotics harmful! Supportive care Watch for hemolytic-uremic syndrome
1-11 days	Relapsing diarrhea, fatigue, weight loss	Weeks-months	*Cyclospora*	Contaminated water, berries, lettuce	Organism-specific stool culture	TMP/SMZ
7 days	Watery diarrhea; crampy abdominal pain; fever; vomiting; relapsing	Days-weeks	*Cryptosporidium*	Contaminated water, vegetables, fruits; unpasteurized milk; ingestion of contaminated water in swimming pools (cysts resistant to chlorine)	Organism-specific stool culture	Supportive
1-4 wk	Diarrhea, bloating, flatulence	Weeks	*Giardia*	Contaminated water—farm wells, streams, lakes	Stool examination for ova and parasites	Metronidazole
1-10 wk	Watery diarrhea with blood and/or mucus, fever, abdominal cramping	Variable; relapses common	*Clostridium difficile*	Antibiotic use, especially cephalosporins and clindamycin	Stool sample for ELISA of toxins	Metronidazole or vancomycin

ELISA, Enzyme-linked immunosorbent assay; ORT, Oral replacement therapy; TMP/SMZ, trimethoprim/sulfamethoxazole.
From Covington C: Diarrhea—a review of common and uncommon issues. Adv Nurse Pract 10:34-39, 2002.

40 years is another alarm symptom, suggesting a condition requiring surgery. Copious bleeding or blood mixed with the stools suggests a more serious cause, such as *ulcerative colitis*. Marked weight loss associated with persistent diarrhea and frothy, foul-smelling stools that sometimes float suggests a pancreatic or small-bowel cause of *steatorrhea* and diarrhea. When acute diarrhea and severe vomiting (out of proportion to the diarrhea) begin 2 to 4 hours after consumption of potentially contaminated foods (especially milk products or meats), *toxic staphylococcal gastroenteritis* should be suspected. The diagnosis is confirmed presumptively if these symptoms also developed in other people who ate the same foods.

In addition to foul-smelling, watery, explosive mucoid stools, patients with giardiasis may have increased flatulence, nausea, and (in severe cases) anorexia and weight loss. Some patients complain of abdominal distention and occasional greasy stools.

Diarrhea associated with perianal excoriation (related to acidic stools), abdominal distention, occasional vomiting, fever, anorexia, and, in children, failure to thrive indicates *lactose intolerance*.

Muscle weakness, lassitude, and hypokalemia can be seen in any patient with protracted, copious diarrhea, but their presence should make the physician suspicious of surreptitious *laxative abuse*, particularly if other components of a hysterical personality are present.

Other associated findings that may suggest the etiology of the diarrhea include arthritis (inflammatory bowel disease), fever (inflammatory bowel disease, lymphoma, amebiasis, and tuberculosis), marked weight loss (malabsorption, cancer, and hyperthyroidism), lymphadenopathy (lymphoma and AIDS), neuropathy (diabetes), and peptic ulcer symptoms (antacid therapy and Zollinger-Ellison syndrome).

PRECIPITATING AND AGGRAVATING FACTORS

Drug-induced diarrhea should be suspected if diarrhea develops after the administration of antibiotics or other drugs. The most commonly implicated antibiotics are ampicillin, tetracycline, lincomycin, clindamycin, and chloramphenicol. The diarrhea ranges from mild and watery with nonspecific crampy abdominal pain and low-grade fever to severe colitis with pseudomembrane formation. *Pseudomembranous enterocolitis* is life-threatening and is of the colonic or dysentery type. It is more common if several antibiotics have been administered but is classically caused by a clindamycin-associated *Clostridium difficile* superinfection. Symptoms may begin during or within 3 months of a course of antibiotic therapy or during/following a hospitalization.

Magnesium-containing antacids, methyldopa, digitalis, beta blockers, systemic anti-inflammatory agents, iron-containing compounds, laxatives, lactulose, colchicine, quinidine, phenothiazine, drugs, prokinetic agents such as metoclopramide or cisapride, and high doses of salicylates can also cause diarrhea.

If the onset of diarrhea is temporally related to acute stress, particularly *emotional stress*, a functional cause is probable. In patients with a functional cause, the onset of diarrhea may be gradual or acute, and the duration protracted.

Ingestion of *contaminated water* or *food* may occur at any time but especially during travel abroad or camping, thus producing *traveler's diarrhea*. All patients with acute diarrhea should be asked about travel, medications, stress, food ingestion, exposure to others with similar symptoms, dairy product consumption, and recent illnesses.

AMELIORATING FACTORS

The diarrhea of lactose intolerance abates with fasting or avoidance of foods that contain lactose. Functional diarrhea is alleviated with decreased stress. If the diarrhea is relieved by antibiotics, bacterial overgrowth may have been the cause. Likewise, if the diarrhea is associated with antibiotic administration, cessation of antibiotics often alleviates the diarrhea.

PHYSICAL FINDINGS

Physical examination must include a careful abdominal examination and in some cases a rectal examination. Fever in association with acute diarrhea suggests an infectious cause. Signs of peritoneal involvement suggest an invasive enteric pathogen. Thyroid enlargement and tremor suggest thyrotoxicosis; and enlarged lymph nodes suggest lymphoma or AIDS. The colon may be tender on palpation in patients with IBS, who may also have abdominal distention. Stools should be examined visually for blood or mucus and microscopically for fecal leukocytes, ova, and parasites. Signs of dehydration such as decreased tissue turgor, postural hypotension, and tachycardia help assess the severity of diarrhea.

DIAGNOSTIC STUDIES

Studies have shown that a specific causative agent cannot be isolated in about 60% of patients with acute gastroenteritis. Examination of patients with persistent, unexplained diarrhea should include a complete blood count and colonoscopic examination with particular attention to the colonic mucosa. Patients with invasive (so-called colonic) diarrhea have an erythematous colonic mucosa that may have ecchymoses, friability, excess mucus, and small ulcerations. These ulcerations must be differentiated from the ragged ulcers of *ulcerative colitis* and the discrete, punched-out ulcers that are almost pathognomonic of *amebic colitis*. Upper endoscopy may be indicated when colonoscopy is negative and the diagnosis is unclear despite persistent diarrhea. Endoscopic biopsies of the small intestine can confirm the diagnosis of celiac disease, though initial evaluation includes a blood test for endomysial and tissue transglutaminase antibodies as well as total IgA. Thyroid stimulating hormone should also be measured in patients with chronic diarrhea. Capsule endoscopy is not usually useful in the diagnosis of diarrhea although it may be helpful when radiologic and endoscopic studies are negative.

Fecal lactoferrin measurement has replaced the study of fecal leukocytes. When results of this study are negative, they usually rules out inflammatory diarrhea and the need for a stool culture. Fecal lactoferrin measurement is a more sensitive test than fecal leukocyte testing. Real-time polymerase chain reaction (PCR) provides a rapid means of identifying bacterial pathogens that cause diarrhea.

Organisms that cause diarrhea by toxin production *(Escherichia coli, Clostridium perfringens, Vibrio cholerae,* and *Staphylococcus)* or by induction of small-bowel lesions (*Giardia* and viruses) may cause a watery stool without fecal leukocytes. Amebic dysentery is usually not associated with fecal leukocytes.

Microscopic examination for ova and parasites may reveal amoeba or *Giardia* cysts in 50% of patients with giardiasis. If neither is found, a *Giardia* antigen test may be obtained. A jejunal biopsy and jejunal or duodenal aspiration may also reveal *Giardia* cysts. Serologic tests for amebiasis are also available. Stool may me assayed for the presence of *Clostridium difficile toxin.*

In patients with diarrhea caused by laxative abuse, proctoscopic examination may reveal melanosis coli. Urine and stool samples may test positive for phenolphthalein. A barium enema may show increased haustral markings.

In patients with lactose intolerance, the stool pH is less than 6.0, stool glucose concentration is greater than 1g/100 mL, and results of a hydrogen breath test are positive.

Flat films, MRI, and abdominal laparoscopy may be useful in special instances.

LESS COMMON DIAGNOSTIC CONSIDERATIONS

Less common causes of diarrhea include amebiasis, pinworm, bacterial overgrowth after abdominal surgery, achlorhydria, gastric stasis (in diabetes), carcinoid syndrome, blind loop syndrome with bacterial overgrowth, inflammatory bowel disease, Crohn's disease, ulcerative colitis, and radiation colitis.

Antidiarrheal drugs can result in obstipation. With obstipation and fecal impaction (which is more common in elderly patients), there may be frequent small, loose, and watery bowel movements without much solid stool. Fecal impaction can usually be diagnosed by rectal examination.

Patients with *inflammatory bowel disease* usually have frequent small stools or diarrhea with the passage of blood, mucus, and occasionally pus. They often have rectal leakage, nocturnal diarrhea, pain, urgency, and early-morning rushes. With the acute form, patients may appear toxic and have malaise, fever, dehydration, and tachycardia. Those with chronic inflammatory bowel disease may have weight loss, anemia, joint pains, and skin lesions (e.g., erythema nodosum).

Intestinal ischemia (bloody diarrhea from ischemic colitis or severe diarrhea from small-bowel ischemia) should be considered in all patients who have experienced shock or a hypotensive episode.

Malabsorption conditions other than lactose intolerance include adult nontropical celiac sprue (actually a gluten sensitivity); intolerance to carbohydrates, cow's milk, or protein; and loss of absorptive surface due to bowel resection or sprue.

Maldigestion results from inadequate bile acid concentration or pancreatic exocrine insufficiency.

Pancreatic islet cell tumors and colorectal carcinoma may present initially with diarrhea. *Colorectal cancer* is more common in middle-aged than elderly patients and may manifest as any change in bowel habits, most often diarrhea alternating with constipation. Diarrhea may be the only presenting symptom, particularly if the lesion is in the cecum or ascending colon.

CHRONIC DIARRHEA IN CHILDREN

The specific time that must elapse for diarrhea to be considered chronic is a matter of controversy. It is generally believed that diarrhea in a child must persist for 1 or more months to be considered chronic. In addition, the child must have either lost weight or failed to gain weight during that period for the situation to be considered clinically significant.

The physician must have a concept of normal stool patterns in children. Breast-fed infants younger than 4 months pass two to four stools daily that are yellow to golden, soft, and have a pH near 5.0; formula-fed infants younger than 4 months have two or three stools daily that are firm and have a pH around 7.0. From ages 4 to 12 months, most children pass one to three stools per day. These stools are darker yellow and firmer. After age 1, children's stools are formed and resemble adult stools in odor and color.

One approach to the differential diagnosis of chronic diarrhea in children is to classify them by type of stool: watery stools, fatty stools, or bloody stools. Watery stools are most often seen in the following situations:

- *Persistent postenteritis* diarrhea (with or without secondary carbohydrate intolerance).
- *Intestinal infections* from viruses, bacteria *(Shigella, Salmonella, E. coli, Yersinia)*, and parasites (particularly *Giardia*).
- *Disaccharidase deficiency;* a *lactose deficiency* secondary to acute gastroenteritis is much more common than a primary lactase deficiency. A sucrase-isomaltase deficiency is rare.

Allergic gastroenteropathies, in which the child is allergic to cow's milk protein or soy protein, may also cause watery diarrhea in infants and children. Other, much less common causes are *Hirschsprung's disease, short-bowel syndrome,* primary immune defects, and diarrhea associated with endocrine disorders.

Fatty stools suggest cystic fibrosis, pancreatic insufficiency, celiac disease, or allergic gastroenteropathy. Rarely, drugs such as neomycin may induce steatorrhea.

Chronic bloody diarrhea suggests *Shigella* or *Salmonella* infection, *dysentery, inflammatory bowel disease* (including ulcerative colitis and Crohn's disease), *amebic dysentery,* or (less often) antibiotic-induced pseudomembranous colitis.

Differential Diagnosis of Diarrhea

CONDITION	NATURE OF PATIENT	NATURE OF SYMPTOMS	ASSOCIATED SYMPTOMS	PRECIPITATING AND AGGRAVATING FACTORS	AMELIORATING FACTORS	PHYSICAL FINDINGS	DIAGNOSTIC STUDIES
Acute Diarrhea							
Viral or bacterial gastroenteritis:	All ages	Abrupt onset, lasts <1 wk No symptoms of other organ involvement Most common cause of diarrhea *Adults*: Benign, self-limiting *Children*: May lead to severe dehydration	Nausea and vomiting Fever Crampy abdominal pain			Hyperactive peristalsis Fever	Stool culture
Rotavirus	Most common in infants younger than 3 yr	Peak incidence in winter					
Salmonella Shigella	Peak incidence in children ages 1-4 yr						Stool culture
Drug-induced:							
Laxatives	Mostly women	Diarrhea Muscle weakness Lassitude			Stop drugs		Proctoscopy Stool sodium hydroxide test for phenolphthalein Barium enema Hypokalemia

Continued

Differential Diagnosis of Diarrhea—cont'd

CONDITION	NATURE OF PATIENT	NATURE OF SYMPTOMS	ASSOCIATED SYMPTOMS	PRECIPITATING AND AGGRAVATING FACTORS	AMELIORATING FACTORS	PHYSICAL FINDINGS	DIAGNOSTIC STUDIES
Antibiotics	Taking antibiotics	Mild, watery diarrhea	Nonspecific, crampy abdominal pain Low-grade fever	Ampicillin Tetracycline Lincomycin Chloramphenicol Clindamycin			
Pseudomembranous enterocolitis	Taking antibiotics, especially clindamycin, recent hospitalization	Severe colitis with pseudomembrane formation Life-threatening diarrhea or colonic or dysenteric type		Use of several antibiotics Classically clindamycin-associated *Clostridium difficile* superinfection			
Other drugs				Iron- or magnesium-containing compounds High doses of: Salicylates Quinidine Anti-inflammatory agents Beta blockers Colchicine Methyldopa Digitalis Phenothiazines			
Toxin-mediated (small-bowel) diarrhea		Abrupt onset of large-volume, watery diarrhea	Nausea, vomiting Increased salivation Crampy abdominal pain General malaise Little or no fever	Contaminated food			

Disease/Cause	Patient	Clinical Features	Symptoms/Signs	Source	Treatment	Other Signs	Diagnostic Tests
Clostridium toxin (botulism)			Neurologic symptoms	Contaminated food			
Staphylococcus toxin		Severe vomiting and diarrhea begin 2-4 hr after eating of contaminated food (especially meat or dairy products)		Contaminated food			
Dysentery syndrome (infectious or colonic diarrhea)	History of prior good health	No symptoms other than gastrointestinal involvement; Acute, watery diarrhea	Fever; Nausea, vomiting; Abdominal cramps; Headache; General malaise; Myalgia				Microscopic stool examination for fecal leukocytes; If leukocytes present, stool culture; If high fever present, blood culture
Chronic Diarrhea							
Inflammatory bowel disease	Adults	Initial episode <2 wk; May recur over months or years	Weight loss; Bloody stools; Fever; Arthralgia	Enteritis; Intestinal infections	Steroids	Fever; Anemia	Proctoscopy; Colonoscopy; Gastrointestinal radiographs
	Children	Diarrhea must persist for >1 mo	Failure to gain weight				
Long-term ingestion of many drugs	Usually adult	Usually watery diarrhea	Those of illness for which drug is being prescribed		Stop drugs		

Continued

Differential Diagnosis of Diarrhea—cont'd

CONDITION	NATURE OF PATIENT	NATURE OF SYMPTOMS	ASSOCIATED SYMPTOMS	PRECIPITATING AND AGGRAVATING FACTORS	AMELIORATING FACTORS	PHYSICAL FINDINGS	DIAGNOSTIC STUDIES
Irritable bowel syndrome (irritable colon, mucous colitis, functional diarrhea)	Most common in young women with children and other stressed people	Chronic or intermittent diarrhea alternates with constipation More frequent and looser stools with onset of pain Hard, marble-like stools alternating with soft bowel movements Typical in morning; seldom at night Rectal urgency	Mucous in toilet bowl or on stool surface Sense of incomplete evacuation	Stress	Reduction in stress Pain relief with defecation	Colon tender on palpation Abdominal distention	
Lactase deficiency	Infants (<1 yr) Adults, especially African and Mediterranean descent Native Americans Asians	Diarrhea	Flatulence Perianal excoriation Abdominal distention Vomiting Fever Anorexia Children: failure to thrive	Lactose load Infectious gastroenteritis	Stop ingestion of lactose		Lactose tolerance test Mucosal biopsy Hydrogen breath test

Diabetes	Diabetic	Uncontrolled, explosive postprandial diarrhea	Neurologic dysfunction	Meals	Antibiotics	Blood sugar Colony count of gastric contents
Giardiasis	Severe in children Adults may be asymptomatic Hikers and campers at higher risk	Foul-smelling, watery, explosive diarrhea Latency period of 1-3 wk Onset may be acute or gradual and may persist from weeks to 6 mo	Mucus in stool Increased flatulence Nausea Anorexia and weight loss Greasy stools Abdominal distention	Drinking water infested with *Giardia lamblia*		Microscopic stool examination for *Giardia* Duodenal aspirate for *Giardia*

Selected References

Agus SG: Approach to a patient with infectious diarrhea, *Mt Sinai J Med* 62:175-177, 1996.

Baldi F, Bianco MA, Nardone G, et al: Focus on acute diarrhoeal disease, *World J Gastroenterol* 15:3341-3348, 2009.

Bramble MG, Record CO: Drug-induced gastrointestinal disease, *Drugs* 15:451-463, 1970.

Chen EH, Shofer FS, Dean AJ, et al: Derivation of a clinical prediction rule for evaluating patients with abdominal pain and diarrhea, *Am J Emerg Med* 26:450-453, 2008.

Gadewar S, Fasano A: Current concepts in the evaluation, diagnosis, and management of acute infectious diarrhea, *Curr Opin Pharmacol* 5:559-565, 2005.

Gore JI, Surawicz C: Severe acute diarrhea, *Gastroenterol Clin North Am* 32:1249-1267, 2003.

Guarderos JC: Is it food allergy? Differentiating the causes of adverse reactions to food, *Postgrad Med* 109:125-134, 2001.

Gunnarsson J, Simrén M: Efficient diagnosis of suspected functional bowel disorders, *Nat Clin Pract Gastroenterol Hepatol* 5:498-507, 2008.

Hyman PE, Milla PJ, Benninga MA, et al: Childhood functional gastrointestinal disorders: neonate/toddler, *Gastroenterology* 130:1519-1526, 2006.

Kolars JC, Fischer PR: Evaluation of diarrhea in the returned traveler, *Prim Care Office Pract* 29:931-935, 2002.

Kroser JA, Metz DC: Evaluation of the adult patient with diarrhea, *Prim Care* 23:629-647, 1996.

Schiller LR: Diarrhea and malabsorption in the elderly, *Gastroenterol Clin North Am* 38:481-502, 2009.

Schiller LR: Chronic diarrhea, *Gastroenterology* 127:287-293, 2004.

Schiller LR: Diarrhea, *Med Clin North Am* 84:1259-1274, 2000.

Swagerty DL, Walling AD, Klein RM: Lactose intolerance, *Am Fam Physician* 65:1845-1850, 1855-1856, 2002.

Dizziness/ Lightheadedness and Vertigo

11

Dizziness is the most common reason why patients older than 75 years visit their doctors. However, most patients who complain of dizziness do not have an ear problem. A careful history is particularly important for these patients. The physician must first determine whether the patient has true vertigo or dizziness/ lightheadedness.

True vertigo is a hallucination of movement. *Objective vertigo* is the illusion that one's surroundings are moving. *Subjective vertigo* is the feeling that, with eyes closed, one's body or head is moving or turning in space.

In contrast, lightheadedness, dizziness, and giddiness represent a sensation of being about to faint *(near-syncope)*; this is not accompanied by true syncope or a feeling of rotation or movement. Some patients describe lightheadedness as a lack of strength or a generalized weakness and may feel that they will pass out if they do not lie down; this symptom usually improves rapidly with recumbency. Lightheadedness, dizziness, and near-syncope must be differentiated from true syncope (not discussed in this chapter), which has more serious implications, especially in elderly patients.

TRUE VERTIGO

Nature of Patient

Most vertiginous episodes in children are benign and self-limiting, except those associated with a seizure disorder. Vertigo is seldom the initial symptom of a seizure; when it is, it may be followed by transitory unconsciousness or amnesia of the event. Although true vertigo is uncommon in children, they may complain of vertigo after an *upper respiratory tract infection* or an *acute viral infection* in which hearing was also disturbed. The most common causes of vertigo in children are *migraine* or *benign paroxysmal positional vertigo*, often referred to as *benign positional vertigo* (BPV). Vertigo may be secondary to acute *viral labyrinthitis*. Children with serous otitis media do not usually complain of dizziness or vertigo but may have nondescript balance disturbances. Vertigo or headaches may develop in children several weeks after a *head injury*. When paroxysmal

127

vertigo occurs in children with a family history of migraine, it may represent a *vestibular migraine.*

In adults, true vertigo is frequently caused by *BPV,* Ménière's syndrome (or disease), and *labyrinthitis.* Ototoxic and salt-retaining drugs, acoustic neuroma, and brainstem dysfunction are less common causes.

To facilitate diagnosis, vertigo can be separated into central and peripheral causes. *Central vertigo* is caused by brainstem or cerebellar lesions and is associated with diplopia, dysarthria, dysphagia, paresthesias, headache, and ataxia. *Peripheral vertigo* is caused by problems of the inner ear or vestibular nerve and can often be diagnosed from the duration of symptoms.

Nature of Symptoms

Although the clinical differential diagnosis of vertigo is best made on the basis of associated symptoms, physical findings, and diagnostic studies, vertigo has some distinguishing features.

Peripheral vertigo is usually severe, has a sudden onset, lasts seconds to minutes, is related to position, is fatigable, and has associated auditory symptoms and horizontal nystagmus.

Central vertigo is mild, has a gradual onset, lasts weeks to months, is not related to position, is not fatigable, and has associated neurologic and visual symptoms and vertical nystagmus.

Recurrent attacks are often associated with *BPV* and *Ménière's syndrome.* *Labyrinthitis* is usually not recurrent. The vertigo associated with *otitis media* has a gradual onset and may persist after the otitis subsides. If the vertigo has been continuous and progressive for several weeks or months, a *mass lesion* should be suspected.

BPV, Ménière's syndrome, and labyrinthitis have varying durations of symptoms. In positional vertigo, symptoms last from seconds to minutes; in *vertebrobasilar insufficiency,* minutes; in Ménière's syndrome, from minutes to hours; and in toxic labyrinthitis, vestibular neuronitis, or brainstem lesion, from days to weeks.

Prior episodes of vertigo may have been correctly diagnosed. However, if the previous physician did not obtain a precise history and perform an appropriate physical examination, prior episodes of vertigo may have been misdiagnosed as "nerves," "tension," or "low blood pressure." Lack of physician awareness of benign paroxysmal positional vertigo is a common cause of the misdiagnosis of dizziness in elderly people.

Associated Symptoms

Tinnitus, ear fullness, and other hearing disturbances are usually present with *Ménière's syndrome,* rare in *labyrinthitis,* and absent in *BPV.* Nausea and vomiting may be present in all. If vertigo is associated with an acute onset of unilateral weakness, problems with coordination, diplopia, or numbness, the vertigo is caused by *brainstem disease,* such as vertebrobasilar insufficiency. Patients with such diseases usually have normal hearing but may have other signs of brainstem dysfunction (e.g., vertical, lateral, or rotatory nystagmus).

Nystagmus is also observed in *Ménière's syndrome* and *BPV*. If the patient has a chronic, progressive, unilateral hearing deficit with tinnitus, facial numbness, or weakness, an *acoustic neuroma* should be suspected. Café-au-lait spots or neurofibromatosis may also be observed in patients with acoustic neuromas. Vertigo may be part of a *migraine* aura or may be a migraine equivalent, which is more common in adolescents.

Precipitating and Aggravating Factors

By definition, positional changes such as head turning, rolling over in bed, bending over and then standing erect, and looking up by extending the neck may precipitate or aggravate BPV. This is usually not the case in Ménière's syndrome, which is thought to have its onset around *menstruation* and during times of *emotional stress*. *Ototoxic drugs* (e.g., streptomycin and aminoglycosides, especially gentamicin and rarely furosemide) may also cause vertigo. Recurrent vertigo may be present when salt-retaining drugs (e.g., steroids or nonsteroidal anti-inflammatory drugs) are ingested.

An acute onset of isolated vertigo suggests a *viral infection* or *middle* or *inner ear lesion*. Repeated vertigo episodes (sometimes associated with nausea and vomiting) over many years suggest Ménière's syndrome or BPV.

Ameliorating Factors

During attacks of BPV, patients may be more comfortable when they are still. Vertigo persists in patients with Ménière's syndrome, otitis, labyrinthitis, and acoustic neuroma even if they do not move.

Physical Findings

The symptoms caused by BPV can be replicated with caloric stimulation or certain postural maneuvers (e.g., a Hallpike maneuver or a modified Hallpike maneuver with body turning). Examination of the eyes for nystagmus is particularly important. Nystagmus occurs in BPV, Ménière's syndrome, and labyrinthitis. Vertical nystagmus occurs only with central causes of nystagmus, and its presence excludes the previously mentioned (labyrinthine) causes of vertigo.

The typical lateral nystagmus of BPV occurs within a few seconds after the patient assumes a provocative posture or performs a provocative maneuver. The nystagmus abates after a few seconds and also fatigues (does not occur) with serial repetition of the maneuver.

No latency or fatigue exists when the nystagmus is caused by a central lesion.

Diagnostic Studies

The reader is referred to the references, particularly the works by Aoki and colleagues (2007) and Sloane and associates (2001). The selection of particular studies (audiometry, cardiovascular testing, neurologic testing, electronystagmography, electroencephalography (EEG), magnetic resonance imaging (MRI), echocardiography, Holter monitoring, vascular imaging) is based on history and physical and diagnostic possibilities.

Less Common Diagnostic Considerations

Less common otologic causes of vertigo include tumors of the middle and inner ear, cholesteatoma, mountain biking, head trauma, and impacted cerumen. Less common neurologic causes of vertigo include cerebellopontine angle tumors, nasopharyngeal carcinoma, brainstem tumors, multiple sclerosis, subclavian steal syndrome, and vertebrobasilar insufficiency (more common in elderly patients). Ramsay Hunt syndrome, Lyme disease, and Wernicke's encephalopathy may cause vertigo in rare instances. Vertigo associated with orthostasis occurs rarely after bariatric surgery.

LIGHTHEADEDNESS/DIZZINESS AND GIDDINESS

Many patients describe lightheadedness/dizziness and giddiness as a sensation of dysequilibrium (worse while standing), nonspecific weakness, or faintness without actually fainting. This sensation may abate when they recline. The most common causes of lightheadedness are *psychological problems, circulatory problems* (sometimes related to *hypotensive drugs*), *arrhythmias,* and *hyperventilation.*

Nature of Patient

When lightheadedness occurs in children, especially those at or near puberty, a *psychological cause* (e.g., stressful home or school environment) should be suspected. Syncope and orthostatic lightheadedness occasionally occur during the adolescent growth spurt. Although it is much less common in children than adults, *hyperventilation syndrome* may produce symptoms of lightheadedness.

When episodes of dizziness are associated with syncope or palpitations, the patient (child or adult) may have *sick sinus syndrome.* Some children and adults experience symptoms of lightheadedness during the tachycardia of *Wolff-Parkinson-White (WPW) syndrome* or *mitral valve prolapse.* Older children should be asked whether they are aware of any rapid or irregular heartbeat during the episode of lightheadedness.

An initial onset of lightheadedness in an elderly patient suggests a *cardiovascular disturbance* or *cerebrovascular insufficiency;* vascular insufficiency secondary to cervical arthritis is less common. Postural dizziness related to *unstable vasomotor reflexes* is more common in elderly people but can be seen at any age. *Dysequilibrium,* a sense of imbalance or unsteadiness especially when standing, is more common in elderly patients. It can be caused by visual, proprioceptive, and cerebellar or motor defects, which occur in patients with stroke, vestibular disease, neuropathy, cerebellar disease, and particularly deconditioning. When a patient frequently complains of transient lightheadedness and no specific cause can be found, it is probably of psychogenic origin.

When a patient rarely complains of lightheadedness, a more thorough history and physical examination should be done. In this patient a psychogenic cause should be a diagnosis of exclusion. When lightheadedness occurs in a patient with a significant psychiatric disorder, *hyperventilation syndrome* or a *reaction to psychotropic agents* should be considered.

Nature of Symptoms

Psychogenic dizziness may be recurrent but is often persistent. Drug-induced giddiness is also persistent. Orthostatic hypotension, reactive hypoglycemia, and arrhythmias cause recurrent episodes of lightheadedness. Psychogenic dizziness and hypoglycemic dizziness are not necessarily related to position.

Associated Symptoms

Patients with *psychogenic dizziness* often have many *functional* complaints. If circumoral or digital paresthesias are present, the dizziness is probably caused by *hyperventilation*. An irregular or rapid heartbeat suggests an *arrhythmia* as the cause of the lightheadedness. Nervousness and sweating indicate *hypoglycemia*.

Precipitating and Aggravating Factors

If giddiness occurs while the patient is standing, *orthostatic hypotension* should be suspected. This is most often induced by antihypertensive drugs, vasodilators used for angina, hypoglycemic agents, and antidepressants. Some patients who have significant systolic pressure reduction, especially elderly people, experience lightheadedness when they assume the erect posture, despite systolic pressure values greater than 120 mm Hg, particularly if the blood pressure has been reduced rapidly with antihypertensive agents. Orthostatic hypotension may also be secondary to severe diabetic or alcoholic neuropathy.

Patients may complain of lightheadedness or unsteadiness due to alcohol or *drug ingestion*. Antihypertensive agents of all types, particularly the more potent drugs, can produce *orthostatic hypotension*, the most common cause of recurrent dizziness and falls in elderly people. Vasodilators such as sildenafil (Viagra) and terazosin, which are used to treat erectile dysfunction and prostatic hypertrophy, respectively, may also cause lightheadedness. Phenytoin, gabapentin, and many psychotropic agents can produce feelings of unsteadiness. Ototoxic drugs (e.g., aminoglycosides, streptomycin, neomycin, quinine, salicylates in high doses) may cause lightheadedness without true vertigo. Dizziness occurs when selective serotonin reuptake inhibitor (SSRI) therapy is discontinued.

If dizziness has a temporal periodicity (middle to late morning, middle to late afternoon, or approximately 2 to 4 hours after eating), *reactive hypoglycemia* should be suspected. The dizziness can be caused by the hypoglycemia itself or hypoglycemia-induced paroxysmal tachycardia. Dizziness on arising in the morning should suggest orthostatic hypotension or hypoglycemia, particularly if the patient is receiving long-acting insulin.

If transient episodes of lightheadedness (without syncope) have been occurring for many years and the history and physical examination do not suggest a specific cause, the patient should be reassured that most likely no serious illness exists. The symptom may be a manifestation of tension, and the patient should be instructed to record associated signs and symptoms as well as precipitating factors until the next visit.

Ameliorating Factors

If lightheadedness abates with recumbency, *orthostatic hypotension* should be suspected. If recurrent lightheadedness and dizziness abate when the patient is on vacation or removed from stressful situations, a *psychogenic cause* is indicated. If ingestion of carbohydrates or rebreathing in a paper bag alleviates the symptom, hypoglycemia or hyperventilation, respectively, should be considered.

Physical Findings

Abnormal physical findings are not usually associated with psychogenic dizziness. Occasionally, the patient can replicate the symptoms of hyperventilation syndrome (dizziness, circumoral numbness) by hyperventilating voluntarily. Patients with reactive hypoglycemia may manifest excessive sweating and tachycardia. Intermittent tachycardia or bradycardia may be observed in patients with WPW syndrome or sick sinus syndrome, respectively. Orthostatic hypotension may be caused by drugs but also by diabetic or alcoholic neuropathy.

Diagnostic Studies

Carotid Doppler ultrasound studies, cerebral angiography, Holter monitoring, magnetic resonance imaging, computed tomography (CT), serum insulin measurements, and tilt test studies may be helpful in selected patients.

Less Common Diagnostic Considerations

Less common diagnostic considerations include cardiac arrhythmias such as bradyarrhythmias, paroxysmal atrial fibrillation, complete heart block, paroxysmal atrial tachycardia, and WPW syndrome (especially in younger patients). Older patients with *subclavian steal syndrome* feel lightheaded after movement of their arms. These patients may have a decreased left carotid pulse, a bruit, or decreased blood pressure in the left arm. Some patients with hemodynamically significant *aortic stenosis* or *idiopathic hypertrophic obstructive cardiomyopathy* may experience lightheadedness, primarily after exertion. Excessive carbon monoxide exposure may cause dizziness. When dizziness or dysequilibrium is associated with neck pain or cervical pathology, cervicogenic dizziness should be suspected.

Differential Diagnosis of Dizziness/Lightheadedness and Vertigo

CONDITION	NATURE OF PATIENT	NATURE OF SYMPTOMS	ASSOCIATED SYMPTOMS	PRECIPITATING AND AGGRAVATING FACTORS	AMELIORATING FACTORS	PHYSICAL FINDINGS	DIAGNOSTIC STUDIES
True Vertigo							
Benign paroxysmal positional vertigo (BPV)	Adults Uncommon in children	Recurrent over many years Not associated with tinnitus or hearing loss Episodes last seconds to minutes	Nausea and vomiting No neurologic defect	Positional changes (e.g., head turning, rolling over in bed)	Some relief if patient is motionless	Nystagmus and vertigo occur seconds after assumption of a provocative posture Lateral or rotatory nystagmus	Symptoms can be replicated by caloric stimulation or certain postural maneuvers Electronystagmography
Otitis media	More common in children	Persistent vertigo	Earache	Upper respiratory infection		Those of otitis media (acute or chronic)	Audiometric testing Tympanogram
Ménière's syndrome (disease)	Adults	Sudden onset of vertigo Not precipitated by sudden movement Recurrent Duration minutes to hours	Tinnitus Hearing loss Ear fullness Nausea and vomiting	Menstruation Emotional stress	Lateral or rotatory nystagmus No nystagmus between attacks Hearing deficit		Audiometric testing
Labyrinthitis (peripheral vestibulopathy)	Any age	Sudden onset of vertigo Lasts days to weeks	Rarely associated with tinnitus Nausea and vomiting Hearing loss possible	May be precipitated by viral infection			Caloric test Postural maneuvers Electronystagmography

Continued

Differential Diagnosis of Dizziness/Lightheadedness and Vertigo—cont'd

CONDITION	NATURE OF PATIENT	NATURE OF SYMPTOMS	ASSOCIATED SYMPTOMS	PRECIPITAT-ING AND AGGRAVATING FACTORS	AMELIORAT-ING FACTORS	PHYSICAL FINDINGS	DIAGNOSTIC STUDIES
Acoustic neuroma	Adults	Gradual onset Persistent vertigo	Chronic, progressive unilateral hearing deficit Tinnitus Facial numbness Weakness Café-au-lait spots			Café-au-lait spots possible Hearing loss Other neuro-logic problems	CT scan
Drugs							
Ototoxic		Persists days to weeks		Streptomycin Aminoglycosides Furosemide	Stop drug		
Salt-retaining		Vertigo recurs when patient is taking drugs		Steroids Phenylbutazone Phenytoin			
Brainstem dysfunction (vertebrobasi-lar insuffi-ciency, stroke, tumors)	Elderly	Acute onset of vertigo Normal hearing Recurrent Progressive with mass lesions	Blurred vision Diplopia Slurred speech Paresthesia Problems with coordination Usually no nausea and vomiting			Vertical, lateral, or rotatory nystagmus	Electroenceph-alography CT scan

Dizziness/Lightheadedness							
Psychogenic	Most common cause of dizziness in children	Recurrent Often persistent Not posture related	Many "functional" complaints	Emotional stress	Stress reduction		
Hyperventilation syndrome	More common in adults Anxious	Recurrent	Circumoral or digital paresthesias	Emotional stress	Rebreathing in paper bag	Hyperventilation infrequent Symptoms replicated by patient hyperventilating voluntarily	
Carbon monoxide poisoning	Any age Often several people living in same house are affected May work in poorly ventilated areas		Headache, nausea, and vomiting	Space heater usage Defective furnace	Breathing 100% O₂ Hyperbaric chamber	Cherry-red lips and nail beds	Carboxyhemoglobin measurement
Reactive hypoglycemia		Recurrent Dizziness has temporal periodicity Onset 2-4 hr after meals	Hypoglycemia-induced paroxysmal tachycardia Trembling Sweating	Carbohydrate ingestion	Temporary relief with carbohydrate ingestion Avoidance of routine excessive carbohydrate ingestion	Sweating Tachycardia	5-hr glucose tolerance test

Continued

Differential Diagnosis of Dizziness/Lightheadedness and Vertigo—cont'd

CONDITION	NATURE OF PATIENT	NATURE OF SYMPTOMS	ASSOCIATED SYMPTOMS	PRECIPITATING AND AGGRAVATING FACTORS	AMELIORATING FACTORS	PHYSICAL FINDINGS	DIAGNOSTIC STUDIES
Hypoglycemia	Diabetic	At peak of insulin action	Trembling, sweating Hunger, tachycardia	Insulin	Carbohydrates Glucagon injection	Sweating, tachycardia	Insulin measurements Blood glucose measurements
Orthostatic hypotension	Elderly Hypertensive Diabetic	Recurrent Giddiness on standing	Occasional syncope	Erect posture Antihypertensive medication	Recumbency	Orthostatic hypotension	
Drugs or alcohol		Persistent lightheadedness or unsteadiness without true vertigo		Phenytoin Psychotropics Ototoxic drugs Vasodilators Discontinuation of selective serotonin reuptake inhibitors	Stop drug(s)		
Sick sinus syndrome	Adults Rare in children	Recurrent dizziness	Syncope Palpitations			Irregular pulse May be normal Bradycardia	Electrocardiography Holter monitoring His bundle study
Wolff-Parkinson-White syndrome		Recurrent	Palpitations			May be normal between attacks	Electrocardiography Holter monitoring His bundle study

CT, Computed tomography.

Selected References

Aoki S, Arai Y, Kikuchi N: Effective maneuver of the positional test: turning head and body together, *Int Tinnitus J* 12:49-50, 2007.

Bhattacharyya N, Baugh RF, Orvidas L, et al: Clinical practice guideline: benign paroxysmal positional vertigo, *Otolaryngol Head Neck Surg* 139(Suppl 4):S47-S81, 2008.

Chan Y: Differential diagnosis of dizziness, *Curr Opin Otolaryngol Head Neck Surg* 17:200-203, 2009.

Chawla N, Olshaker JS: Diagnosis and management of dizziness and vertigo, *Med Clin North Am* 90:291-304, 2006.

Erbek SH, Erbek SS, Yilmaz I, et al: Vertigo in childhood: a clinical experience, *Int J Pediatr Otorhinolaryngol* 70:1547-1554, 2006.

Hoffman R, Einstadter D, Kroenke E: Evaluating dizziness, *Am J Med* 107:468-478, 1999.

Kapoor WN: Syncope in older persons, *J Am Geriatr Soc* 42:426-436, 1994.

Lawson J, Fitzgerald J, Birchall J, et al: Diagnosis of geriatric patients with severe dizziness, *J Am Geriatr Soc* 47:12-17, 1999.

Lewis RF: Vertigo: some uncommon causes of a common problem, *Semin Neurol* 16:55-62, 1996.

Linstrom CJ: Office management of the dizzy patient, *Otolaryngol Clin North Am* 25:745-780, 1992.

Neuhauser H, Lempert T: Vestibular migraine, *Neurol Clin* 27:379-391, 2009.

Sloane PD, Coeytaux RR, Beck RS, Dallara J: Dizziness: state of the science, *Ann Intern Med* 134:823-832, 2001.

Tusa RJ: Dizziness, *Med Clin North Am* 93:263-271, 2009.

Tusa RJ, Saada AA, Niparko JK: Dizziness in childhood, *J Child Neurol* 9:261-274, 1994.

Waterston J: Vertigo: a practical approach to diagnosis and treatment, *Aust Fam Physician* 28:883-887, 1999.

White J: Benign paroxysmal positional vertigo: how to diagnose and quickly treat it, *Cleveland Clin J Med* 71:722-728, 2004.

Earache

12

Primary otalgia (earache) is ear pain due to a problem in the ear. Referred otalgia is pain in the ear not due to an ear problem. It is nonotogenic ear pain. Otalgia is usually a sign of an acute or chronic infection of the external auditory canal or mastoid or an acute infection of the middle ear. These infections can be easily identified with careful examination.

Other common causes of ear pain are acute serous otitis media, eustachitis, acute otitic barotrauma, mastoiditis, traumatic perforation of the tympanic membrane, foreign bodies, and referred pain, such as that from temporomandibular joint (TMJ) dysfunction, impacted third molars, periodontal abscess, or recent dental work. About 50% of referred ear pain is caused by a dental problem.

If otologic examination fails to show the source of the pain, referred pain should be considered. Because the ear is innervated partially by sensory branches of the vagus nerve (Arnold's nerve), glossopharyngeal nerve (Jacobson's nerve), trigeminal nerve (auriculotemporal nerve), facial nerve, and branches of cranial nerves (CNs) II and III, pathologic conditions such as infection and malignant disease of the upper aerodigestive tract (carcinoma of the larynx, hypopharynx, oropharynx, and base of the tongue) and odontogenic disease can also cause otalgia (Fig. 12-1).

NATURE OF PATIENT

Otitis externa occurs more frequently in adults, particularly elderly diabetic patients, and in patients with seborrheic dermatitis or psoriasis of the scalp. Necrotizing otitis externa (a necrotizing osteomyelitis of the skull) occurs in diabetic and immunocompromised patients. Swimmer's ear is common in people who swim frequently but also occurs in those who clean their ears with cotton swabs, paper clips, or towel tips or by other means.

Otitis media is more common in children, particularly those younger than 8 years. Various studies suggest that 20% of all children have at least three episodes of otitis media in their first year of life and that two thirds of all children have at least one episode before age 2 years. After upper respiratory infection

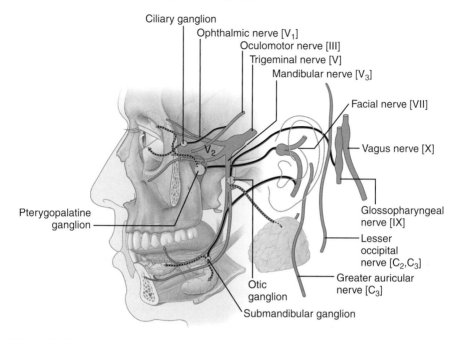

Figure 12-1. Nerve supply to the ear. (From Beddoe GM: Otalgia. Am Fam Physician 11:108-110, 1975.)

(URI) and tonsillopharyngitis, otitis media is the third leading reason for pediatric office visits. Premature children on respirators are at higher risk, as are those with cleft palate and Down syndrome.

Serous otitis is also more common in children. It is usually not associated with severe pain, except when an acute infection results in acute otitis media. Serous otitis media is often asymptomatic but frequently detected on routine audiometric testing of schoolchildren, because it is the most common cause of hearing deficiencies in children.

Local causes of ear pain predominate in children, whereas the incidence of referred pain increases with age. One study showed that 60% of patients (mean age, 36 years) referred to an ear, nose, and throat clinic had referred pain to their ears. In 80% the ear pain was caused by *cervical spine lesions, TMJ dysfunction,* or *dental pathology. Impacted third molars* are more common in women between ages 15 and 25 and may cause referred ear pain. In elderly patients, *malignant lesions* of the oropharynx and larynx can cause referred otalgia.

Referred pain to the ear does not rule out a local painful process. *Barotrauma* should be considered in patients who have recently traveled by air and in scuba-diving enthusiasts. Pain from direct trauma can result from a blast or a slap on the ear and in *ear picking.*

NATURE OF SYMPTOMS

Otitis externa is easily differentiated from otitis media in that patients with otitis externa find movement or pressure on the pinna extremely painful. In addition, they may have itching and tender swelling of the outer ear canal. *Bilateral pain* in the ears is more suggestive of otitis externa. When bilateral ear pain occurs in young children, bacterial infection of otitis media is more likely, and antibiotics may be indicated. Bilateral pain virtually rules out a referred source of the pain. The pain of otitis media has been described as a rapid-onset, deep-seated, severe pain that often prevents the patient from sleeping. Children who are too young to talk may present with irritability, restlessness, fever, poor feeding, or rubbing of the affected ear. Frequently, the patient has a history of a recent URI.

Serous otitis and *eustachitis* are not usually associated with a severe earache, but patients with these disorders may have some intermittent discomfort and may state that they hear crackling or gurgling sounds. Severe pain in and especially behind the ear occurs with *acute mastoiditis.* The patients have exquisite tenderness when pressure is applied over the mastoid process.

The pain of *barotrauma* may be severe and persistent, and superimposed otitis media occasionally develops. The pain is most frequently experienced during descent in an airplane, especially if the patient has a concurrent URI with eustachian tube dysfunction. The pain may be excruciating.

Patients with *impacted cerumen* may also complain of severe pain in the ear, or they may have only a vague sensation of discomfort sometimes associated with impaired hearing. On questioning, the patients may admit to a long-standing problem with cerumen accumulation in the ears, with exacerbation leading to visits to the physician.

The pain of *TMJ dysfunction* is usually intermittent and often worse in the morning if associated with *night grinding.* The pain may also occur toward the end of the day, especially if it is secondary to tension-induced bruxism (see Chapters 13 and 17).

ASSOCIATED SYMPTOMS

The usual sequence of symptoms in *otitis media* is a blocked feeling in the ear, pain, fever, headache, irritability, rhinitis, and anorexia. Children may have vomiting, diarrhea, listlessness, ear tugging, and discharge if the tympanic membrane perforates. Some relief of pain and fever occurs with perforation. Patients with *serous otitis* are usually well and afebrile. They frequently present with impaired hearing as the only complaint, although they may also complain of a feeling of fullness in the ear, popping or crackling sounds, or tinnitus.

Symptoms typically associated with *TMJ dysfunction* include vertigo, tinnitus, headache, and a jaw click.

PRECIPITATING AND AGGRAVATING FACTORS

Otitis externa is often precipitated by excess moisture (swimmer's ear), trauma (ear picking), or dermatitis, and is usually due to bacterial (90%) or fungal (10%) infections. *Otitic barotrauma* is aggravated by URIs, hay fever, middle ear effusion, and stuffy nose. It is often precipitated by an increase in atmospheric pressure, such as occurs with descent in an airplane. *Eustachitis* is often precipitated by pharyngitis or URI, which may cause mechanical or functional obstruction of the eustachian tube; air in the tube is reabsorbed, and the drum is retracted. *Acute otitis media* often precedes acute mastoiditis by 10 to 14 days. Pain in the ear that is referred from the second and third spinal nerves may be worse with flexion of the neck. Otalgia exacerbated by swallowing suggests *Eagle's syndrome*, an elongated styloid process. When ear pain develops soon after dental procedures, the pain is often due to *TMJ dysfunction* caused by the dental procedure.

AMELIORATING FACTORS

The pain of *barotrauma* and *eustachitis* may be alleviated somewhat by chewing, Valsalva's maneuver, and nasal decongestants. *TMJ pain* may be eased by a dental bite appliance.

PHYSICAL FINDINGS AND DIAGNOSTIC STUDIES

The physical findings in otitis externa, otitis media, and serous otitis are well known (see references) and are not described here.

The physician must perform an accurate, complete examination of the eardrum to rule out otitis media. If an adequate view is obstructed because of wax accumulation or secondary external ear canal infection, otitis media cannot be ruled out; it can be excluded only if the entire drum is normal and there is no conductive hearing loss. In serous otitis, serous or glutinous fluid accumulates in the middle ear space. The eardrum may look abnormal because of the effusion, or it may be injected with noticeable radial vessels. With serous otitis and eustachitis the tympanic membrane may be retracted and show decreased mobility on pneumatic otoscopy (Fig. 12-2). Impedance tympanometry (Fig. 12-3) helps to confirm the diagnosis. New models of acoustic reflectometers are useful in detecting middle-ear fluid in children. Bullae on the tympanic membrane (bullous myringitis) are frequently seen in patients with a mycoplasma infection.

When the patient complains of ear pain, has a fever and noticeable swelling behind the ear, or experiences tenderness on palpation over the mastoid process, *acute mastoiditis* is probable. The tympanic membrane is often red, bulging, and immobile because of associated otitis media. It should be suspected whenever discharge from the middle ear is continuous for more than 10 days.

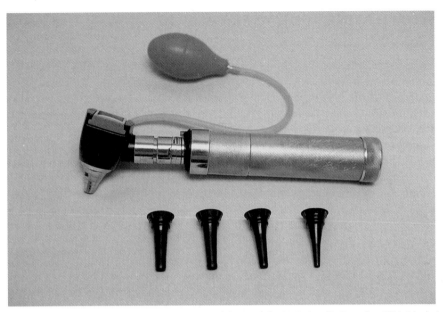

Figure 12-2. Pneumatic otoscopy. (From Seidel HM, Ball JW, Dains JE, Benedict GW: Mosby's Guide to Physical Examination, 5th ed. Mosby, St. Louis, 2003, p 73.)

Computed tomography (CT) scans and radiographs are helpful in establishing the diagnosis.

Whenever a patient complains of pain in the ear and findings in the ear canal and drum are normal, referred pain is most probable.

The most common cause of referred ear pain is of dental origin and includes caries, periapical infections, and impacted teeth. Because the glossopharyngeal nerves provide sensory innervation to the middle ear mucosa, posterior part of the external auditory canal, and eustachian canal as well as the pharynx, tonsils, and posterior third of the tongue, conditions such as tonsillitis, pharyngitis, peritonsillar abscess, and retropharyngeal abscess can give rise to referred otalgia. Another common cause of referred pain to the ear is *TMJ dysfunction.* It may be either *acute,* resulting from opening the mouth extremely wide, or *chronic,* resulting from malocclusion or arthritis of the TMJ, which occurs more frequently in patients with *rheumatoid arthritis.* Malocclusion or enlarged masseter muscles caused by bruxism may be apparent on physical examination. In addition, the patient often has tenderness on palpation over the TMJ. Occasionally, the examiner may hear clicking or palpate crepitus over the TMJ.

Patients with *impacted third molars* may have trismus and pain when pressure is applied above and behind the angle of the mandible. The diagnosis can be confirmed by dental radiographs. Magnetic resonance imaging (MRI) and CT are useful in diagnosing osteomyelitis of the external canal as well as tumors causing primary and secondary otalgia.

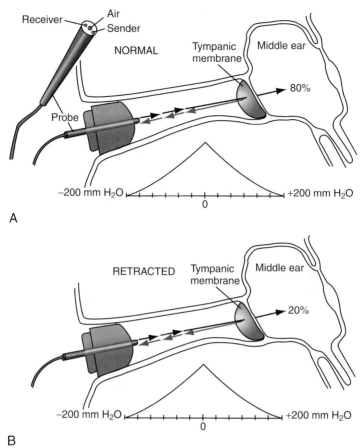

Figure 12-3. Theory of tympanometry. **A,** Normal. Low-frequency (220-Hz) probe tone is emitted from tiny aperture in probe tip and is directed to tympanic membrane. When tympanic membrane is stiffened by positive or negative pressure, a greater amount of sound energy is reflected off membrane and directed back down ear canal. Small microphone housed in probe assembly reads amount of reflected sound energy. When tympanic membrane is in a neutral position, pressure in middle ear is equal to that of atmospheric pressure and is thus in its most mobile position. Here, most of sound energy from probe tone is absorbed by tympanic membrane into middle ear, and the least amount is reflected back down ear canal. **B,** Retracted. Retracted tympanic membrane reflects negative pressure in middle ear relative to atmospheric pressure. Most compliant position of membrane (peak of tympanogram) is found when artificially induced negative pressure is introduced from manometer of instrument. Thus, pressure point at which peak of tympanogram occurs represents an indirect measure of middle ear pressure. Note that greater sound energy is reflected off tympanic membrane until pressure introduced down ear canal is equal to that in middle ear (in this case, −200 mm H_2O). (From Schwartz RH: New concepts in otitis media. Am Fam Physician 19:91-98, 1979.)

Differential Diagnosis of Earache

CONDITION	NATURE OF PATIENT	NATURE OF SYMPTOMS	ASSOCIATED SYMPTOMS	PRECIPITATING AND AGGRAVATING FACTORS	PHYSICAL FINDINGS AND DIAGNOSTIC STUDIES
Otitis media	Children, especially <8 yr	Pain is unilateral, deep, and severe	Irritability Restlessness Fever Poor feeding Ear feels full	URI	Tympanic membrane inflamed and bulging Decreased light reflex
Serous otitis media	Children and adults	Not usually painful Unilateral	Decreased hearing Crackling and gurgling sounds	URI	Fluid behind tympanic membrane
Eustachitis					Tympanic membrane shows decreased mobility Decreased conductive hearing Impedance tympanometry
Otitis externa	Adults Diabetic patients Patients with seborrhea "Ear pickers" Swimmers	Often bilateral			Pain on manipulation of pinna
Otitic barotrauma		Pain may be severe	URI Nasal stuffiness	Worse on airplane descent	Tympanic membrane retracted

Condition	Population	Symptoms	Associated findings	Diagnostic findings
Mastoiditis		Pain in and behind ear	Fever, Drainage from middle ear ≥ 10 days	Otitis media 10-14 days previously	Exquisite pain with pressure on mastoid process, Swelling behind ear, Radiograph of mastoid, MRI
Foreign body	Children	Pain or vague discomfort	May impair hearing	Foreign body or cerumen in ear
Impacted cerumen	Adults	Rarely bilateral	Recurrent problem	Normal otologic findings
Referred otalgia, as with TMJ dysfunction, dental problems, and tumors	Adults (increases with age)	TMJ dysfunction intermittent and often worse in morning	Resemble those of TMJ dysfunction: vertigo, tinnitus, jaw click; Pain referred from infected tooth may be worse with hot or cold foods	TMJ arthritis, Malocclusion or bruxism, Impacted molar
Bullous myringitis	Usually adults	Unilateral or bilateral	URI, Cough, Pneumonia	Bullae on tympanic membrane

MRI, Magnetic resonance imaging; TMJ, temporomandibular joint; URI, upper respiratory infection.

LESS COMMON DIAGNOSTIC CONSIDERATIONS

Pain in the ear can be caused by *infections* such as impetigo, insect bites, chondrodermatitis nodularis chronica helicis (an exquisitely tender nodule of the helix seen in older adults), perichondritis of the pinna, and gouty tophi (which usually are not painful). Rarely, *tumors* of the middle ear and meatus can produce nonremitting pain. Relapsing polychondritis is multiorgan and most frequently involves cartilage in the ear bilaterally.

Patients with *herpes zoster oticus (Ramsay Hunt syndrome)* have severe pain in one ear for several days, after which vesicles appear on the auricle or in the meatus. These vesicles may also appear on the tympanic membrane and occasionally on the palate. Concurrent with the vesicles, there is usually a complete lower motor neuron lesion of CN VII that is associated with pyrexia, constitutional disturbances, deafness, tinnitus, vertigo, and nystagmus.

Drugs such as mesalamine and sulfasalazine may cause otalgia.

If otalgia develops in a child within 2 weeks of orthodontic treatment and otologic findings are normal, TMJ dysfunction should be considered, especially if otalgia recurs after orthodontic therapy. In infants and children, gastroesophageal reflux may rarely cause referred otalgia. Studies in children have now shown that *Helicobacter pylori* may cause otitis media with effusion. Reflux esophagitis is assumed to be the route of infection. Pain referred to the ear can occur from CN V lesions, dental caries, abscesses of lower molars, trigeminal neuralgia, sinusitis, and parotid pathology. **Acute and subacute thyroiditis affecting one lobe may refer pain to the ear on the affected side.** Ear pain can be referred from CNs IX and X in lesions of the vallecula, posterior third of the tongue, tonsils, larynx, migraine, glossopharyngeal neuralgia, and carotidynia (persistent sore throat with normal pharynx, ear pain aggravated by swallowing, and tenderness over the carotid bulb).

Selected References

Ely JW, Hansen MR, Clark EC: Diagnosis of ear pain, *Am Fam Physician* 77:621-628, 2008.
Ingvarsson L: Acute otalgia in children: findings and diagnosis, *Acta Paediatr Scand* 71:705-710, 1982.
Leung AKC, Fong JHS, Leong AG: Otalgia in children, *J Natl Med Assoc* 92:254-260, 2000.
Licameli GR: Diagnosis and management of otalgia in the pediatric patient, *Pediatr Ann* 28: 364-368, 1999.
Majumdar S, Wu K, Bateman ND, et al: Diagnosis and management of otalgia in children, *Arch Dis Child Educ Pract Ed* 94:33-36, 2009.
McCormick DP, Chandler SM, Chonmaitree T: Laterality of acute otitis media: different clinical and microbiologic characteristics, *Pediatr Infect Dis J* 26:583-588, 2007.
Osguthorpe JD, Nielsen DR: Otitis externa: review and clinical update, *Am Fam Physician* 74: 1510-1516, 2006.
Ramakrishnan K, Sparks RA, Berryhill WE: Diagnosis and treatment of otitis media, *Am Fam Physician* 76:1650-1658, 2007.
Shah RK, Blevins NH: Otalgia, *Otolaryngol Clin North Am* 36:1137-1151, 2003.

Teppo H, Revonta M: Comparison of old, professional and consumer model acoustic reflectometers in the detection of middle-ear fluid in children with recurrent acute otitis media or glue ear, *Int J Pediatr Otorhinolaryngol* 71:1865-1872, 2007.

van den Aardweg MT, Rovers MM, de Ru JA, et al: A systematic review of diagnostic criteria for acute mastoiditis in children, *Otol Neurotol* 29:751-757, 2008.

Yilmaz T, Ceylan M, Akyön Y, et al: *Helicobacter pylori*: a possible association with otitis media with effusion, *Otolaryngol Head Neck Surg* 134:772-777, 2006.

Facial Pain

13

Because doctors can usually differentiate headache from other causes of facial pain, the differential diagnosis of headache is discussed in Chapter 17. Typically, by the time patients consult a physician for facial pain, they already have visited a dentist several times. This fact illustrates the diagnostic difficulty.

The most common causes of facial pain are dental and oral diseases, and TMJ dysfunction. Other causes of facial pain include *eye disease* (glaucoma); *nose* or *sinus disease* (sinusitis); vascular pain such as *migraine* and *temporal arteritis; neurologic pain,* such as *trigeminal neuralgia (TGN); sphenopalatine neuralgia (SPN); glossopharyngeal neuralgia* (GPN), *herpes zoster, postherpetic neuralgia,* referred pain, rarely from *angina pectoris* and occasionally from *muscle contraction headaches;* and psychogenic pain, such as that seen with *atypical facial pain, hysteria,* and *depression.* Another means of classifying facial pain is by its components: neuropathic, myofascial, migrainous, or supraspinous.

Because pain is a symptom and cannot be seen or easily measured, the evaluation and diagnosis must depend on the patient's description; therefore, historical details that the clinician elicits are important. A patient's reaction to pain can be seen and may indicate the severity of the pain.

With chronic pain the initial symptoms may have been psychologically based, further complicating the diagnostic process. Depressed, anxious, or neurotic people often seek help for organic causes of facial pain more frequently than other people. In addition, chronic or recurrent episodes of facial pain can lead to depression and anxiety.

Facial neuralgias are rare in children. Dental pain is more common than TGN. TGN, glossopharyngeal neuralgia, Bell's palsy, and cluster headache very rarely occur in children.

NATURE OF PATIENT

TGN is more common in patients older than 50 years. If facial pain occurs in a younger patient (less than age 40), TGN is less likely, and other conditions that can mimic tic douloureux should be considered. These include *multiple sclerosis, acoustic neuroma,* and *trigeminal neuroma,* especially if the upper division (pain in the forehead or eye) is involved or the symptoms are unilateral.

Glaucoma is more common in elderly persons; it affects 2% of those older than 40 years. It is more common in farsighted than nearsighted people.

TMJ dysfunction is more common in female patients older than 40 years, particularly if they are edentulous or have worn posterior teeth or poorly fitting dentures, but it can accompany severe malocclusion or mandibular trauma at any age. Patients with rheumatoid arthritis appear to have a higher incidence of TMJ dysfunction.

Atypical facial pain is most common in women between ages 30 and 50; 60% of these patients have a similar family history. Such pain tends to occur in people with a history of high stress, drug addiction, low self-esteem, impotence or frigidity, marital or family conflicts, or prior episodes of anxiety or depression. The typical patient is an edentulous, haggard-looking, middle-aged woman. She may have a history of concomitant psychiatric illness as well.

Facial pain from *sinusitis* can occur at any age but is less common in children and teenagers.

NATURE OF SYMPTOMS

The mnemonic PQRST is helpful in dealing with painful conditions. *P* represents precipitating or palliating factors; *Q* refers to the quality of the pain (sharp or stabbing, burning or stinging, aching, boring, or throbbing); *R* stands for radiation and original location of pain; *S* stands for severity (score of 1-10 or how the pain compares with prior painful experiences); and *T* stands for timing, including initial onset, duration, frequency, seasonal, daily, and whether nocturnal or diurnal.

The quality of dental pain is often severe, throbbing, and poorly localized. Excruciating, lancinating, stabbing, paroxysmal pain is characteristic of the *trigeminal, sphenopalatine,* and *glossopharyngeal* neuralgias. The pain of *glaucoma* is described as dull and frontally located. However, the pain of *acute narrow-angle glaucoma* can cause severe pain of abrupt onset. Myofascial pain is often described as deep, continuous, and producing a dull ache.

Pain is relatively uncommon in patients with chronic or subacute sinusitis; it is typically seen with episodes of *acute sinusitis,* which may be superimposed on subacute sinusitis. Sinusitis pain is usually dull and relatively constant; it may occasionally be described as throbbing. This pain is usually located over the affected sinus or behind the orbit. However, with sphenoid sinusitis, pain may present at the vertex of the head and may radiate to the neck and orbit. Sinusitis pain is usually unilateral but can be bilateral.

Neuralgia pains usually have a sudden onset. A typical attack may consist of two to three stabbing pains over 1 minute. Episodes may become more frequent with time, and several attacks may occur in a single day, with spontaneous remission for weeks or months. The pain may be recurrent, but it is usually paroxysmal and instantaneous. Although the actual pain may last only a few seconds and then disappear, some patients experience a gradual transition from lancinating pain to a vague ache or burning. TGN pains usually occur during the day, whereas glossopharyngeal pains often develop at night. Over time the episodes of TGN may become more frequent and may occur one or more times daily. These pains seldom awaken patients from sleep.

The pain of *glaucoma* may be precipitated by dark rooms. The timing is gradual in onset, although the pain of acute narrow-angle glaucoma can begin suddenly and may manifest as a dramatic emergency. The timing of the pain of sinusitis is gradual in onset and can last for days to weeks if not adequately treated.

Most causes of facial pain, including dental problems, TGN, sinusitis, glaucoma, and TMJ dysfunction, manifest as unilateral pain; occasionally, all can be bilateral or alternating. The pain of *TGN* is located over the course of one of the three divisions of the fifth cranial nerve. It is usually unilateral but is bilateral in 5% to 10% of patients. The bilateral attacks tend to be more common in certain families and possibly more common in women. TGN most often occurs along the distribution of the second (maxillary branch) or third (mandibular branch) division and seldom over the first division (ophthalmic branch). Most patients report that the pain is on the surface, not deep inside the head, as is more common with sphenopalatine ganglion neuralgia. **Both the lancinating nature of neuralgia pain and the tendency to be remittent and associated with trigger areas distinguish it from the more chronic pain of sinus infection, dental abscesses, and glaucoma.**

The anatomic distribution of the pain helps differentiate neuralgia from *atypical facial pain,* which is not confined to an anatomic distribution of any cranial or cervical nerve. The entire side of the head as well as the face, neck, or throat may be involved.

The pain of *subacute glaucoma* usually causes frontal headaches, whereas the pain of *acute glaucoma* is often described as pain in the eye or just behind the eye radiating to the head, ears, or teeth. The pain of *sinusitis* corresponds in location to the sinus involved. Patients with *maxillary* sinusitis usually complain of pain over the cheek or under the eye; the pain of *frontal* sinusitis is above the eyes or in the forehead; and the pain of *ethmoid* sinusitis is most often supraorbital and may occasionally radiate to the vertex of the head. Sphenoid sinusitis and ethmoid sinusitis seldom occur as isolated phenomena; they are usually associated with other forms of sinusitis.

The pain of *TMJ arthritis* or *dysfunction* is normally located in the TMJ area, although it may be referred to the ear or temples, thus simulating the pain of a tension headache. **Any time a patient complains of pain in the ear and physical findings in the ear are normal, the physician should palpate over the TMJ, question the patient for other signs and symptoms of TMJ dysfunction, and consider other causes of referred otalgia.** The pain of TMJ dysfunction may radiate to either the teeth or the ear.

ASSOCIATED SYMPTOMS

Involuntary facial contractions may occur with the severe pain of *TGN,* which may cause a chronic painful syndrome associated with sleeplessness, weight loss, anxiety, depression, and rarely a suicidal tendency. Patients with *sinusitis* often have or recently had symptoms of an upper respiratory infection. Patients with *atypical facial pain* are frequently depressed and emotional, with a significant affective component to their illness. Patients with *cluster headaches* (Horton's headache, histamine cephalalgia) have ipsilateral lacrimation or rhinorrhea.

In the patient who sees halos or rainbows around lights, has temporary obscuring of vision, and experiences pain in and around the eye, *glaucoma* should be suspected. Occasionally such a patient also complains of nausea and vomiting, which sometimes lead to the erroneous diagnosis of migraine headaches.

The associated symptoms of *TMJ dysfunction* include jaw clicking or popping, crepitation, tinnitus, vertigo (rarely), pain in the ear, jaw clenching (bruxism), neckache, and headache. Patients may report that it is difficult to open the mouth widely because it elicits these symptoms.

PRECIPITATING AND AGGRAVATING FACTORS

Dental pain may increase with ingestion of hot, sweet, or acidic foods. *Neuralgia* pains are often induced by the touching of trigger points or by temperature extremes. *Sphenopalatine neuralgia* may be precipitated by sinusitis or a postnasal drip. Coughing and sneezing may exacerbate sinus pain. Erect posture may worsen pain caused by *maxillary sinusitis,* whereas recumbency exacerbates *frontal sinus* pain.

Darkness and drugs, which cause pupillary dilatation, often precipitate the pain of *glaucoma.* Bruxism and opening the mouth widely may aggravate *TMJ pain.* Mastication and temperature extremes may exacerbate dental pain. Acidic foods and mastication may precipitate pain from a sialolith. Pain in the jaw brought on by exertion suggests *angina pectoris,* especially in older patients.

AMELIORATING FACTORS

Sinus pain is often relieved by postural changes; some sinuses drain better when the patient is erect, whereas others drain more effectively in recumbency. Because frontal sinuses drain better when erect, the pain of *frontal sinusitis* lessens as the day progresses. In contrast, the pain of *maxillary sinusitis* improves with recumbency, because the maxillary sinuses drain better in this position.

Effective relief of pain with carbamazepine (Tegretol) suggests that the pain is caused by *neuralgia.* Phenytoin also relieves neuralgic pain but is seldom effective in patients with migraine headaches. Patients with *atypical facial pain* rarely obtain relief from anything other than psychotherapy or antidepressants.

The pain of *TMJ dysfunction* is occasionally relieved by anti-inflammatory agents and muscle relaxants. Depending on the cause, bite plates or correction of a malocclusion may be helpful. This may correct the malalignment of the TMJ but not necessarily the arthritic changes in the joint, whether primary or secondary changes to the malocclusion. Therefore, even extensive dental work does not always completely relieve TMJ pain.

PHYSICAL FINDINGS

The physician must conduct a meticulous examination of the eyes, ears, nose, nasopharynx, mouth, and hypopharynx to determine the source of facial pain. The physical examination is usually normal in patients with atypical facial pain and the various neuralgias. Rarely, patients with TGN may have a sensory deficit over the division involved and pupillary inequality. If the TGN is atypical or bilateral or occurs in patients younger than age 50, the physical examination should focus on findings that could be caused by a basilar artery aneurysm, multiple sclerosis, or cerebellar dysfunction. Patients with long-standing, undiagnosed *neuralgia* may be partially or completely toothless; extractions may have been performed to relieve pain thought to be of dental origin.

The physical findings in *glaucoma* include increased intraocular pressure as determined by tonometry, a dilated pupil, and conjunctival injection. In the early stages of simple glaucoma, the patient does not usually notice any pain, obscuring of vision, halos, or visual field cuts. The patient with subacute glaucoma may have the vision temporarily obscured and may see halos or rainbows around lights.

Patients with *acute glaucoma* may have marked conjunctival injection; therefore, acute glaucoma is part of the differential diagnosis of the patient with a *red eye*. Other physical findings include edema of the eyelids; a hazy and *steamy* cornea; decreased corneal sensation; an injected, discolored iris; and a pupil that is mildly dilated and occasionally vertically oval. The intraocular tension is raised, and the eye is hard to the touch and tender on gentle palpation.

Acute glaucoma can be differentiated from iritis (which may be painful) and conjunctivitis by the appearance of the cornea and the pupil. In conjunctivitis and iritis, the cornea is clear and sensitive (Table 13-1). In conjunctivitis the pupil is active, whereas in iritis it is small and fixed. In both conjunctivitis and iritis, intraocular tension is normal.

Patients with *acute sinusitis* have ipsilateral nasal fullness and pain over the affected sinus that is exacerbated by palpation or percussion. Transillumination over the affected sinus is impaired. Patients may complain of toothaches or tenderness on percussion of the upper teeth because the roots of these teeth are close to the floor of the maxillary sinus. Because maxillary sinusitis is so common, it is occasionally misdiagnosed as hay fever or chronic allergic rhinitis, and vice versa.

Fewer physical findings and symptoms are associated with *subacute* or *chronic sinusitis*. Patients with subacute sinusitis may complain of headache, postnasal drip, or purulent discharge from the nose or posterior pharynx when the sinus ostia permit drainage in this subacute phase. Patients with chronic sinusitis may have a mucopurulent discharge that is unresponsive to medical management. They may complain of vague ear pain or hearing loss that is secondary to serous otitis. They often have a sore throat secondary to postnasal drip.

Patients with *TMJ dysfunction* may experience pain with palpation of the joint when they open and close the mouth. The TMJ can be palpated in the preauricular area or through the external auditory canal. The masseter muscles

Table 13-1. Points of Distinction between Conjunctivitis, Iritis, and Acute Glaucoma

SITE	CONJUNCTIVITIS	IRITIS	ACUTE GLAUCOMA
Conjunctiva	Conjunctival vessels bright red and injected; movable over subjacent sclera; injection most marked away from corneoscleral margin; color fades on pressure	Ciliary vessels injected, deep red or bluish red; most marked at corneoscleral margin; color does not fade on pressure	Both conjunctival and ciliary vessels injected
Cornea	Clear, sensitive	Clear, sensitive	Steamy, hazy, insensitive
Anterior chamber	Clear; normal depth	Aqueous turbid; slightly shallow	Very shallow
Iris	Normal color	Injected, swollen, adherent to lens, muddy-colored	Injected
Pupil	Black, active	May be filled with exudate	Dilated, fixed, oval
Intraocular tension	Normal	Small, fixed Normal	Raised

From Hart FD, editor: French's Index of Differential Diagnosis, 10th ed. Baltimore, Williams & Wilkins, 1973.

may be prominent in patients who grind their teeth. Auscultation over the joint may reveal a clicking sound with opening and closing of the mouth.

Tenderness on palpation of the temporal artery suggests *temporal arteritis*. Pain on palpation of the carotid bulb suggests *carotidynia*.

Cervical lymphadenopathy or neurologic deficits should suggest an intracranial or local *tumor*.

DIAGNOSTIC STUDIES

All patients with *unexplained* facial pain should be evaluated with dental, sinus, and skull radiographs or computed tomography (CT) scans; tonometry; measurement of the erythrocyte sedimentation rate, which is elevated in patients with temporal arteritis; and thorough examination of the nose, nasopharynx, larynx, oropharynx, and hypopharynx.

The radiographic findings in *chronic sinusitis* may be normal or may show haziness of the sinus cavity or thickening of the sinus mucosa. Generally, CT scans are preferred in the evaluation of the paranasal sinuses. Likewise, in *acute sinusitis*, radiographic findings can be normal in the earliest stage and become abnormal later. In other words, positive radiographic findings are confirmatory, although negative findings do not absolutely rule out acute or chronic sinusitis. The findings of nasal endoscopy and a modified CT scan of the sinuses may be abnormal and explain facial pain despite normal radiographic findings. The absence of radiographic changes significantly decreases the likelihood of chronic, recurrent sinusitis.

Radiographic findings in *TMJ dysfunction* include the loss of the TMJ space, thinning or loss of lamina over the condylar head or glenoid fossa, flattening of the condylar head, and spur formation. Routine mandibular radiographs may be normal, but CT scans or magnetic resonance imaging (MRI) may show arthritic changes in the TMJ.

LESS COMMON DIAGNOSTIC CONSIDERATIONS

Eagle's syndrome is suggested by vague facial pain; neuralgia and headache; neck or throat pain radiating to the ipsilateral ear; and aching or sharp stabbing pain on swallowing, head movement, yawning, or coughing. This syndrome is related to an elongated styloid process or calcified stylohyoid ligament, which is present in 4% of the population. Only 4% of those with an elongated styloid process have symptoms. The diagnosis may be confirmed radiographically.

Symptoms of burning, constant, and persistent pain affecting the upper division or any other division of the trigeminal nerve that begins after a recognized bout of herpes may signal *postherpetic neuralgia*. This is most common in older patients who, after a bout of TGN, continue to have local neuralgia pain with intermittent exacerbations.

Pain that usually occurs at night (in contrast to TGN, which usually occurs during the day) should suggest the possibility of *glossopharyngeal neuralgia*. Patients (usually older) describe the pain as stabbing, jolting, burning, or continuous. The pain may last seconds to minutes, and attacks tend to occur in clusters, lasting from days to months. The pain is often localized to the posterior half of the tongue, the tonsils, and the pharynx, although it may radiate to the ear, the neck, and/or the jaw. This diagnosis should be suspected if the pain begins at night or if it is triggered by swallowing; talking; yawning; or eating spicy, salty, or bitter foods. Its incidence is quite rare compared with that of TGN.

When a patient complains of constant unilateral burning or aching in the region of the mandible, maxilla, or frontotemporal area and if the pain is described as "deep" instead of "on the surface," the problem may be *sphenopalatine neuralgia* (Sluder's syndrome). It can be differentiated from trigeminal and glossopharyngeal neuralgia because it is usually a constant pain. It will last hours to days, and nasal mucosa may be inflamed ipsilaterally. It often develops in patients who have sinusitis or postnasal drip. A diagnosis may often be made by anesthetization of the sphenopalatine ganglion. Cocaine or other topical anesthetics can be used on the tip of a nasal swab, which is inserted straight back through the nares after the nasal mucosa is shrunk.

The presentation and differential diagnosis of *temporal arteritis* are described in Chapter 17. If a patient complains of dull, aching pain in the lower jaw (either unilateral or bilateral) that occurs with physical exertion, it may be *atypical referred anginal pain*. Rarely, craniofacial pain (throat, either mandible, left TMJ, and teeth) may be the only manifestation of cardiac ischemia. This is more common in women who often have atypical pain during

Differential Diagnosis of Facial Pain

CONDITION	NATURE OF PATIENT	NATURE OF PAIN	ASSOCIATED SYMPTOMS	PRECIPITATING AND AGGRAVATING FACTORS	AMELIORATING FACTORS	PHYSICAL FINDINGS	DIAGNOSTIC STUDIES
Neuralgia							
Trigeminal	Age >50 yr	Lancinating Stabbing Sudden onset Usually occurs in daytime On surface Usually unilateral Maxillary or mandibular division more common		Touching of trigger points Extremes of temperature	Carbamazepine Phenytoin	Tenderness at trigger points	
Glossopha-ryngeal		Paroxysmal Recurrent Often nocturnal					
Sphenopala-tine		Constant Pain "in deep"	Postnasal drip				
Sinusitis		Dull Constant Over affected sinus or behind orbit Recurrent or chronic Gradual onset or chronic	Nasal stuffi-ness Mucopuru-lent nasal discharge Upper respiratory infection	Upper respiratory infection Coughing and sneezing Frontal sinusitis pain worsens when patient is recumbent Maxillary sinusitis pain may worsen when patient is erect	Maxillary pain eases when patient is recumbent Frontal pain lessens when patient is erect	Tender on palpation or percus-sion Decreased transillumi-nation Nasal congestion	Sinus radiographs Nasal endoscopy Sinus CT

Continued

Differential Diagnosis of Facial Pain—cont'd

CONDITION	NATURE OF PATIENT	NATURE OF PAIN	ASSOCIATED SYMPTOMS	PRECIPITATING AND AGGRAVATING FACTORS	AMELIORATING FACTORS	PHYSICAL FINDINGS	DIAGNOSTIC STUDIES
Glaucoma	Age >40 yr Farsighted	Dull Severe with acute narrow angle Usually unilateral	Nausea and vomiting			Increased ocular tension Pupil dilated	Tonometry
Acute		Orbital Severe Sudden onset	Halos or rainbows around light Temporary visual obscuration	Darkness Drugs that dilate pupils (e.g., sympathomimetics, psychotropics, anticholinergics)		Conjunctival injection Steamy cornea	
Subacute		Frontal Dull Gradual onset					
TMJ dysfunction	Age >40 yr Those with rheumatic arthritis	Recurrent or chronic Usually unilateral over TMJ Felt in ear, temple, or teeth Worse in morning in "night grinders"	Tinnitus Clicking Crepitation of TMJ Bruxism	Bruxism Opening mouth widely	Bite plates Correction of malocclusion	Tender on palpation over TMJ Malocclusion Prominent masseter muscles	Radiographs, MRI, and tomograms of TMJ
Cluster headache (see Chapter 17)		Eye pain Frontal headaches	Ipsilateral lacrimation and rhinorrhea				

Condition	Patient	Clinical Features	Associated Features	Precipitating Factors	Signs	Treatment	Diagnostic Findings
Temporal arteritis (see Chapter 17)			Headache Transient blindness		Temporal artery tender on palpation		Elevated ESR
Tumors of nasopharynx	Elderly	Constant pain in nose, ethmoid, midface					Skull radiographs and CT scans
Atypical facial pain	Women Anxious Similar family history Often depressed	Pain does not follow any cranial or cervical nerve Hemicrania	Significant affective component			Psychotherapy Antidepressants	Normal
Dental abscess	Any age	Chronic pain in teeth, jaw, or maxillary region		Temperature extremes Mastication	Sensitive to hot or cold Tender on percussion over teeth		Dental radiographs

CT, Computed tomography; ESR, erythrocyte sedimentation rate; MRI, magnetic resonance imaging; TMJ, temporomandibular joint.

an acute myocardial infarction. The diagnosis is confirmed if the jaw pain is relieved by administration of sublingual nitroglycerin. Pain or dysesthesia that is located in the nasal cavity, in the ethmoid or supraorbital region, or deep in the midface and is not attributable to one of the more common causes of facial pain should suggest the possibility of *neoplasm,* particularly if the patient is elderly.

Barodontalgia, sensitivity, or pain in a tooth caused by a change in pressure may occur in divers and flyers.

The triad of facial pain, cochleovestibular dysfunction, and skin changes in the ear and external ear canal suggest compatibility with subacute herpes zoster or the Ramsay Hunt syndrome (herpes zoster oticus).

Pain in the eye is caused most often by TGN, postherpetic neuralgia, sinus disease, or cluster headaches. Less common occurrences of referred pain to the eye can be observed in patients with hypertension, temporal arteritis, orbital tumors, and ophthalmoplegic migraine (pain with a third nerve palsy), which may be caused by an intracranial aneurysm. Direct causes of pain in the orbit include herpetic keratitis, herpes zoster of the ophthalmic branch, narrow-angle glaucoma, acute iritis, and keratoconjunctivitis sicca.

Sialolithiasis may be present if the patient complains of submandibular or parotid pain that is worse on chewing or swallowing, particularly with tenderness or swelling in the salivary glands. Exacerbation of the pain and swelling after instillation of lemon juice into the oropharynx or ingestion of lemon juice confirms the diagnosis.

Lyme disease may manifest as symptoms of TMJ and dental pain, facial pain, facial nerve palsy, or headache.

Selected References

Benoliel R, Eliav E: Neuropathic orofacial pain, *Oral Maxillofac Surg Clin North Am* 20:237-254, 2008.

Casale M, Rinaldi V, Quattrocchi C, et al: Atypical chronic head and neck pain: don't forget Eagle's syndrome, *Eur Rev Med Pharmacol Sci* 12:131-133, 2008.

Cooper BC, Cooper DL: Recognizing otolaryngologic symptoms in patients with temporomandibular disorders, *J Craniomandib Pract* 11:260-267, 1993.

Grazzi L, Usai S, Rigamonti A: Facial pain in children and adolescents, *Neurol Sci* 26(Suppl 2): s101-s103, 2005.

Jones N: Classification and diagnosis of facial pain, *Hosp Med* 62:598-606, 2001.

Keith DA: Differential diagnosis of craniofacial pain, *Cranio Clin Int* 1:173-184, 1991.

Kreine M, Okeson JP, Michaelis V, et al: Craniofacial pain as the sole symptom of cardiac ischemia: a prospective multicenter study, *J Am Dent Assoc Jan* 138:74-79, 2007.

Montgomery MT: Extraoral facial pain, *Emerg Clin North Am* 18:577-600, 2003.

Okeson JP: Nonodontogenic toothache, *Northwest Dentistry* 79:37-44, 2000.

Schoenen J: Differential diagnosis of facial pain, *Acta Neurol Belg* 101:6-9, 2001.

Siccoli MM, Bassetti CL, Sándor PS: Facial pain: clinical differential diagnosis, *Lancet Neurol* 5:257-267, 2006.

Thaller SR, Thaller JL: Head and neck symptoms: is the problem in the ears, face, neck or oral cavity? *Postgrad Med* 87:75-77, 80, 83-86, 1990.

Zakzewksa JM: Diagnosis and management of non-dental orofacial pain, *Dent Update* 34:134-139, 2007.

Fatigue

Fatigue has been defined as a feeling of overwhelming, sustained exhaustion with a decreased capacity for physical and mental work not relieved by rest.

Fatigue is the seventh most common complaint in primary care. It can be the presenting symptom of almost any disease. Thorough history and physical examination will establish a diagnosis in about 85% of patients. If, in addition to experiencing fatigue, the patient complains of localizing symptoms such as abdominal pain or hemoptysis, the diagnosis is easier. Specific attention can then be focused on abdominal or chest causes, respectively. If the patient's only complaint is fatigue, the diagnosis is more difficult.

Fatigue is often confused (by patients and doctors alike) with excessive daytime sleepiness. Fatigue is more likely to be called weariness, weakness, and depleted energy, whereas excessive daytime sleepiness may be called drowsiness, decreased alertness, and sleep propensity ("I can always go to sleep"). In fact, in one study of patients with obstructive sleep apnea, the patients usually complained of fatigue, tiredness, and lack of energy rather than sleepiness.

Fatigue can be categorized as acute, chronic, or physiologic. *Acute fatigue* is most often a prodrome or sequela of an acute viral or bacterial infectious process. Heart failure and anemia may also manifest as a sudden onset of fatigue.

Chronic fatigue (of weeks' to months' duration) can be caused *by depression; chronic anxiety or stress; chronic infection, especially infectious mononucleosis, hepatitis, or tuberculosis; cancer; rheumatoid arthritis, fibromyalgia,* and other rheumatologic disorders; *heart failure; sleep apnea; serum electrolyte abnormalities* (hyponatremia, hypokalemia, hypercalcemia); *chronic lung disease; or anemia.* Prescribed and over-the-counter drugs are common and frequently unrecognized causes of chronic fatigue, especially in patients older than 45 years. These drugs include antihistamines, tranquilizers, psychotropics, hypnotics, and antihypertensives (particularly reserpine, methyldopa, clonidine, and beta blockers).

Patients with *physiologic fatigue* usually recognize the cause of their fatigue and usually do not consult a physician about it. Physiologic fatigue can result from overwork (either physical or mental) and insufficient or poor-quality sleep, which may be caused by depression, caffeine, drugs, alcohol, or chronic pain.

In about 50% of patients who present with fatigue, the cause is functional (*depression, anxiety,* or a *somatoform disorder*); in the other 50% an organic cause exists. The physician must recognize that multiple causes of fatigue may be present. For example, a patient who complains of fatigue may demonstrate the signs and symptoms of depression and may also have hepatitis, infectious mononucleosis, or bronchogenic carcinoma.

Depression as a cause of fatigue *is not a diagnosis of exclusion.* Innumerable diagnostic tests to rule out all possible organic causes should **not** be performed before the diagnosis of depression is made. Instead, if thorough history and physical examination do not reveal clues to an organic cause but do uncover symptoms of depression, depression is the probable cause of the fatigue.

NATURE OF PATIENT

Fatigue is an uncommon complaint in children and young adults. When it is the presenting symptom, it is usually caused by a prodrome or sequela of an *acute infectious process.* Chronic fatigue in adolescents is most often related to *infectious mononucleosis, hepatitis, substance abuse, depression,* and/or *chronic anxiety.*

Depression in children seldom manifests as lowered mood or fatigue; instead, the children present with somatic complaints such as headache and *acting out.* Depression often manifests in children as hyperactivity, withdrawal, eating problems, school troubles, sleep disturbances, or vague physical complaints. When fatigue is associated with acting-out behavior (e.g., substance abuse, sexual misconduct) in adolescents, depression may be the underlying culprit. Illnesses such as cancer, chronic lung disease, heart disease, and leukemias are uncommon in children and adolescents.

As in younger patients, the most common cause of *acute* fatigue in adults is *infection,* followed by *depression* and *anxiety.* The incidence of fatigue has been reported to be higher in women than men. Life events such as childbirth and menopause may be responsible, although more women than men are diagnosed with depression as causing their fatigue.

There is a greater prevalence of fatigue in patients older than 65 years than in the general population.

In adult patients, particularly the elderly, serious *organic illnesses,* such as circulatory and pulmonary diseases, anemia, cancer, and endocrine abnormalities, are more likely to manifest as fatigue. In elderly patients, the chief complaint of *masked hyperthyroidism* may be fatigue. Patients with this condition do not necessarily show tachycardia, tremors, and other classic signs of hyperthyroidism. Weakness may be caused by diuretic-induced hypokalemia, psychotropic agents, alcoholism, and neuropathies. **Sleep apnea, which is more common in obese patients and patients who snore, may lead the patient to complain of fatigue, not sleepiness.**

Because fatigue is such a common symptom of depression in adults, the physician must recognize that the signs and symptoms of depression vary not only with age but also with gender and socioeconomic status (Table 14-1). Men more

TABLE 14-1.   Discriminators of Depression by Socioeconomic Class

	LOWER CLASS	MIDDLE CLASS	HIGHER-CLASS
Affective	Hopelessness Self-accusation Crying Dissatisfaction Guilt Depressed mood	Loneliness Helplessness Guilt Crying Anxiety, tension Depressed mood	Decreased social life Pessimism Dissatisfaction Anxiety, tension
Somatic	Palpitation Headache Anorexia Early awakening	Decreased libido Urinary complaints Trouble falling asleep Headache Anorexia Early awakening	Fatigue Insomnia

Data from Rockwell DA, Burr BD: The tired patient. J Fam Pract 5:853-857, 1977; and Schwab J, Bralow M, Brown J: Diagnosing depression in medical patients. Ann Intern Med 67:695-707, 1967.

often demonstrate depression as guilt, feelings of helplessness, pessimism, and depressed moods. Early signs of depression in women include headache, insomnia, and withdrawal from social activities. Depressed patients of lower socioeconomic class are likely to have depressed moods, feelings of guilt, hopelessness, and dissatisfaction, and crying spells. They may complain of palpitations, loss of appetite, early awakening, and headaches. Depressed middle class patients state that they feel sad or blue, guilty, helpless, lonely, or anxious. They may complain of crying spells, initial insomnia, early awakening, loss of appetite, headache, and decreased libido. Patients of the upper socioeconomic class more often complain of fatigue, insomnia, anxiety and tension, dissatisfaction, and decreased interest in work and social life.

About 90% of patients with *fibromyalgia* are women. They usually complain of fatigue, nonarticular rheumatism, and nonrestorative sleep.

NATURE OF SYMPTOMS

The following historical clues suggest fatigue of *organic* origin: It is of shorter duration, related to exertion, *not* present in the morning but increasingly evident as the day goes on, relieved by rest, and progressive rather than fluctuating over time. Other obvious organic symptoms or signs may be present. The fatigue may be related to a specific muscle group (e.g., weakened arms or drooping eyelids, as in myasthenia gravis). Fatigue that increases over several months suggests a progressively deteriorating condition such as anemia or cancer.

Most cases of chronic fatigue in which an organic cause is not initially apparent are probably caused by psychosocial factors. Fatigue of *functional* origin is usually of longer duration than that of organic origin; it is often present and may be worse in the morning but improves gradually as the day progresses; and it is usually not related to exertion. The cause of functional fatigue may become apparent during the history taking, especially if the onset of symptoms correlates with emotional stresses, including doubts about job security, major life changes, and significant loss (e.g., death of a spouse, loss of a job, or amputation of a limb). Fatigue that tends to be worse in the morning, even while the patient is in bed, and improves as the day progresses suggests *depression*. Fatigue that is constant over weeks or months, is not aggravated by effort, is associated with numerous somatic complaints, and shows no diurnal variation is probably caused by *chronic anxiety*.

Physiologic fatigue that does not represent a pathologic process should be expected in the following situations: prolonged physical activity without adequate rest; insufficient or poor-quality sleep; dieting; sedentary lifestyle; pregnancy and the postpartum period; and prolonged mental stress.

ASSOCIATED SYMPTOMS

Fatigue associated with dyspnea on exertion or shortness of breath suggests *chronic cardiorespiratory disease*. Fatigue associated with a low-grade fever suggests an *infectious process* such as hepatitis, tuberculosis, or subacute bacterial endocarditis (SBE). *Inflammatory diseases* may also present with fatigue and a low-grade fever. Patients with these conditions may also present only with fatigue and no fever.

In adults complaining of fatigue who also have vague gastrointestinal (GI) symptoms (e.g., constipation, bloating, indigestion), skin disorders, and chronic pain syndromes, *depression* may be the cause. Fatigue associated with restlessness, irritability, sweating, palpitations, and paresthesias is probably caused by *chronic anxiety, stress,* or (rarely) *hyperthyroidism*.

When fatigue is associated with breathlessness, anorexia, weight loss, and pallor, *anemia* should be suspected. If these symptoms are accompanied by numbness in the legs or arms, *pernicious anemia* should be considered. If fatigue is associated with shortness of breath, swelling of the ankles, or paroxysmal nocturnal dyspnea, *congestive heart failure* should be suspected. The presence of diffuse musculoskeletal pain and several tender points suggests *fibromyalgia*.

When chronic fatigue is associated with headache and upper respiratory complaints, *sick building syndrome* should be suspected. The patient with such symptoms usually works in a modern office building with an impervious outer shell, inoperable windows, and inadequate ventilation.

PRECIPITATING AND EXACERBATING FACTORS

Identifying a precipitating factor is often crucial in the diagnosis of fatigue. Initiation of medications, increased workload, insomnia, loss of a job, and family problems can all be precipitating factors. If the onset of fatigue is associated with psychosocial problems, the cause may be chronic anxiety or stress; in such cases a minimal additional stress may exacerbate anxiety and result in a new complaint of fatigue. However, patients with organic disease may erroneously attribute their fatigue to a psychosocial problem.

Postpartum fatigue may be a symptom of medical or psychiatric illness, but it must be distinguished from severe tiredness, which typically occurs after delivery. Postpartum fatigue may be caused by thyroid disorders, anemia, infections, depression, and cardiomyopathy.

Sleep disorders may lead a patient to complain of fatigue or tiredness.

AMELIORATING FACTORS

Intermittent fatigue reduced by rest is probably *physiologic*. Fatigue from organic disease is constant and relieved only by sleep and decreased activity. If fatigue improves on weekends and vacations, *chronic stress* related to employment may underlie the fatigue. The symptoms of *sick building syndrome* (fatigue, headache, upper respiratory complaints) may also abate promptly when the patient leaves the workplace. Fatigue from chronic anxiety or depression is often relieved by exercise and often improves as the day progresses. *Drugs* are causal if fatigue disappears after they are stopped. If fatigue abates after a viral illness, the *viral infection* likely caused the fatigue or tiredness.

PHYSICAL FINDINGS

The most critical component in examining a patient complaining of fatigue is a thorough history that focuses on the onset of symptoms, relation to exertion, family and social history, a full systemic review, and questions about abuse of drugs or other substances.

Physical findings may provide clues about the cause of fatigue. Coarse hair, loss of the outer third of the eyebrows, a hoarse voice, a doughy consistency to the skin, and myoclonic reflexes (particularly the *hung-up* ankle jerk) all suggest *hypothyroidism*. Tachycardia; tremors; fine hair; and warm, moist palms suggest *hyperthyroidism*. Conjunctival or skin pallor suggests *anemia*. Signs of avitaminosis, such as a smooth, glossy tongue and cheilosis, suggest a *nutritional deficiency*. Distended neck veins, rales at the lung bases, tachycardia, gallop, and edema suggest that *congestive heart failure* is the cause of fatigue. Auscultation of a midsystolic click or a late systolic murmur suggests *mitral valve prolapse;* this is a fairly common condition in which patients often complain of fatigue that is most commonly a manifestation of *anxiety*.

When associated with splenomegaly or hepatomegaly, adenopathy (particularly posterior cervical adenopathy) suggests *infectious mononucleosis*. Hepatomegaly (with or without jaundice) and pruritus suggest *hepatitis*, and diffuse adenopathy suggests a *lymphoma*, such as *Hodgkin's disease*, or *acquired immunodeficiency syndrome* (AIDS). An enlarged liver with ascites and spider angiomata suggests *cirrhosis*. Increased bruising sometimes associated with pallor suggests a platelet deficiency, which may be part of some other *hematologic problem*.

Differential Diagnosis of Fatigue

TYPE	NATURE OF PATIENT	NATURE OF SYMPTOMS	ASSOCIATED SYMPTOMS	AMELIORATING FACTORS	PHYSICAL FINDINGS	DIAGNOSTIC STUDIES
Physiologic						
Prolonged physical activity Overwork Inadequate sleep Dieting Pregnancy and postpartum period Sedentary lifestyle	Usually recognizes cause of fatigue and does not complain to physician about it			Rest		Results within normal limits
				Increased physical activity		
Functional	May appear depressed	Fatigue on arising; may diminish during day Onset with emotional stress (job insecurity, major life change, significant loss) Often chronic	Insomnia Vague GI symptoms Chronic pain			
Depression				Improvement in life situations	"Flat" affect	
Anxiety			Numerous somatic complaints Irritability Breathlessness	Removal of stress	No physical abnormalities	
Emotional stress		Of longer duration than that of organic origin Often present or worse in morning Improves during day Unrelated to exertion	Irritability Breathlessness	Removal of stress	No physical abnormalities	

Organic Illnesses	Of shorter duration than that of functional origin. Related to exertion. Not present in morning but worsens during day. Often related to onset of physical ailment (hypothyroidism)	Symptoms of disease causing fatigue: dyspnea on exertion (cardiorespiratory disease), fever (infections), muscle weakness (myasthenia), cold intolerance	Signs of organic pathology causing fatigue: pallor (anemia), rales (pulmonary congestion), weight loss (cancer), tachycardia (hyperthyroidism)	If diagnosis not clinically apparent: CBC with differential, urinalysis, serum glucose SMA-22, ESR, chest x-ray, PPD test, monospot test, thyroid function tests, serum electrolytes
Acute				
Viral or bacterial infections	Most common cause of acute fatigue in all age groups. Fatigue usually subsides in 2 weeks	Fever	Signs of particular infection	CBC with differential. Cultures
Depression	Common cause of fatigue in adults	Sleep disturbances	No physical abnormalities	
Anxiety	Tense, nervous	Somatic complaints	May be signs of mitral valve prolapse	
Drugs and medications		Bizarre behavior. Drowsiness	Bradycardia from methyldopa and beta blockers	

Continued

Differential Diagnosis of Fatigue—cont'd

TYPE	NATURE OF PATIENT	NATURE OF SYMPTOMS	ASSOCIATED SYMPTOMS	AMELIORATING FACTORS	PHYSICAL FINDINGS	DIAGNOSTIC STUDIES
Organic illnesses:						
Anemia		May have acute onset but increases progressively over time	Breathlessness Anorexia and weight loss Pallor Numbness of extremities (with pernicious anemia)		Conjunctival or skin pallor	Hemoglobin, hematocrit
Hypothyroidism			Weight gain cold intolerance		Coarse hair Loss of outer third of eyebrow Hoarse voice "Doughy" skin Myoclonic reflexes (especially "hung-up" ankle jerk)	Thyroid function tests
Serious organic illnesses (e.g., cancer, endocrine disorders)	Rare in children Most common in elderly		Depends on organic illness			

Chronic

Depression (not a diagnosis of exclusion)	Does not manifest as fatigue in children. Often overlooked in elderly. Adolescents may present with somatic complaints and acting-out behavior (e.g., abuse, sexual misconduct). Most common cause of chronic fatigue in adults	In adults, worse in the morning and improves as day progresses. Signs and symptoms may vary with age, gender, and socioeconomic status	*Children:* Somatic complaints. Acting out. Hyperactivity. School, eating, and sleeping problems. Withdrawal. *Adults:* Feelings of guilt, helplessness, pessimism, sadness, loneliness, anxiety, dissatisfaction. Decreased libido. Insomnia. Early awakening. Weight loss and decreased appetite. Social withdrawal. Crying spells. Headache. Vague GI symptoms. Skin disorders. Chronic pain syndromes	"Flat" affect	Physician should *not* perform multiple diagnostic studies to rule out all possible organic causes before diagnosing depression
Medications	Users of anti-histamines, psychotropics, tranquilizers, antihypertensives (reserpine, methyldopa, clonidine, beta blockers)	Onset correlates with beginning of drug ingestion	Cessation of drugs		

Continued

Differential Diagnosis of Fatigue—cont'd

TYPE	NATURE OF PATIENT	NATURE OF SYMPTOMS	ASSOCIATED SYMPTOMS	AMELIORATING FACTORS	PHYSICAL FINDINGS	DIAGNOSTIC STUDIES
Sleep apnea	Often obese	May complain of fatigue, tiredness, lack of energy rather than sleepiness	Snoring Awakening in morning not feeling well rested	Sleeping on side	Large uvula Relaxed soft palate	Sleep studies
Chronic anxiety or stress		Constant over weeks or months Shows no diurnal variation Is not aggravated by effort May be precipitated by psychosocial factors	Somatic complaints Restlessness Irritability Sweating Palpitations Paresthesias		With mitral valve prolapse, possible midsystolic click or late systolic murmur	
Organic illnesses						
Congestive heart failure Cancer Chronic infection	Adults		Vary with illness		Vary with illness	
Mononucleosis	Most common in adolescent and young				Posterior cervical adenopathy Hepatomegaly Splenomegaly	Monospot test

Hepatitis	Most common in alcoholics and IV drug users			Hepatomegaly with or without jaundice	Abnormal liver function and hepatitis antigen values
Fibromyalgia	Adults, usually female	Fatigue may be severe; may occur after minimal exertion	Insomnia Nonrestorative sleep Nonarticular rheumatism	Often relieved by tricyclic antidepressants, trazodone or pregabalin	Hyperalgesic tender sites: low cervical/lumbar spine, suboccipital muscles, lateral epicondyle, medial fat pad of knee	Abnormal sleep, EEG

CBC, Complete blood count; EEG, electroencephalogram; ESR, erythrocyte sedimentation rate; GI, gastrointestinal; IV, intravenous; PPD, purified protein derivative (tuberculin); SMA-22, comprehensive (22-item) metabolic blood test.

Fever suggests an *infectious process*. Rales at the lung apices suggest *pulmonary tuberculosis*. Low blood pressure associated with increased skin pigmentation suggests *adrenal insufficiency*. Polyarticular arthritis suggests *rheumatoid arthritis*, whereas migratory arthritis suggests a *connective tissue disorder*.

Multiple (at least eight) hyperalgesic sites, usually in the neck, back, or trunk, suggest *fibromyalgia*. The tender points are in the middle of the supraspinatus muscle; midpoint of the upper trapezius; pectoralis insertion just lateral to the second costochondral junction; low cervical interspinous ligaments (C4-C6); low midlumbar interspinous ligaments (L4-S1); lateral epicondyle; upper outer quadrant of the buttock (gluteus medius muscle); and medial fat pad of the knee.

DIAGNOSTIC STUDIES

Laboratory tests seldom yield the cause of chronic fatigue. However, when the diagnosis is not readily apparent, the following laboratory tests should be performed: complete blood count (CBC) with differential, urinalysis, measurements of serum glucose, thyroid stimulating hormone (TSH), and erythrocyte sedimentation rate (ESR), comprehensive (22-item) metabolic blood test (SMA-22), and determination of T-cell subsets; tests for human immunodeficiency virus (HIV); and chest radiograph. When the patient has a normal erythrocyte sedimentation rate, serious organic disease is probably not present. Depending on the diagnostic considerations, other laboratory tests may be indicated, such as a tuberculin test, a monospot test, and serum electrolyte evaluation. Sleep studies may be indicated if sleep apnea or other sleep disorders are suspected. In patients with chronic fatigue, an abnormal laboratory finding does not necessarily indicate the cause.

LESS COMMON DIAGNOSTIC CONSIDERATIONS

The less common causes of fatigue include neoplasia, connective tissue diseases (e.g., disseminated lupus erythematosus, polymyalgia rheumatica, temporal arteritis), metabolic states (e.g., uremia, hypokalemia, hyponatremia), endocrine disorders (e.g., hypothyroidism, hyperthyroidism, hypoglycemia, Addison's disease, diabetes), malnutrition with or without malabsorption, chronic pain, chronic neurologic disorders (e.g., myasthenia gravis, post-polio syndrome, multiple sclerosis, Parkinson's disease), and chronic infections (e.g., acquired immunodeficiency syndrome , brucellosis, subacute bacterial endocarditis, post-virus fatigue syndrome). *Chronic fatigue syndrome* (CFS), also called *benign myalgic encephalomyelitis*, can be totally disabling.

Selected References

Bennett R: Fibromyalgia, chronic fatigue syndrome, and myofascial pain, *Curr Opin Rheum* 10: 95-103, 1998.

Cahill CA: Differential diagnosis of fatigue in women, *J Obstet Gynecol Neonatal Nurs* 28:81-86, 1999.

Cavanaugh RM: Evaluating adolescents with fatigue: ever get tired of it? *Pediatr Rev* 23:337-348, 2002.

Chervin RD: Sleepiness, fatigue, tiredness, and lack of energy in obstructive sleep apnea, *Chest* 118:372-379, 2000.

Darbishire L, Ridsdale L, Seed PT: Distinguishing patients with chronic fatigue from those with chronic fatigue syndrome: a diagnostic study in UK primary care, *Br J Gen Pract* 53:441-445, 2003.

Doherty M, Jones A: Fibromyalgia syndrome, *Br Med J* 310:386-389, 1995.

Harrison M: Pathology testing in the tired patient-a rational approach, *Aust Fam Physician* 37: 908-910, 2008.

Pigeon WR, Sateia MJ, Ferguson RJ: Distinguishing between excessive daytime sleepiness and fatigue: toward improved detection and treatment, *J Psychosom Res* 54:61-69, 2003.

Poluri A, Mores J, Cook DB, et al: Fatigue in the elderly population, *Phys Med Rehabil Clin North Am* 16:91-108, 2005.

Ponka D, Kirlew M: Top ten differential diagnoses in family medicine: fatigue, *Can Fam Physician* 53:892, 2007.

Ruffin MT, Cohen M: Evaluation and management of fatigue, *Am Fam Physician* 50:625-632, 1994.

Shen J, Barbera J, Shapiro CM: Distinguishing sleepiness and fatigue: focus on definition and measurement, *Sleep Med Rev* 10:63-76, 2006.

Wessely S: Chronic fatigue: symptom and syndrome, *Ann Intern Med* 134:838-843, 2001.

Zala J: Diagnosing myalgic encephalomyelitis, *Practitioner* 283:916-919, 1989.

Fever

This chapter emphasizes fever as the presenting problem rather than fever of unknown origin (FUO). **Classically, FUO is a temperature greater than 101° F** that occurs on several occasions during a 3-week period in an ambulatory patient or during a 1-week period in a hospitalized patient. Some suggest that the fever must persist for only 10 to 14 days in an outpatient. The cause of the fever should not be apparent, even after a complete history, physical examination, complete blood count (CBC) with differential, urinalysis, 27-item blood chemistry analysis (SMA-27), cardiogram, chest radiograph, monospot test, and intermediate-strength purified protein derivative (tuberculin [PPD]) test.

In most febrile patients, a diagnosis is readily apparent or becomes evident within a few days. FUO is usually caused by a common disorder that displays atypical manifestations or is a benign, self-limiting illness for which no specific cause is found. Nevertheless, it is still important for the physician to search for occult sources of infection, especially if a response to antibiotics is possible.

Normal oral temperature is 98.6° F (37° C) plus or minus about 1° F. Body temperature shows normal diurnal variation; the lowest point is registered in the early-morning hours, and the highest is reached in the late afternoon.

Acute fevers are caused most often by *upper respiratory infections* (URIs), *tonsillitis, viral syndromes* (e.g., influenza, gastroenteritis), *drug reactions,* and *genitourinary* (GU) *tract infections* (e.g., cystitis, pyelonephritis, prostatitis). Less often, acute fevers accompany meningitis, intra-abdominal abscess, and other forms of sepsis.

Chronic low-grade fevers are caused most often by *hepatitis, tuberculosis* (TB), *infectious mononucleosis* (especially in children and young adults), *lymphomas,* and *occult neoplasms* (especially in elderly patients). If the source of a fever is not readily apparent on the basis of history, symptoms, or physical examination, the possibility of *drug fever* (particularly from penicillins, cephalosporins, antituberculosis agents, sulfonamides, macrolides, aminoglycosides, methyldopa, procainamide, and phenytoin), *sinusitis, dental abscess, prostatitis, TB, infectious mononucleosis* (especially with associated fatigue), and *hepatitis*

172

(both anicteric and icteric) should be considered. Cocaine, Ecstasy, and amphetamine abuse may also cause hyperpyrexia.

When recurrent fever occurs at *regular intervals* (21-28 days) in a child, the most likely cause is PFAPA syndrome (periodic fever, aphthous ulcers, pharyngitis, and adenopathy). When recurrent fever occurs at *irregular intervals* in a child, the most common causes include repeated viral infections; repeated bacterial or occult bacterial infections, especially urinary tract infections; and inflammatory bowel disease, especially Crohn's disease.

Less common causes of fever without a readily apparent cause from presenting symptomatology include neoplasms, abdominal abscess, multiple pulmonary emboli, diverticulitis, subacute bacterial endocarditis (SBE), osteomyelitis, and thrombophlebitis.

NATURE OF PATIENT

The most common cause of fever in children is a viral URI. Young children usually have signs or symptoms of a respiratory infection but may show only fever. Other viral causes of fever in children are chickenpox (varicella), "slapped cheek disease" (erythema infectiosum,) roseola infantum, papulovesicular acro-located syndrome (PALS), and enteroviral infections. Common causes of fever in children who have no localizing signs or symptoms at the time of examination include *URIs, gastroenteritis, tonsillitis, otitis media, urinary tract infections (UTIs), measles,* and *roseola.* A true FUO in a child has serious implications. In one study, 41% of children with true FUO were found to have a chronic or fatal disease. Fever in children younger than 3 months may be the only indication of a serious disease. Unexplained fever in adolescents may be a manifestation of *drug abuse* or *endocarditis.* Severe, acute respiratory disease (SARS) seems to occur more frequently in young adults, for whom the average age is 40 years.

A history of UTI, sinusitis, prostatitis, and recurrent pneumonia on the same side increases the likelihood that the current febrile episode may be similar to those in the past.

In the absence of physical signs or symptoms suggesting the cause of fever, the physician should question the patient specifically about occupational history, exposure or contact with animals (e.g., bird flu, Lyme disease), chemicals, drug ingestion, travel away from the patient's usual residence (SARS, malaria, typhoid, and rickettsial infections). Fever from unusual infections is more common in immunocompromised patients and in those with human immunodeficiency virus (HIV) infection. In febrile, elderly patients who lack signs or symptoms that suggest a cause, *TB, occult neoplasm, temporal arteritis,* and *recurrent pulmonary emboli* must be considered. **Febrile response to infections is often diminished or absent in elderly patients,**

In the postoperative patient, fever may be caused by infection, atelectasis, or a reaction to anesthesia or medications.

NATURE OF SYMPTOMS

Contrary to common belief, studies have shown that the fever pattern is not likely to be helpful diagnostically, although the magnitude may. Temperatures above 105° F (40.5° C) suggest *intracranial pathology, factitious fever, pancreatitis, or UTI,* especially with shaking chills. When severe hyperthermia is associated with muscle rigidity, the following causes should be suspected: Ecstasy, cocaine, or other sympathomimetic agents, serotonin syndrome, antipsychotic drugs, drugs with strong anticholinergic properties, and inhalational anesthetics. Other causes are thyrotoxicosis, tetanus, strychnine poisoning, and central nervous system (CNS) infections. A mild fever suggests *URI* or a *flulike syndrome.* Low-grade fever (especially when associated with fatigue) may be the initial manifestation of *tuberculosis, infectious mononucleosis,* or *hepatitis.* The fever range may also be helpful. A narrow range of fever, without spikes or chills, may be seen in lymphomas such as *Hodgkin's disease, lymphatic leukemia,* and *hypernephroma.*

A fever in an emotionally disturbed patient who is otherwise in good health and is employed in a health care–related position, has no weight loss, and demonstrates no related or proportional increase in pulse rate should make the physician suspect a factitious cause. Some investigators report that this situation is more likely in female patients. If a factitious cause is suspected, a simultaneous measurement of urine and rectal temperature should be obtained. **The temperature of the urine normally approximates rectal temperature, and a factitious cause should be suspected if the rectal temperature is significantly (usually more than 2.7° C)** higher than the urine temperature. Other clues to a factitious cause include failure of temperature to follow a diurnal pattern, rapid defervescence without sweating, high temperature without prostration, and high temperature without weight loss or night sweats.

Drug fevers usually occur about 7 to 10 days after initial administration but reappear rapidly with subsequent administration.

ASSOCIATED SYMPTOMS

The following clues may help the physician differentiate viral from bacterial infections. If the fever is high and there appears to be a sparsity of systemic symptoms (e.g., aches, pains, malaise, backache, fatigue), with the more specific findings limited to the pharynx, abdomen, or chest, a *bacterial infection* is more likely. However, if a relatively low-grade fever of less than 101.5° F (38.5° C) is associated with systemic complaints (e.g., aches, pains, backache, fatigue, and headache) and the localizing findings are sparse, a *viral infection* is more likely. For example, the combined findings of a temperature of 103° F (39.4° C); a red, sore throat; hoarseness; and possible dysphagia suggest bacterial pharyngitis. A viral cause is more likely if the temperature is less than 101° F (38.3° C); the pharynx is injected and edematous but little evidence of follicular tonsillitis is present; and the patient complains of aches, pains, myalgia, and headache. Influenza syndrome is characterized by a sudden onset of cough and fever, headache, sore throat, myalgia, nasal congestion, weakness, and anorexia.

When a rash is associated with fever, the rash may be a viral exanthem (e.g., rubella, rubeola, varicella) or a clue to a more serious illness (e.g., Rocky Mountain spotted fever, meningococcemia, thrombocytopenia, Lyme disease, infectious mononucleosis, erythema multiforme, vasculitis).

Fever (>100.3° F), *absence of cough, myalgia, diarrhea, absolute lymphopenia, low platelet counts*, and *travel to affected areas should suggest SARS.*

Shaking chills suggest bacteremia frequently due to *pyelonephritis*. When fatigue is associated with a low-grade fever, *infectious mononucleosis or TB* is likely. Persistent fever after a URI, occasionally associated with a frontal headache, should suggest *sinusitis*.

When fever is associated with arthritis or endocarditis, the physician should suspect disseminated gonococcal infection, or *Lyme disease*. If fever is associated with generalized musculoskeletal pain, the physician must consider rheumatologic or autoimmune disorders.

PRECIPITATING AND AGGRAVATING FACTORS

Contact with people with URI or influenza or a local endemic increases the likelihood of *URI* or *influenza*. These two conditions are particularly common in the winter and late summer.

In women, a marked increase in sexual activity may precipitate *cystitis* or *urethritis*, referred to as *honeymoon cystitis*. In men, a sudden decrease in sexual activity, particularly after an increase in sexual relations (e.g., during a vacation), may precipitate *prostatitis*.

The pain of *sinusitis* may be exacerbated by bending forward, coughing, sneezing, or blowing the nose. Medications and over-the-counter drugs may also cause fever.

PHYSICAL FINDINGS

In addition to conducting a careful, thorough physical examination, the physician should pay special attention to certain areas when evaluating a patient whose chief complaint is fever. Relative bradycardia, or a large dissociation between the fever and pulse rate, suggests a drug fever, factitious fever, or (rarely) typhoid. *Drug fever* should also be suspected if the patient looks *inappropriately well* for the severity of the fever. The sinuses should be percussed and transilluminated for evidence of *sinusitis*. The throat should be examined for signs of *bacterial* or *viral infection* as well as the enanthema of *measles* or *infectious mononucleosis*. Carious teeth should be tapped for signs of *periapical abscess*. All lymph nodes should be palpated. Rectal examination must be performed for evidence of a *perirectal abscess* or *prostatitis*.

If an obvious source of fever is not made apparent through the history or physical examination, attention should be focused on sources of fever that initially manifest without any clue other than fever. This is particularly true in children. Because significant physical findings and symptoms other than fever may be absent in young children, the physician may use the following clues to assess the severity of the illness: decreased playfulness, decreased alertness, reduced motor ability, respiratory distress, and dehydration. Fever may be seen as an early manifestation of many illnesses, ranging from *teething* to *roseola.* If the source of the fever in a child is not apparent, a urinalysis should be performed; pyuria and albuminuria may be the only manifestations of a UTI.

In teenagers and young adults, *infectious mononucleosis* should be suspected if the fever is associated with any one or more of the following: pharyngitis (either exudative or nonexudative), enanthema on the soft palate, posterior cervical or generalized adenopathy, hepatosplenomegaly, and exanthema. If these patients are given ampicillin, a rash similar to that seen after administration of penicillin may develop. If this occurs in patients with proven infectious mononucleosis, the likelihood of true penicillin sensitivity is small.

DIAGNOSTIC STUDIES

Laboratory tests useful in determining the cause of a fever include complete blood count with differential (particular attention should be given to monocytes and atypical lymphocytes) neutrophil counts; absolute lymphopenia; thick and thin blood smears for malaria; a monospot test; measurement of erythrocyte sedimentation rate (ESR); urinalysis; a 22-item blood chemistry analysis (SMA-22); antistreptolysin titer; a tuberculin test (purified protein derivative [PPD] skin test); tests for antinuclear antibodies and febrile agglutinins; and cultures of blood, urine, pharynx, and stools. Computed tomography (CT) scans; sonograms; technetium Tc99m pertechnetate, gallium, and indium-111 scans; and special radiographic studies may be helpful in some cases.

The procalcitonin test is very useful in separating bacterial infections from viral and invasive nonbacterial infections. It is particularly helpful in such infections them in febrile children (between 1 and 36 months of age) and adults.

LESS COMMON DIAGNOSTIC CONSIDERATIONS

The many uncommon illnesses that cause fever include subacute bacterial endocarditis, acute bacterial endocarditis, bacteremia, meningitis, encephalitis, systemic lupus erythematosus, vasculitis, disseminated fungal infection, severe head injury (neurogenic fever), actinomycosis (including pelvic actinomycosis, often related to a retained intrauterine device), systemic calcium pyrophosphate deposition disease (pseudogout), myocarditis, lung abscess, osteomyelitis, encephalitis, neoplasms in any location, retroperitoneal lesions, lymphomas, connective tissue disorders, inflammatory bowel disease, diverticulitis, periodic fever, metal fume fever, factitious fever, malaria, rat-bite fever, and pulmonary emboli (Table 15-1). Periorbital edema associated with fever may be due to local or systemic infections or anaphylaxis.

TABLE 15-1.   Causes of Fever of Unknown Origin in Adults*

CATEGORY	PETERSDORF AND BEESON	SHEON AND VAN OMMEN	HOWARD ET AL	GLECKMAN ET AL	ESPOSITO AND GLECKMAN
Infection	36	21	37	18	36
Tuberculosis	11	5	4	6	8
Abdominal abscess	4	3	9	6	11
Hepatobiliary	7	0	7	0	6
Endocarditis	5	8	9	0	8
Pyelonephritis	3	0	4	0	0
Other	6	5	4	6	3
Neoplasm	19	17	31	9	24
Lymphoma/ Carcinoma	6	7	22	9	14
Renal	1	0	2	0	4
Pancreatic	2	0	0	0	1
Hepatobiliary	0	2	0	0	3
Unknown primary	2	2	2	0	2
Other	8	6	5	0	0
Connective tissue disorder	15	13	19	9	25
Giant cell arteritis	2	0	4	3	17
Systemic vasculitis	0	6	5	3	6
Lupus erythematosus	5	5	3	0	0
Still's disease	0	0	1	3	0
Rheumatic fever	6	2	0	0	1
Other	2	0	6	0	1
Miscellaneous	23	10	8	29	10
Pulmonary emboli	3	0	0	9	5
Factitious fever	3	0	0	0	0
Periodic disease	5	0	0	3	3
Drugs	1	0	2	0	2
Inflammatory bowel disease	0	4	4	3	0
Other	11	6	2	14	0
Undiagnosed	7	39	5	35	5

*All values are expressed as a percentage of total cases.
From Esposito AL, Gleckman RA: A diagnostic approach to the adult with fever of unknown origin. Arch Intern Med 139:575-579, 1979.

Differential Diagnosis of Fever

TYPE	NATURE OF PATIENT	NATURE OF SYMPTOMS	ASSOCIATED SYMPTOMS	PRECIPITATING AND AGGRAVATING FACTORS	PHYSICAL FINDINGS	DIAGNOSTIC STUDIES
Acute						
URI Viral	Any age	Oral temperature usually <101.5° F	Signs of URI Possible systemic symptoms	Contact with people with URI Local epidemic	Cough Oropharynx injected but not beefy red	Procalcitonin
Bacterial	More common in children	Often high fever, >101° F	Marked signs of URI Few systemic symptoms Children restless		Pharyngotonsillar exudate Pulmonary findings	Positive culture or rapid strep screen
Other viral syndromes:						
Influenza	Any age	Usually mild fever	Muscle aches, cough, headache			
Gastroenteritis	Any age	Usually mild fever	Nausea Vomiting Cramps Diarrhea			
Viral exanthems	Children	Usually mild fever			Enanthem in some instances Rash Adenopathy	
Drug reactions	Taking prescription, recreational, or over-the-counter drug	Often high fever	Occasional rash Muscle rigidity with Ecstasy, cocaine, and methamphetamines		Fever abates when patient stops taking drug	
Urinary tract infection	More common in adults	Often high fever with chills	Backache Urinary frequency and urgency	Obstructive uropathy	Costovertebral angle tenderness	Urinalysis Urine culture

Condition	Age/Population	Fever pattern	Symptoms	Sexual frequency	Physical findings	Diagnostic tests
Prostatitis			Dysuria Backache	Marked change in sexual frequency	Prostate tenderness	Culture of prostate secretions
Bacterial sepsis		Often high fever with chills				Blood culture WBC with differential count
Chronic						
Hepatitis	More common in IV drug users	Usually low-grade fever	Fatigue Jaundice Anorexia		Hepatomegaly Liver tender on percussion Jaundice	Liver function tests Hepatitis antigens
Tuberculosis	More common in diabetics	Usually low-grade fever			Chest findings	Chest radiograph Tuberculin test
Infectious mononucleosis	Teenagers Young adults	Usually low-grade fever	Fatigue		Enanthema Pharyngitis Adenopathy (especially postcervical) Splenomegaly	Monospot test
Neoplasm	Elderly adults	Usually narrow fever range	Weight loss			
Occult infection (sinusitis, dental abscess, prostatitis, fungal infections, diverticulitis, SBE, osteomyelitis, inflammatory bowel disease)		Usually low-grade fever	Depends on cause		Depends on cause	Many, including radionuclide scanning

Continued

Differential Diagnosis of Fever—cont'd

TYPE	NATURE OF PATIENT	NATURE OF SYMPTOMS	ASSOCIATED SYMPTOMS	PRECIPITATING AND AGGRAVATING FACTORS	PHYSICAL FINDINGS	DIAGNOSTIC STUDIES
Drug reaction	Taking prescription, recreational, or over-the-counter drug		Occasional rash		Fever abates when drug discontinued	CBC may show hematologic abnormality
Factitious fever	May be emotionally disturbed Associated with health care	Usually >105° F Can be low-grade fever	No weight loss Pulse rate not proportional to fever	Emotional stress	Disparity between rectal or oral temperature and urine temperature	

CBC, Complete blood count; IV, intravenous; SBE, subacute bacterial endocarditis; URI, upper respiratory infection; WBC, white blood cell.

Neuroleptic malignant syndrome (NMS) from antipsychotic medications (e.g., phenothiazines, risperidone, haloperidol) may present with fever or even malignant hyperthermia. The fever may begin at the onset of treatment or after long-term administration. Other associated symptoms of NMS are severe muscle rigidity, tremors, diaphoresis, and elevated creatine kinase levels.

Fever may develop in patients (often of African, Eastern Mediterranean, or Southeast Asian descent) who have a *glucose-6-phosphate dehydrogenase deficiency* who have received sulfonamides, nitrofurantoins, phenacetin, antimalarials, or quinidine.

Cytomegalovirus disease, malignant histiocytosis, juvenile rheumatoid arthritis, Crohn's disease, and cryptic hematoma have been found to cause occult fevers.

Recurrent fevers can be caused by recurrent viral or bacterial infection, UTIs, inflammatory bowel disease, and (in children) PFAPA syndrome.

Selected References

Agrawal A, Timothy J, Thapa A: Neurogenic fever, *Singapore Med J* 48:492-494, 2007.

Blair JE: Evaluation of fever in the international traveler, *Postgrad Med* 116:13-29, 2004.

Browne GJ, Currow K, Rainbow J: Practical approach to the febrile child in the emergency department, *Emerg Med* 13:426-435, 2001.

Chen S-Y, Su C-P, Ma MH-M, et al: Predictive model of diagnosing probable cases of SARS in febrile patients with exposure risk, *Ann Emerg Med* 43:1-5, 2004.

Feder HM: Periodic fever, aphthous stomatitis, pharyngitis, adenitis: a clinical review of a new syndrome, *Curr Opin Pediatr* 12:253-256, 2006.

Hedad E, Weinbroum AA, Ben-Abraham R: Drug-induced hyperthermia and muscle rigidity: a practical approach, *Eur J Emerg Med* 10:149-154, 2003.

John CC, Gilsdorf JR: Recurrent fever in children, *Pediatr Infect Dis J* 21:1071-1077, 2002.

Johnson DH, Cunha BA: Drug fever, *Infect Dis Clin North Am* 10:85-91, 1996.

McKinnon HD, Howard T: Evaluating the febrile patient with a rash, *Am Fam Physician* 62:804-814, 2000.

Monto A, Gravenstein S, Elliott M, et al: Clinical signs and symptoms predicting influenza infection, *Arch Intern Med* 21:3243-3247, 2000.

Norman DC, Yoshikawa TT: Fever in the elderly, *Infect Dis Clin North Am* 10:93-99, 1996.

Norris B, Angeles V, Eisenstein R, et al: Neuroleptic malignant syndrome with delayed onset of fever following risperidone administration, *Ann Pharmacother* 40:2260-2264, 2006.

Ponka D, Kirlew M: Top ten differential diagnoses in family medicine: fever, *Can Fam Physician* 53:1202, 2007.

Sakr Y, Sponholz C, Tuche F, et al: The role of procalcitonin in febrile neutropenic patients: review of the literature, *Infection* 36:396-407, 2008.

Schlossberg D: Fever and rash, *Infect Dis Clin North Am* 10:101-110, 1996.

Forgetfulness

16

Forgetfulness and loss of memory are common complaints, particularly in elderly patients. Often their families raise the issue. *Age-associated memory impairment* (AAMI) is an impairment in episodic memory that occurs in older patients without evidence of dementia. *Age-associated cognitive decline* (AACD) has now been described as a more severe impairment than AAMI. Patients with AACD have more extensive cognitive impairment than their contemporaries. The condition is more likely to progress to Alzheimer's disease than AAMI. Gradual loss of memory in otherwise healthy elderly individuals is so common that it was previously referred to as *benign senescent forgetfulness* (BSF). Nevertheless, patients are usually concerned that it might be an early sign of *Alzheimer's disease* (AD).

The most common causes of forgetfulness are *AAMI*, AACD, depression, alcohol, substance abuse, medications (particularly psychotropic drugs), and *Parkinson's disease*. Forgetfulness can also be caused by dementia, especially AD, frontotemporal dementia, and Lewy body dementia.

When patients complain of forgetfulness, particularly if they appear to be unreliable, it is essential to seek out someone more reliable, such as a friend or spouse, who can confirm the details of the patient's forgetfulness. **Although loss of memory and concentration may have a functional rather than organic origin, the clinician must not assume one or the other without an adequate assessment. This assessment must include adequate history, physical examination, and especially a mental status examination or a computerized test for mild cognitive impairment.**

NATURE OF PATIENT

When adolescents or young adults complain of forgetfulness, memory impairment, or loss of concentration, the most likely causes are *severe anxiety, depression, alcohol abuse,* and *substance abuse.* In a middle-aged person who is not suffering from depression, a sudden onset of forgetfulness should suggest an organic cause such as *alcohol abuse, drug abuse,* administration of *psychotropic agents, brain tumor,* or the onset of a *dementing process.*

In a healthy patient older than 50 years, gradual impairment of memory is probably caused by *AAMI* when it manifests as problems with everyday activities

182

such as misplacing objects and forgetting the names of persons, multiple items to be purchased, or tasks to be done. In this age group a sudden loss of memory is more likely to reflect a serious etiology, including *stroke (cerebrovascular accident [CVA]), intracranial hemorrhage,* and *brain lesions (e.g., tumor, normal pressure hydrocephalus).* AD tends to have a familial incidence. A gradual onset of cognitive impairment and/or dementia may be caused by multi-infarctions, hypothyroidism, Parkinson's disease, alcoholism, subdural hematoma, and normal pressure hydrocephalus.

Repeated *head trauma* (e.g., that experienced by boxers) may cause memory loss. If the patient is an alcoholic or substance abuser or has a history of treatment with psychotropic drugs, particularly tranquilizers and hypnotics, impaired memory and concentration can result.

NATURE OF SYMPTOMS

It is particularly important to note whether the onset of memory impairment was sudden or gradual. A sudden onset may suggest administration of *psychotropic agents* (e.g., benzodiazepines, hypnotics), a *grieving process, stroke (cerebrovascular accident),* or *head trauma.* A gradual onset (or sudden onset less frequently) suggests *depression, progressive dementia, AD, Parkinson's disease,* or a *deteriorating medical disorder* (e.g., cardiac, respiratory, renal, or liver disease). **Loss of concentration, which may be confused with memory impairment, is a cardinal symptom of depression.**

ASSOCIATED SYMPTOMS

Feelings of sadness, impaired concentration, anhedonia, insomnia, and decreased libido suggest that the forgetfulness is probably caused by *depression,* although other major psychiatric disorders can also cause memory loss. Severe headaches, often worse with coughing and sometimes associated with vomiting, suggest the possibility of a *brain tumor.* Resting tremor, bradykinesia, festinating gait, and masked facies suggest that *Parkinson's disease* may be the cause of the memory loss. A progressive decrease in cognitive skills suggests a dementing process such as *AD* or *multi-infarct dementia.* If the patient has signs of infection, meningitis, or inflammatory brain disease, the sudden loss of memory may be caused by *viral, bacterial,* or *fungal brain disease,* especially in patients with *acquired immunodeficiency syndrome (AIDS).*

PRECIPITATING AND AGGRAVATING FACTORS

Depression is probably the most common precipitating cause of forgetfulness and impaired concentration. This may come on spontaneously or may be precipitated by bereavement or other severe loss. *Infectious, inflammatory,* or *neoplastic brain disease* may also precipitate memory loss. A single *head injury* resulting in a period of unconsciousness for more than 1 hour may cause a sudden memory loss. *Alcohol abuse, substance abuse,* and *psychotropic agents,* particularly hypnotics and benzodiazepines, may also precipitate a loss of memory. In some cases the administration of benzodiazepines to alleviate symptoms of bereavement may cause the continuation of forgetfulness after the normal grieving process has ended. *Multiple cerebral infarcts,* as seen in multi-infarct dementia, can manifest as a progressive loss of memory, as can the onset of other dementing diseases such as *AD* and *Parkinson's disease.*

AMELIORATING FACTORS

Most often, simple reassurance by a physician that the symptoms do not represent a major debilitating condition such as AD or Parkinson's disease will alleviate much of the patient's concern, even though minimal forgetfulness persists. In other patients, simple mnemonics, writing a list of things to be done, and other methods to diminish the effects of memory loss often help, particularly in individuals with *AAMI.* Treatment of depression with antidepressants usually alleviates the symptoms of forgetfulness and impaired concentration. Likewise, stopping any medications or over-the-counter drugs that might interfere with memory or concentration may also be helpful.

PHYSICAL FINDINGS

While taking a history and performing a physical examination, the physician should carefully observe the patient's general appearance and behavior, looking specifically for a depressed affect or abnormal behavior. In addition, the patient should be questioned carefully about mood, diurnal variations in mood, suicidal ideation, sleep disturbances, loss of weight, decreased libido, anorexia, and low self-esteem.

A physical examination must include a mental status examination. Memory and concentration can be examined by determining the patient's cognitive state. The physician asks patients to subtract 7 from 100, then from 93, etc. (serial 7s), determines their digit span (ability to remember a series of numbers), and asks them to recite the months of the year in reverse. Recent memory can be tested by determining the patient's 5-minute recall of an address. Standardized tests for memory, orientation, and concentration include the Wechsler Memory Scale and the Gresham Ward questionnaire.

The physician should also look for signs of progressive medical disorders, such as *renal, cardiac, pulmonary,* or *hepatic disease.*

DIAGNOSTIC STUDIES

Diagnostic studies for a patient with memory loss should include standardized tests to determine mental status and memory capabilities. Certain psychological tests, such as the Mini-Mental State Examination (MMSE) (or, preferably,

Differential Diagnosis of Forgetfulness

CONDITION	NATURE OF PATIENT	NATURE OF SYMPTOMS	ASSOCIATED SYMPTOMS	PRECIPITATING AND AGGRAVATING FACTORS	AMELIORATING FACTORS	PHYSICAL FINDINGS	DIAGNOSTIC STUDIES
Age-associated memory impairment	Older than 50 yr	Gradual onset	Difficulty remembering names and tasks to be done Misplacing objects		Reassurance Making lists Other memory-assisting techniques	Healthy	Mental status examination in all patients
Depression	All ages	Usually a gradual onset	Loss of concentration Anhedonia Decreased libido Low self-esteem	Grieving process Severe loss	Antidepressant medications	Depressed affect Weight loss	Serial 7s Gresham Ward Questionnaire Wechsler Memory Scale
Alcohol and substance abuse	All ages, especially adolescents and young adults	Usually a sudden onset					Toxicology screen
Medications	All ages	Usually a sudden onset		Ingestion of psycho-tropic agents (e.g., benzodiazepines, hypnotics)	Stopping of all medications, including over-the-counter drugs		
Alzheimer's disease, multi-infarct dementia, other progressive dementing processes	Older patients	Gradual onset Progressive	Progressive decrease in cognitive skills			Disheveled appear-ance Abnormal behavior	CT MRI PET Mini-Mental Status Exam

Continued

Differential Diagnosis of Forgetfulness—cont'd

CONDITION	NATURE OF PATIENT	NATURE OF SYMPTOMS	ASSOCIATED SYMPTOMS	PRECIPITATING AND AGGRAVATING FACTORS	AMELIORATING FACTORS	PHYSICAL FINDINGS	DIAGNOSTIC STUDIES
Parkinson's disease	Older patients	Gradual onset Progressive	Resting tremor			Resting tremor Bradykinesia Festinating gait Masked facies	
Other intracranial pathology	All ages	Sudden onset	Severe headache Nausea Fever	Stroke (CVA) Infection AIDS Brain tumor Severe head trauma Repeated head trauma			CT Lumbar puncture
Normal-pressure hydrocephalus	All ages	Gradual onset	Urinary incontinence Dementia Parkinsonian-like gait		Neurosurgical procedures may stop progression	Abnormal gait Incontinence	CT Spinal tap

AIDS, Acquired immunodeficiency syndrome; CT, computed tomography; CVA, cerebrovascular accident; MRI, magnetic resonance imaging; PET, positron emission tomography.

a computer assessment of mild cognitive impairment, which is more sensitive) and the Kendrick Cognitive Tests for the Elderly (KCTE), may help to discriminate dementia from functional illness, particularly depression. Non-contrast computed tomography (CT) is cost effective and may show ventricular and sulcal dilatation in patients with AD, but 20% of normal elderly patients may demonstrate a similar picture. Magnetic resonance imaging (MRI) is often helpful in the early differentiation of patients with AD and multi-infarct dementia from those with AAMI. Serum electrolyte measurements, thyroid function tests, and vitamin B12 and folate evaluations may be indicated. Apolipoprotein E (apo E4) genotyping is a promising test for the early detection of AD.

In the early stages of memory loss, it may be impossible to determine whether the patient has early AD or AAMI. Serial examinations may be the most efficient way to make the correct diagnosis.

LESS COMMON DIAGNOSTIC CONSIDERATIONS

Korsakoff's syndrome, herpes simplex encephalitis, normal-pressure hydrocephalus, and multi-infarct dementia can cause mild to severe memory impairment.

Selected References

Anonymous: Aging-getting forgetful: is it dementia? *Harvard Health Letter* 27:6-7, 2002.

Barrett AM: Is it Alzheimer's disease or something else? 10 disorders that may feature impaired memory and cognition, *Postgrad Med* 117:47-53, 2005.

D'Esposito M, Weksler ME: Brain aging and memory: new findings help differentiate forgetfulness and dementia, *Geriatrics* 55:55-58, 61-62, 2000.

Karlawish JHT, Clark CM: Diagnostic evaluation of elderly patients with mild memory problems, *Ann Intern Med* 138:411-419, 2003.

Kelley RE, Minagar A: Memory complaints and dementia, *Med Clin North Am* 93:389-406, 2009.

Pokorski RJ: Differentiating age-related memory loss from early dementia, *J Insur Med* 34:100-113, 2002.

Ross GW, Bowen JD: The diagnosis and differential diagnosis of dementia, *Med Clin North Am* 86:455-476, 2002.

Saxton J, Morrow L, Eschman A, et al: Computer assessment of mild cognitive impairment, *Postgrad Med* 121:177-185, 2009.

Weaver CJ, Maruff P, Collie A, et al: Mild memory impairment in older healthy adults is distinct from normal aging, *Brain Cogn* 60:146-155, 2006.

Headache

17

Primary headaches, such as migraine, tension, and cluster (a form of trigeminal, autonomic, and cephalgia) headaches, are usually recurrent or chronic. *Secondary headaches* include those secondary to stroke, tumor, infection, rarely sinusitis, fever, and other serious conditions that tend to be constant. About 80% of Americans experience some form of headache each year. Fifty percent of these patients have severe headaches, and 10% to 20% consult a physician with headache as the chief complaint. The most common type of headache is the *muscle contraction,* or *tension-type,* headache. About 10% of the population has *vascular* headaches. Headaches caused by acute *sinusitis* are also fairly common. Less common causes of headaches include *glaucoma,* short-term use of *medications* (nitrates, vasodilators, sildenafil) and medication overuse (long-term administration or the sudden withdrawal of analgesics, triptans, and ergot derivatives), *temporal arteritis* (more common in elderly patients), *cervical arthritis, temporomandibular joint* (TMJ) *dysfunction,* and *trigeminal neuralgia.*

Eye strain and hypertension are uncommon causes of headaches. Most patients with hypertension do not have headaches, and most patients with headaches do not have hypertension. When headaches and hypertension coexist, the headaches are usually not related to the hypertension.

To establish a correct diagnosis, the physician must first differentiate acute headaches from recurrent and chronic headaches. Most common headaches are recurrent; and a few are chronic. Acute headaches are often the most serious (subarachnoid hemorrhage, transient ischemic attack, and *thunderclap headache*). Acute, recurrent headaches are usually due to migraine. The physician should first elicit the *temporal profile* of the particular headache and a history of prior headaches. The examiner must ask any patient who complains of headaches about the number and types of headaches, age and circumstances at the time the headaches began, any family history of headaches, the character of the pain (e.g., location of pain, frequency of attacks, duration of headache, time of onset of attack), any prodromal symptoms, associated symptoms, precipitating factors, emotional factors, previous medical history (especially past illnesses, concurrent disease, recent trauma or surgery), allergies, and responses to medication.

An organic disorder should be suspected if the patient has an isolated, severe headache; consistently localized head pain that prevents sleep; headaches associated with straining; headaches accompanied by neurologic signs or symptoms; a change in usual headache pattern; or a chronic, progressively severe headache.

NATURE OF PATIENT

Tension headaches, *vascular* headaches (including migraine), and headaches due to *temporal arteritis* are significantly more common in women, as are pseudotumor cerebri and subarachnoid hemorrhage. *Cluster* headaches are much more common in men (male-to-female ratio, 9:1).

In children as well as adults, the most common type of headache is due to *tension* or muscle contraction. These headaches are usually of psychogenic origin and are often induced by situational (home, family, school, or work) problems. Although most children with tension headaches may be suffering from simple anxiety or stress, the headache may also be a manifestation of depression, particularly if it is associated with mood change, withdrawal disturbances, aggressive behavior, loss of energy, self-deprecation, or weight loss. **If a headache has been present continuously for 4 weeks in the absence of neurologic signs, it is probably psychogenic in origin.** Migraine headaches are recurrent.

Studies of young children with *chronic* headaches have revealed that only a small fraction had an organic cause. In children and adolescents, organic headaches are caused most often by non–central nervous system infections, fever, trauma, and migraine. In children, acute headaches may be the presenting symptoms of a *febrile illness* such as pharyngitis or otitis media.

Children up to age 7 years have a 1.4% incidence of *migraine;* among patients aged 17 years, the incidence is 5%. Migraine headaches in young children are usually bilateral and of short duration, and associated symptoms are infrequent. Population studies indicate a 12% incidence of migraine in postpubescent males and up to a 20% incidence in postpubescent females. Despite these studies, the physician must realize that 20% of all adults who experience migraine headaches have onset of symptoms before age 5, and 50% have onset of migraine symptoms before age 20. **Although combination headaches (tension and migraine) are common in adults, they are rare in children and their frequency increases with adolescence. Cluster headaches are also rare in children.**

Sinus headaches are uncommon in children, but they may occur in young patients, particularly in association with persistent rhinorrhea, cough, otitis media, or allergies. The maxillary sinus is most frequently involved in children. Likewise, headaches of ocular origin are uncommon in children, although the possibility of *astigmatism, strabismus,* or *refractive error* must be considered. This possibility is particularly important if the headaches appear to be related to reading or schoolwork or if they occur late in the afternoon or evening.

Increased intracranial pressure should be suspected if a child who complains of headache has other signs of neurologic dysfunction or projectile vomiting without nausea or if the headache is precipitated or exacerbated by coughing or straining. Causes of increased intracranial pressure in children include tumors (headache usually progressive and chronic), *pseudotumor cerebri, hydrocephalus* (detected by serial head measurements), *subdural hematoma* (more common in battered children or after trauma), and *brain abscess* (which may be a complication of otitis media). *Malingering* can be the cause of headaches in children as well as adults.

In *classic migraine (migraine with aura)* the aura and prodrome are prominent, and the headaches are throbbing and unilateral. The patient often goes to sleep and, on awakening, frequently finds that the headache has disappeared. *Common migraine (migraine without aura)* occurs more frequently than classic migraine. In common migraine the aura may be vague or absent. The prodrome may be vague and manifested only by personality change or malaise, nausea, and vomiting. Common migraine headaches are less often unilateral than classic migraine headaches.

Cluster headaches are extremely rare in children, although they may occur in teenagers. Cluster headaches have their highest frequency in the fourth to sixth decades of life. A family history of *vascular, sinus*, or *sick* headaches is present in most patients with migraine. A positive family history is not usually present in patients with cluster headaches. Most patients with vascular headaches have a history of headaches caused either by tension or vascular problems. Prior diagnoses may be incorrect because of an inadequate or incomplete history.

Because the incidence of significant disease causing headaches increases with age, the onset of headaches in patients after age 50 years requires careful evaluation and differential diagnosis. **Fewer than 2% of patients older than 55 years experience new, severe headaches. If patients older than 55 years have an acute onset of an unrelenting headache that lasts for hours or days, significant disease such as tumor, meningitis, encephalitis, or temporal arteritis should be suspected.** Headache may precede the onset of a neurologic deficit. Occasionally, a sudden, new onset of headaches in elderly people strongly suggests *cerebral ischemia* and *impending stroke* as well as *arteritis*.

In patients older than 50 years, only a few conditions cause chronic, severe headaches; they are temporal arteritis, cluster headaches, mass lesions, posttraumatic headaches, cervical arthritis, Parkinson's disease, medications, and depression. **Depression is a common cause of chronic headache in patients older than 50 years, but these patients usually experienced chronic headaches before age 50 as well.** Although it is uncommon, temporal arteritis occurs more frequently in elderly women; it should be suspected in elderly patients older than 60 years who have unilateral chronic head pain, unexplained low-grade fever, proximal myalgia, a greatly elevated erythrocyte sedimentation rate (ESR), or an unexplained decrease in visual acuity.

Other, less common causes of headache in elderly patients are congestive heart failure, glaucoma, trigeminal neuralgia, and TMJ dysfunction. Iritis, cerebrovascular insufficiency, cerebral hemorrhage, subdural hematoma, and meningitis are even less common but more serious causes of chronic headache.

NATURE OF PAIN

The time of onset may be a helpful clue to diagnosis. A headache that awakens the patient suggests headaches of sudden onset, such as a subarachnoid hemorrhage. Morning headache suggests increased intracranial pressure. Other causes of morning (awakening) headaches include medication overuse, depression, carbon monoxide exposure, epilepsy, and, occasionally, migraine. Tension headaches occur in the late afternoon.

The type, severity, and location of pain are important in the differentiation of the cause of headaches (Tables 17-1 to 17-3). *Tension (muscle contraction)* headaches are usually dull, not throbbing, steady, and of moderate but persistent intensity. If a patient with chronic tension headaches awakens with a headache, its severity may increase as the day progresses and then decrease toward evening. The pain of *migraine* headaches is severe, initially throbbing, and, later, boring. The severity of this pain increases rapidly and steadily. The pain of *cluster* headaches is much more severe and more stabbing and burning in quality than that of the usual vascular or tension headaches. The pain of acute *sinus* headache is usually described as severe, throbbing, and pressure-like. It may be unilateral, often located in the frontal ethmoid or suborbital region.

Common migraine headaches are usually unilateral but may be bilateral. Most often they are located in the frontotemporal or supraorbital region. *Classic migraine* headaches are unilateral. Cluster headaches are unilateral and periorbital in any given cluster; the pain is described as in the eye and radiating to the front of the face or the temporal regions. Tension headaches are most often occipital, suboccipital, and bilateral, and patients describe the pain as similar to that caused by a constrictive band around the head or as tightness of the scalp. These headaches may radiate down the back of the head and neck. The pain of sinus headaches is usually over the involved sinus or sinuses: maxillary, ethmoid, and/or frontal. Some patients with *ethmoid sinusitis* present complaining of pain behind the eye that intensifies with coughing or sneezing.

Classic migraine headaches usually last for 2 to 8 days. Common migraine headaches last from 4 hours to several days. The onset of most migraine headaches is gradual. Tension headaches usually persist all day for several days; some patients state that these headaches are constant. Cluster headaches have a much shorter duration than tension headaches or migraines; most last from 20 to 60 minutes.

Patients with *trigeminal neuralgia* usually complain of facial pain, but occasionally their presenting symptom is headache (see Table 17-3). This pain is usually short, sharp, severe, and stabbing. Each episode lasts less than 90 seconds, but repeated pain persists for 2 to 3 minutes.

Headaches caused by *mass lesions* are persistent but intermittent, whereas headaches due to intracranial infections are usually constant.

Pain in the temporoparietal or periauricular region or dental pain often associated with a *jaw click* suggests TMJ dysfunction.

TABLE 17-1.   Causes of Headaches by Location

AREA OF PAIN	POSSIBLE CAUSE
Generalized	Muscle tension
	Hypertension
	Arteriosclerosis or anemia
	Central nervous system tumor
	Head trauma or chronic subdural hematoma
	Systemic: uremia, thyrotoxicosis
Frontal:	
Upper	Muscle tension
	Frontal ethmoid sinusitis
	Rhinitis
Midfacial	Dental disease, maxillary sinusitis, nasal disease
	Ocular or vascular disease, tumor
	Neurologic (cranial nerve) or vascular degenerative disease
Lateral:	
Temporal	Muscle tension
	Temporomandibular joint disorders, myofascial disease
	Vascular: arteritis, migraine, cluster headache
Facial or ear	Pharyngeal disease (referred pain)
	Otologic or dental disease; Ramsay Hunt syndrome
	Myofascial disease
Vertex	Sphenoid or ethmoid disease
	Hypertension
	Muscle tension
	Central nervous system, nasopharyngeal neoplasm
Occipital	Uremia
	Fibromyositis
	Subarachnoid hemorrhage
	Hypertension
	Muscle tension

From Schramm VL: A guide to diagnosing and treating facial pain and headache. Geriatrics 35:78-90, 1980.

Headache Patterns

The common varieties of headaches have a typical pattern for each patient. A change in the pattern should suggest the development of a new problem. If a patient who usually has tension headaches in the occipital region or in a band-like region around the head begins to have unilateral headaches associated with nausea and vomiting, migraine headaches may have developed as an additional

TABLE 17–2. Diagnosis of Tension Headache versus Migraine by History

CHARAC-TERISTICS	TENSION (MUSCLE CONTRACTION) HEADACHE			MIGRAINE* TYPE OF VASCULAR HEADACHE	
	DESCRIPTION	PERCENTAGE OF PATIENTS		DESCRIPTION	PERCENTAGE OF PATIENTS
		1970s†	1950		1950
Laterality	Bilateral	86	90	Unilateral	80
Locus	Occipital	25	—	Supraorbital frontal region	55
	Occipital and suboccipital	26	—		
	Frontal and occipital/frontal	61	<50		
Quality of head pain	Nonthrobbing	73	70	Throbbing or pulsating	80
Onset of head pain	Severity increases gradually	81	—	Severity increases rapidly in classic, steadily in common	
Frequency	≤8 mo	54	—	<1 wk	60
	Constant or daily	—	50		
Duration	≤7 hr	50	—	<12 hr	50
	1-12 hr	—	33		
	1-3 hr	—	10		
Prodromes	None	88	90	Present	75
Autonomic symptoms	None	75	90	Present	50
Age at onset	15-24 yr	52	—	Before 20 yr	55
	Before 20 yr	—	30		
Family history	No	54	60	Yes	65

*Percentages for common and classic combined.
†Percentages calculated from data of 1420 tension headache patients in three multicenter studies.
From Friedman AP: Characteristics of tension headache. Psychosomatics 20:451-457, 1979.

problem. *Migraine* headaches recur at irregular intervals and have no specific pattern; they may recur once or twice weekly or once a year. They often occur around the menstrual period.

The pattern of *tension* headaches varies with the cause of tension. They most often occur daily but may also occur several times a week. **A patient with chronic tension headaches may awaken in the morning with a headache but rarely has**

TABLE 17–3. Factors in Neuralgia and Vascular Pain

FACTOR	TYPICAL NEURALGIA	ATYPICAL NEURALGIA	MIGRAINE	CLUSTER HEADACHE	TEMPORAL ARTERITIS
Age	50-70 yr	30-50 yr	15-30 yr	30-50 yr	50-70 yr
Gender	Equal	Predominantly female	About equal	Predominantly male	Predominantly female
Family history	Not significant	In 60% of cases	Frequent	In 20% of cases	Not significant
Pain location	Usually limited to one cranial nerve	Deep, diffuse, crosses sensory boundaries	Unilateral head and face	Unilateral face and orbit	Distribution of cranial artery, but multiple locations possible
Pain duration	Short, paroxysmal, seconds to minutes	Fluctuating, hours to days	Minutes to hours	Minutes to hours	Fluctuating, persistent
Pain type	Sharp, localized	Aching, drawing, pulling	Progressive, dull, boring, and then throbbing	Repetitive burning or intense throbbing	Intense, deep-boring, or throbbing
Precipitating factors	Touch, wind, others	Variable	None	None	None
Trigger zone	Usual	No	No	No	Artery tenderness only
Autonomic nervous system or other signs or symptoms	Unusual	Occasional lacrimation, flushing	Nausea, photophobia, scotomata, hemianopsia, paresthesia	Common: lacrimation, rhinorrhea, flushing, congested nose, and conjunctival injection Occasional: ipsilateral Horner's syndrome	Fever, malaise Anorexia Progressive decreased visual acuity

Effect of drugs:

Vasoconstrictors	None	Occasional relief	Relief	Relief	None
Analgesics	Inadequate	Relief with narcotic	Not adequate	Not adequate	Variable
Local anesthetics	Relief	Occasional relief	None	None	None
Steroids	None	None	None	None	Gradual relief
Effect of surgery:					
Cranial nerve	Generally effective	Not effective	None	None	None
Biopsy	None	None	None	None	Diagnostic

From Schramm VL: A guide to diagnosing and treating facial pain and headache. Geriatrics 35:78-90, 1980.

headache at night. A specific form of muscle contraction headache is caused by *bruxism* (grinding of the teeth). Patients may present with a constant headache on awakening if they are *"night grinders."* Typically, *hypertensive* headaches also occur in the morning after nighttime recumbency and are usually throbbing in nature.

The frequency patterns of *cluster* headaches are diagnostic because these types of headaches usually occur in close succession. They often occur at approximately the same time of day for 3 to 8 weeks and may recur one to three times a day. They may have an inexplicable remission for months or years and an equally inexplicable recurrence. Although early-morning onset (1 to 5 AM) is typical of cluster headaches, some attacks occur during the day. If they happen at night, which is rare, they are possibly related to rapid eye movement during sleep. *Sinus* headaches also often begin in the morning and progressively worsen but tend to improve toward evening.

Migraine headaches have prodromes, which are uncommon in cluster headaches; occasionally, some patients experience a burning sensation on the forehead before the onset of pain. The classic migraine prodrome occurs 15 to 30 minutes before the headache. It is abrupt in onset, lasts for 10 to 15 minutes, and is often contralateral to the headache. Visual auras include a variety of scotomata, transient blindness, blurred vision, and hemianopsia. Nonvisual auras may include weakness, aphasia, mood disturbances, and photophobia. In contrast to classic migraine, common migraine usually has no specific aura. When prodromes are present, they vary widely and may manifest as psychic disturbances, fatigue, gastrointestinal symptoms, or mood changes.

ASSOCIATED SYMPTOMS

With *classic migraine* the most common associated symptoms are anorexia, nausea, vomiting, sonophobia, photophobia, and irritability. Less common symptoms are dizziness, fluid retention, abdominal pain, and sleepiness. The symptoms associated with *common migraine* include all those associated with classic migraine as well as fatigue, chills, diarrhea, and urticaria. Cyclic abdominal pain or vomiting in children and motion sickness in adults are typically seen in patients with migraine headaches.

Pain in the posterior cervical region that is exacerbated by neck extension is often seen in patients with *tension* headaches, who are frequently tense, anxious, significantly depressed, and fatigued. Patients with chronic tension headaches seem to be more emotionally involved in their headache symptoms; they seem to focus on their symptoms more than patients with migraines. In addition, the intensity of the affective disturbance is more marked in those with tension headaches than those with migraine.

Patients with acute *sinus* headaches may complain of toothaches; this complaint indicates a maxillary infection. Pain in the eye suggests ethmoid sinusitis. Nasal discharge, percussion tenderness over the sinus area, and upper respiratory infection (URI) symptoms are often present. A *nasal* or *sinus neoplasm* may be present if the physician suspects a sinus headache that does not improve after approximately 2 weeks of appropriate therapy (including antibiotics and nasal decongestants) and if there is blood-tinged rhinorrhea. These symptoms recur despite therapy, and sinus radiographs may show evidence of bone destruction.

The symptoms associated with *cluster* headaches are significantly different and help the physician establish the diagnosis. Patients may complain of injection of the involved eye, a blocked nose with rhinorrhea, and marked ipsilateral lacrimation. They may have ipsilateral Horner's syndrome. About 25% of patients with cluster headaches have peptic ulcer disease.

Sick building syndrome should be suspected if fatigue and upper respiratory complaints are associated with the headache and the patient works in an inadequately ventilated building with an impervious outer shell.

Fever suggests an infection, such as meningitis, encephalitis, brain abscess, or extracranial infection.

Organic brain disease should be suspected if one or more of the following signs or symptoms are noted:

1. Intermittent or continuous headache that progressively increases in frequency and severity.
2. Headache that is exacerbated by coughing or straining at stool.
3. Headache that is worse in the morning (note that sinus and hypertensive headaches may also be worse in the morning).
4. Vomiting.
5. Headache that disturbs sleep.
6. Inequality of pupils.
7. Signs of cranial trauma.
8. Seizures.
9. Confusion.
10. Recent onset of neurologic deficit.
11. Papilledema.
12. Onset of severe headaches after age 50 years.

PRECIPITATING AND AGGRAVATING FACTORS

A helpful first question is "What were you doing when your headache started?" Although migraine headaches may be precipitated by *menstruation,* their frequency increases as estrogen levels fall. Migraine headaches are often precipitated by emotional stress. Less frequently, they are precipitated by fatigue, bright lights, fasting, hypoglycemia, foods rich in tyramine (e.g., aged cheeses, sour cream, wine), odors, exercise, weather changes, and high altitude.

Patients may have a history of headaches that are caused by ingestion of certain foods and beverages (e.g., chocolate, yogurt, buttermilk, and wine). Headaches may be precipitated by foods that contain nitrites (*hot dog headache*) or monosodium glutamate (*Chinese restaurant syndrome*). *Alcohol* and *caffeine* are frequent offenders, as is *caffeine withdrawal. Medications* such as reserpine, vasodilators, H_2-receptor blockers, indomethacin, angiotensin-converting enzyme (ACE) inhibitors, nitrates, beta blockers, calcium channel blockers, sildenafil, and oral contraceptives may also cause headaches. Some patients who have been heavy users of ergot drugs to control migraine may experience migraine headaches when these therapeutic agents are stopped. Sinusitis rarely causes headaches.

Tension headaches can be precipitated by emotional or physical stress; extended periods of mental concentration; and prolonged, somewhat abnormal positions of the neck. Some muscle contraction headaches may occur with cessation of analgesics or tranquilizers used in their treatment. Dental malocclusion may stimulate contraction of the muscles of mastication, thus causing spasm of the muscles and headache. Poorly fitting dentures, particularly if they have been worn for 10 or more years, may also lead to tension headaches.

Cluster headaches may be precipitated by short naps, alcohol ingestion, nitroglycerin, tyramine, and emotional stress. *Sinus* headaches may be aggravated by coughing or sneezing, but this is also true of other types of headache, especially those of vascular origin. Eye pain due to *glaucoma* is often precipitated by darkness or sympathomimetic drugs, which cause pupillary dilatation.

AMELIORATING FACTORS

If the patient states that ergot-containing drugs or triptans improved the acute headaches, a vascular cause is probable. Severe headaches relieved by aspirin or indomethacin suggest trigeminal autonomic cephalgia. Likewise, relief with nasal decongestants and antibiotics suggests a sinus cause. A headache that is severe, is associated with nausea, vomiting, scotomata, or aura, and is relieved by sleep is probably migraine. Medication-overuse headaches are relieved on cessation of the medication.

PHYSICAL FINDINGS

In patients with *tension* or *migraine* headaches, the physical findings seldom contribute to the differential diagnosis. Patients with *trigeminal neuralgia* may have a trigger point. During an attack of *cluster* headache, ipsilateral lacrimation and rhinorrhea may occur. Patients with acute *sinus* headaches may have a mucopurulent or blood-tinged nasal discharge. In addition, they may have tenderness on percussion or palpation over the involved sinus, which may also demonstrate impaired transillumination.

The presence of fever suggests an *infectious process* as the cause of the headache. Severe *hypertension* may suggest that the headaches are of hypertensive origin, although most patients with hypertension do not have headaches. Tenderness on palpation over the temporal artery suggests *temporal arteritis* as a cause.

When nuchal rigidity is found, *meningitis* or *subarachnoid bleeding* should be suspected. Nuchal rigidity must be differentiated from the stiff neck seen in cervical arthritis (more common in elderly patients). In patients with true nuchal rigidity, the neck is stiff throughout the arc as the examiner flexes it but not in extension or lateral rotation. In contrast, with *cervical arthritis*, the early phase of neck flexion is supple; this finding is followed by a sudden boardlike rigidity, with resistance in other directions of movement as well.

A patient with *psychogenic* or *conversion* headaches may describe the pain in very vivid terms and with much affect; the patient does not really appear to be in great pain.

Pain localized to one or both eyes with increased intraocular pressure indicates *glaucoma*. The presence of a jaw click or point tenderness on palpation over the TMJ suggests that the headache may be due to TMJ dysfunction.

Most patients with headaches do not exhibit any abnormalities on neurologic examination. However, transient ipsilateral Horner's syndrome may be seen with some migraine headaches.

DIAGNOSTIC STUDIES

Only a few laboratory tests help in the differential diagnosis of headaches. Imaging studies are rarely useful in common tension or migraine headaches. A noncontrast computed tomography (CT) scan is generally the best initial imaging test, especially if a subarachnoid hemorrhage is suspected. Radiographs or CT scans may confirm *acute sinusitis* if a typical fluid level exists in one or more of the sinuses. Patients may experience sinus headaches and still have normal sinus radiographic findings. A lumbar puncture should be performed promptly if meningitis is suspected. The ESR is greatly elevated with *temporal arteritis*. A biopsy of the arterial wall showing giant-cell infiltration is pathognomonic of arteritis. CT scans and lumbar puncture may be needed if a subarachnoid hemorrhage is suspected. **Positron emission tomography (PET) and functional magnetic resonance imaging (MRI) are rarely helpful in making a diagnosis in patients with primary headaches, except in those with a recent change in headache patterns, seizures, or focal neurologic signs or symptoms.**

If the sudden onset of headache occurs in patients older than 50 years, the physician must make a difficult decision regarding whether to perform lumbar puncture. The procedure is indicated in suspected cases of *cerebral hemorrhage* or *bacterial encephalitis*, but it is dangerous in patients with mass lesions or increased intracranial pressure. Noninvasive tests such as CT and magnetic resonance imaging should be done first if intracranial disease is suspected. Arteriograms may show vascular abnormalities and mass lesions.

LESS COMMON DIAGNOSTIC CONSIDERATIONS

Migraine equivalents include cyclic vomiting, paroxysmal vertigo in children, *migraine sans migraine*, monocular scintillating scotomata, and blindness without headache. A chronic cluster-like headache may be secondary to a prolactinoma. The pain responds to high doses of verapamil.

Differential Diagnosis of Headache

TYPE	NATURE OF PATIENT	NATURE OF SYMPTOMS	ASSOCIATED SYMPTOMS	PRECIPITATING AND AGGRAVATING FACTORS	AMELIORATING FACTORS	PHYSICAL FINDINGS	DIAGNOSTIC STUDIES
Tension (muscle contraction) headaches	Most common cause of headache at any age More common in females	Recurrent or chronic Usually of psychogenic origin *Children:* May be manifestation of stress, anxiety, or depression *Adults:* Usually dull and nonthrobbing, with persistent low intensity May last a few days Severity may increase as day progresses and then decrease toward evening Usually occipital, suboccipital, and bilateral Described as constrictive band around head or tightness of scalp Rarely awakens patient from sleep	Fatigue	Emotional or physical stress Abnormal neck positions (especially neck extension) Prolonged mental concentration Withdrawal of analgesics or tranquilizers Dental malocclusion or poorly fitting dentures Bruxism (nighttime grinding of teeth) Withdrawal of analgesics used chronically to treat headaches	Stress reduction		

Vascular headaches	Affect 10% of U.S. population More common in women Family history of headaches	Recurrent or chronic		Coughing Sneezing	Ergot-containing drugs Beta blockers Triptans
Common migraine: migraine headache without aura	More frequent in children	Recurrent or chronic Aura and prodrome vague or absent Gradual onset Lasts up to 72 hr Not always unilateral Usually in frontotemporal or supraorbital region	Those of classic migraine General malaise Fatigue Chills Diarrhea Urticaria Motion sickness		Sleep Triptans
Classic migraine: migraine headache with aura	More common in women Incidence: 1.4% in children (age <7 yr) 5% in children at age 17 yr 17% in post-pubescent males 20% in post-pubescent females 50% of adults with migraines have symptoms before age 20 yr	Recurrent or chronic Prominent aura Prodrome: Has abrupt onset Lasts 15-20 min Precedes headache by 15-30 min Often contralateral to headache Headache: Severe Throbbing Unilateral Gradual onset Intensity increases steadily and rapidly Lasts 2-8 days	Visual auras (scotomata, transient blindness, blurred vision, hemianopsia) Nonvisual auras (weakness, aphasia, mood disturbances, photophobia) Nausea and vomiting Anorexia Sonophobia Photophobia Irritability Dizziness Fluid retention Abdominal pain Sleepiness	Menstruation Emotional stress Fatigue Bright lights High altitude Weather changes Exercise Certain foods Fasting Hypoglycemia	Sleep Triptans

Continued

Differential Diagnosis of Headache—cont'd

TYPE	NATURE OF PATIENT	NATURE OF SYMPTOMS	ASSOCIATED SYMPTOMS	PRECIPITATING AND AGGRAVATING FACTORS	AMELIORATING FACTORS	PHYSICAL FINDINGS	DIAGNOSTIC STUDIES
Cluster headaches	Highest incidence in fourth to sixth decades Rare in children Much more common in men than women (9:1) Family history of cluster headaches uncommon Recur at same time(s) of day, 1-3 times per day, for 3-8 wk Typical early-morning onset	Recurrent or chronic Pain more severe, stabbing, and burning than in vascular or tension headache Unilateral and periorbital in any given cluster May radiate to front of face or temporal regions Duration 20-60 min	25% of patients have peptic ulcer disease Injection of involved eye Rhinorrhea Marked ipsilateral lacrimation May be ipsilateral Horner's syndrome	Short naps Alcohol Nitroglycerin Tyramine Emotional stress		Ipsilateral lacrimation and rhinorrhea	
Headaches due to febrile illnesses	Common cause of headache in children	Headache may be only presenting symptom in children	Fever	Pharyngitis, especially with otitis media		Fever	

Sinusitis (see Chapter 13)	Uncommon in children	*Children:* Maxillary sinus most often involved. *Pain:* Severe, throbbing, and intense pressure. Usually over involved sinus. Begins in morning, progressively worsens during day, improves toward evening	Persistent rhinorrhea. Otitis media. Allergies. Symptoms of upper respiratory infection. Toothache with maxillary involvement. Eye pain with ethmoid involvement	Coughing. Sneezing	Treatment of sinus infection	Mucopurulent or blood-tinged nasal discharge. Percussion tenderness over involved sinuses	Transillumination of sinuses. Sinus radiographs or CT
Depression	Common cause of headache in patients >50 yr	Constant, chronic headache	Those of depression		Treatment of depression		
TMJ dysfunction (see Chapter 13)	Adults	Usually pain in TMJ or ear, but may manifest as headache (temporoparietal)	Bruxism	Opening mouth too wide		Jaw clicks. Point tenderness on palpation over TMJ. Prominent masseter muscle	Radiograph of TMJ. MRI of TMJ
Temporal arteritis	Most common in elderly women	Unilateral, chronic headache	Unexplained low-grade fever. Proximal myalgia. Decreased visual acuity			Tenderness on palpation over temporal artery	ESR greatly elevated

Continued

Differential Diagnosis of Headache—cont'd

TYPE	NATURE OF PATIENT	NATURE OF SYMPTOMS	ASSOCIATED SYMPTOMS	PRECIPITATING AND AGGRAVATING FACTORS	AMELIORATING FACTORS	PHYSICAL FINDINGS	DIAGNOSTIC STUDIES
Cervical arthritis	Most common in elderly people	Occipital or nuchal headache				Stiff neck Early phase of flexion is supple but followed by sudden board-like rigidity with resistance in other directions	Radiograph of cervical spine
Trigeminal neuralgia (see Chapter 13)	Adult	Pain is short, episodic, sharp, severe, and stabbing Each episode lasts <90 sec but recurs for 2-3 min	Pain in face along distribution of one division of nerve	Trigger point Extremes of temperature		Possible trigger point	
Increased intracranial pressure		Progressive, chronic headache	*Children* Neurologic dysfunction Projectile vomiting without nausea	Coughing Sneezing		Papilledema	CT scan Increased cerebrospinal fluid pressure
Glaucoma (see Chapter 13)		Frontal headache	Patient sees halos Pain in eye	Darkened areas Drugs that dilate pupils		Increased intraocular pressure Marked "cupping" of optic discs	Tonometry

CT, Computed tomography; *ESR*, erythrocyte sedimentation rate; *MRI*, magnetic resonance imaging; *TMJ*, temporomandibular joint.

Patients with *glaucoma* may complain of pain in one or both eyes and describe a visual halo around objects. Headaches often develop in a darkened environment. Intraocular pressure is increased, occasionally with tenderness on palpation over the globe.

Exertional headaches usually have an acute onset and are often precipitated by sexual activity, exercise, or cough. Hemicrania continua is uncommon and often misdiagnosed. It lasts more than 3 months, is unilateral, continuous, and often associated with conjunctival infection, lacrimation, rhinorrhea, ptosis, and/or miosis, and complete relief may be achieved with indomethacin.

Eyestrain is a diagnosis that is often applied incorrectly. Headache from eyestrain is unusual. It tends to occur in people who perform work that requires close vision. In addition, the headaches tend to occur after a prolonged period of using the eyes. *Chronic daily headaches* are usually due to *chronic migraine*, although they may result from medication overuse or drug rebound.

Systemic causes of headaches include uremia, occult carbon monoxide poisoning, sick building syndrome, thyrotoxicosis, severe anemia, brain tumors, chronic subdural hematoma, subarachnoid hemorrhage, and ocular disease. Tumors of the eye, ear, nose, and throat may also manifest as headache. Occult carbon monoxide poisoning may result from faulty furnaces or kitchen stoves at home, and propane space heaters at workplaces (warehouse worker's headache).

Trigeminal autonomic cephalgia includes paroxysmal hemicrania, *SUNCT syndrome* (short-lasting [5-250 seconds], unilateral, neuralgiform headache with conjunctival infection, tearing, and rhinorrhea), and cluster headache. SUNCT syndrome occurs more often in males. It shares features with cluster headaches and trigeminal neuralgia, but SUNCT syndrome appears to be rare.

The key to diagnosing headaches consists of a careful, detailed clinical history; headache diary; and neurologic examination. The physician must take time to observe the patient and evaluate the whole patient in relation to the family and environment which is helpful in determining the underlying cause of headache. The physician should try to avoid the use of habituating drugs in the treatment of patients with chronic headaches.

Selected References

Clinch CR: Evaluation of acute headaches in adults, *Am Fam Physician* 63:685-692, 2001.

Davenport R: Diagnosing acute headache, *Clin Med* 4:108-112, 2004.

Diener H-C, Limmroth V: Medication-overuse headache: a worldwide problem, *Lancet Neurol* 3:475-483, 2004.

Dodick DW: Thunderclap headache, *Curr Pain Headache Rep* 6:226-232, 2002.

Evans RW: Diagnostic testing for the evaluation of headaches, *Neurol Clin* 14:1-25, 1996.

Flippen CC: Pearls and pitfalls of headache, *Semin Neurol* 21:371-376, 2001.

Friedman DI: Headache and the eye, *Curr Pain Headache* 12:296-304, 2008.

Go S: Nontraumatic headaches in the emergency department: a systematic approach to diagnosis and controversies in two big ticket entities, *Mo Med* 106:156-161, 2009.

Green MW: A spectrum of exertional headaches, *Med Clin North Am* 85:1085-1092, 2001.

Hecherling PS, Leikin JB, Maturen A, et al: Predictors of occult carbon monoxide poisoning in patients with headache and dizziness, *Ann Intern Med* 107:174-176, 1987.

Johnson CJ: Headache in women, *Prim Care Clin Office Pract* 31:417-428, 2004.

Jones NS: Sinus headaches: avoiding over- and mis-diagnosis, *Expert Rev Neurother* 9:439-444, 2009.

Larner AJ: Not all morning headaches are due to brain tumours, *Pract Neurol* 9:80-84, 2009.

Maizels M: The patient with daily headaches, *Am Fam Physician* 70: 2299-2306, 2313-2314, 2004.

May A: New insights into headache: an update on functional and structural imaging findings, *Nat Rev Neurol* 5:199-209, 2009.

Miles R: The GP strategy for headaches in children, *Practitioner* 244:618-622, 625-626, 2000.

Pinto A, Arava-Parastatidis M, Balasubramaniam R: Headache in children and adolescents. J Can Dent Assoc 75:125–131.

Purdy RA: Clinical evaluation of a patient presenting with headache, *Med Clin North Am* 85: 847-861, 2001.

Rothner AD: Headaches in children and adolescents, *Child Adolesc Psychiatr Clin North Am* 8:727-745, 1999.

Ryan RE, Pearlman SH: Common headache misdiagnoses, *Prim Care Clin Office Pract* 31:395-405, 2004.

Salawu FK, Olokoba AB, Danburam A: A review of trigeminal autonomic cephalgias: diagnosis and treatment, *Niger J Med* 18:17-24, 2009.

Heartburn, Indigestion, and Dyspepsia

18

Heartburn and indigestion are common presenting complaints. Because these symptoms are often vague, it is difficult for the physician to determine a precise cause, and treatment is frequently ineffective.

Heartburn is a sensation of burning, warmth, or heat in the retrosternal region between the xiphoid and the manubrium that occasionally radiates toward the jaw or (rarely) the arms. Water brash (regurgitation of fluid) may be present.

Dyspepsia is a separate entity. *Functional dyspepsia,* which is similar to indigestion, is defined, by Rome III criteria, as epigastric pain or burning, postprandial fullness, or early satiety without underlying organic disease. Episodic or persistent abdominal symptoms, often related to feeding, are thought to result from disorders of the proximal portion of the digestive tract. Dyspeptic symptoms include upper abdominal discomfort, postprandial fullness, early satiety, anorexia, belching, nausea, heartburn, vomiting, bloating, borborygmi, dysphagia, and abdominal burning. These symptoms are usually related to eating and occur during the day but rarely at night. Children often present with persistent or recurrent upper abdominal pain.

The most common causes of heartburn and indigestion include *reflux esophagitis* (with or without hiatal hernia), ingestion of *drugs* (e.g., aspirin, nonsteroidal anti-inflammatory drugs [NSAIDs], bisphosphonates, metformin, antibiotics, digitalis, potassium or iron supplements, theophylline derivatives), *gastritis, nonulcer dyspepsia,* excessive consumption of *food* or *alcohol, chronic active gastritis, gallbladder disease, pregnancy, aerophagia,* and *functional gastrointestinal* (GI) *disorder.* Although patients with tumors of the GI tract may complain of heartburn or indigestion, neoplasms are not common causes of these symptoms.

This chapter focuses on indigestion and heartburn *not* associated with abdominal pain. Conditions associated with abdominal pain are discussed in Chapters 1 and 2.

NATURE OF PATIENT

Dyspeptic symptoms have organic or, most often, functional causes. Younger patients are less likely to have organic causes of indigestion, whereas older patients are more likely to have serious organic causes. The most common functional GI disorders in children are functional dyspepsia, irritable bowel syndrome, and functional abdominal pain. Children rarely complain of indigestion or heartburn, although vague abdominal discomfort may affect children who experience *malabsorption* or *food intolerance*. Helicobacter pylori infection is unusual in children. With these conditions, certain foods may cause crampy abdominal pain or diarrhea. Weight loss with significant malabsorption may be noted. When children complain of distention or awareness of peristalsis and gurgling, they often have *functional GI disease*. If these complaints are intermittent and not disabling, the patient is otherwise healthy, and the results of the physical examination are normal, an emotional cause should be suspected. Questioning the child may reveal depression or other emotional problems. These problems frequently occur with external environmental stress such as divorce, the birth of a sibling, illness in the family, starting school, and problems with a boyfriend or girlfriend.

In adults, heartburn is almost always caused by *reflux esophagitis*. This is more common in pregnant women, particularly during the later months. Patients with esophagitis may complain of severe heartburn that is relieved by alkali and aggravated by recumbency. Although *hiatal hernia* is three times more common in multiparous patients than primigravid women, **symptoms of heartburn are caused by esophageal reflux and not by the hiatal hernia.** Pregnant patients have delayed gastric emptying, increased intra-abdominal pressure, and increased estrogen levels, all of which facilitate esophageal reflux. From 30% to 50% of adults demonstrate hiatal hernias on radiographs; only 5% of this population report symptoms of heartburn.

Dyspepsia due to gastritis occurs frequently in patients who ingest large quantities of *alcohol* or *drugs* such as salicylates, corticosteroids, NSAIDs, theophylline, quinidine, and some antibiotics.

Travelers and campers who become infested with *Giardia* may experience only bloating, nausea, and upper abdominal discomfort. These dyspeptic symptoms may persist for months, with only occasional episodes of diarrhea.

About 50% of all diabetic patients, whether or not they are insulin dependent, have delayed gastric emptying *(diabetic gastroparesis)*. Many of these patients complain of pain, nausea, vomiting, or postprandial fullness *(diabetic dyspepsia)*. In addition to these symptoms, the delayed gastric emptying may contribute to erratic absorption of oral hypoglycemic agents and thus poor blood glucose control.

Elderly patients are more likely to complain of atypical symptoms of gastroesophageal reflux disease (GERD) and vague feelings of indigestion, possibly related to bloating. Many of the symptoms of indigestion and abdominal bloating are caused by excessive *intestinal gas* and *disordered motility*. Virtually all intestinal gas is the result of bacterial fermentation, although the amount of discomfort is not necessarily proportional to the amount of gas in the intestines. The complaints of indigestion and bloating are more common in elderly patients because of their relative gastric and intestinal stasis, hypomotility of the gut, altered intestinal bacteria, increased incidence of constipation, and lack of exercise, all of which tend to facilitate the production of intestinal gas. Elderly patients with *gastritis* or *duodenal ulcers* are usually infected with *H. pylori*. *H. pylori*–negative gastritis is usually caused by NSAID ingestion.

Tense and *anxious* patients are more likely to be aware of normal intestinal movement and are also more likely to complain about these feelings. Many patients with *gallbladder disease, irritable bowel syndrome,* and *ulcers* complain of vague abdominal discomfort and occasional distention.

NATURE OF SYMPTOMS

Heartburn is a burning sensation that occurs in the xiphisternal region, with occasional proximal radiation. It may vary in intensity from a mild feeling of warmth to extreme pain. Occasionally, the pain may be indistinguishable from that of severe angina pectoris; therefore, it is important for the physician to note that heartburn has *no relation to physical activity*. The pain is usually caused by esophageal spasm, is intermittent over several minutes, and recurs over long periods. Pain may radiate into the neck and occasionally into the arms, back, or jaw. In one study, the pain radiated to the back in 40% of patients with proven *esophageal reflux* but radiated to the arms or neck in only 5%.

Initially, the pain of heartburn is felt only after heavy meals or while the patient is lying down or bending over. In more advanced cases, the pain is more easily provoked, lasts longer, and is accompanied by *dysphagia*.

Patients with *gastritis* may have abdominal pain, vague indigestion, or heartburn as a presenting complaint. Epigastric discomfort that is worse after eating, loss of appetite, a sense of fullness, nausea, and occasional vomiting are also common complaints in patients with gastritis. These same symptoms may be seen in patients with nonulcer dyspepsia caused by *H. pylori*. Studies have shown that symptoms alone cannot differentiate dyspeptic patients without ulcer as having *H. pylori* or not.

Heartburn is also a common complaint in patients with *bile gastritis*, which often occurs after gastric resection or pyloroplasty. Bile refluxes into the stomach and subsequently into the distal esophagus, causing heartburn. Some patients who have *peptic ulcer disease* complain not of the classic symptoms but only of vague indigestion that is sometimes relieved by vomiting.

The symptoms in patients with *functional GI disorders* are often vague and nonspecific. Patients do not obtain consistent relief with any medication or therapeutic regimen. Other symptoms of anxiety are often present, with no evidence of systemic disease or weight loss despite a long history of vague symptoms. Because various patients with organic pathology (e.g., peptic ulcer, gallbladder disease, colonic tumors) may also have vague symptoms, a specific workup is required in some cases. When these vague symptoms occur in a young adult, it is unlikely that a malignant process is present. Likewise, if the symptoms have been present for many years without any significant progression or evidence of systemic disease, a major disease process is unlikely.

Other distinguishing characteristics often help the physician differentiate functional from organic pain. With *functional* illness, patients may have severe and continuous pain but no significant weight loss. The patients often give exaggerated descriptions of their pain and have a significant emotional investment; they may come into the office with a list of their symptoms. With *organic* disease, the pain, though severe, is often periodic and may be associated with weight loss.

ASSOCIATED SYMPTOMS

Patients with *peptic esophagitis* frequently have chest pain. They may complain of heartburn or chest pain when esophageal spasm occurs. Some patients complain only of substernal pain, which may radiate into the neck, jaw, or upper arms. When water brash is associated with heartburn, *gastroesophageal reflux* is most likely. When nocturnal pain is associated with abdominal pain and dyspepsia, *peptic ulcer* is likely. **If dyspepsia is continuous, exacerbated by food, and in particular associated with anorexia and weight loss, gastric cancer is more likely.**

Belching secondary to *aerophagia* is often seen in patients with reflux esophagitis and those with functional GI disease. If indigestion is associated with nausea, right upper quadrant (RUQ) pain, or pain in the right shoulder (particularly the inferior angle of the right scapula), *duodenal loop distention* or *cholelithiasis* should be considered. Hematemesis suggests *peptic ulcer disease* or *variceal bleeding*, regardless of how vague the other symptoms are.

PRECIPITATING AND AGGRAVATING FACTORS

In many patients with symptoms caused by *reflux esophagitis*, coronary artery disease (CAD) or anxiety have been previously diagnosed. **Clues to the correct diagnosis of esophagitis are that the pain is not usually brought on by exercise, frequently occurs in the recumbent position, and is often relieved by antacids. Despite these clues, chest pain caused by reflux esophagitis is often induced by exercise, and CAD and** gastroesophageal reflux disease **often coexist.** Anything that distends the lower third of the esophagus, irritates its mucosa, or reduces lower esophageal pressure can precipitate reflux esophagitis. This includes recumbency, acidic foods, gastric stasis, large meals, and fatty foods, which delay gastric emptying. Several studies show that in addition to gastric juices, bile and other duodenal juices may play a role in the pain of reflux esophagitis.

Conditions that increase intra-abdominal pressure (e.g., pregnancy, marked ascites) can facilitate regurgitation of gastric or duodenal contents into the distal esophagus. Caffeine frequently causes heartburn in susceptible people. Certain spices, carminatives (e.g., oil of spearmint and peppermint), garlic, onions, chocolate, fatty foods, alcohol, and carbonated beverages may reduce lower esophageal pressure and thus facilitate reflux. Cigarette smoking also reduces lower esophageal pressure and stimulates gastric acidity. Certain drugs, particularly theophylline derivatives, isoproterenol, and anticholinergics, lower esophageal pressure and may precipitate reflux and heartburn. Other precipitating factors are straining; recumbency; lifting; and ingestion of orange juice, tomato juice, and spicy foods and drinks.

In some patients who swallow air, chew gum, or eat rapidly, heartburn develops as a result of belching and subsequent regurgitation of gastric juices into the distal esophagus. Although some patients with hiatal hernia have heartburn or chest pain, a hiatal hernia does not establish the presence of esophagitis.

AMELIORATING FACTORS

In general, avoidance of precipitating factors reduces and may eliminate the discomfort. In addition, raising the head of the bed (by tilting the entire bed, not merely using another pillow), retiring with an empty stomach, sucking on antacid tablets, eating small but frequent meals, following a low-fat diet, and avoiding tight garments may help.

The pain of *peptic esophagitis* is frequently relieved by antacids, which reduce gastric acidity and reestablish more normal lower esophageal sphincter pressure, thus reducing reflux. The physician must remember that the pain of peptic esophagitis may be relieved by nitrates, typically thought to relieve only the pain of angina pectoris. **Relief of substernal pain by nitroglycerin does not necessarily establish the diagnosis of angina pectoris, because this drug can also relieve the pain of lower esophageal spasm.** Patients with peptic esophagitis who obtain inadequate relief from the usual therapeutic measures (antacids, proton-pump inhibitors, H2-blockers, pro-motility agents) may receive additional relief from nitroglycerin. **If the pain is relieved by ingestion of viscous lidocaine (Xylocaine Viscous), it is probably caused by peptic esophagitis.** Some authorities suggest using this procedure as a diagnostic tool, although false-positive results may occur among patients with chest pain of coronary origin. Therefore, this test is useful but does not rule out CAD with absolute certainty.

Once the diagnosis of serious disease is excluded, patients with vague symptoms of indigestion and functional GI complaints should be treated with reassurance and occasionally anxiolytics. If the symptoms of the dyspepsia are relieved by ingestion of bismuth salts (e.g., Pepto-Bismol), antibiotics, or both, an *H. pylori* infection should be suspected.

PHYSICAL FINDINGS

Most patients who complain of indigestion or heartburn demonstrate no abnormal physical findings. Auscultation of peristalsis in the chest should suggest a large diaphragmatic *hernia*. Mild, diffuse abdominal tenderness associated with abdominal distention is sometimes observed with *pancreatitis* or *excessive swallowed air* in the intestinal tract. A succussion splash can often be elicited in patients with *gastric dilatation*, whether reflex or secondary to pyloric obstruction.

Some patients with *gastritis* have tenderness on abdominal palpation, whereas others may have no physical findings other than midepigastric tenderness on percussion. The same is true for those with *peptic ulcer disease*. Patients with *cholelithiasis* may have no symptoms but occasionally have RUQ tenderness on palpation or percussion. In some patients with *gallbladder hydrops*, a dilated gallbladder is palpable or ballotable.

DIAGNOSTIC STUDIES

Endoscopy is the most reliable diagnostic technique for establishing the cause of upper GI symptoms, although most patients with vague symptoms do not require this invasive procedure. Early endoscopy should be recommended if the dyspeptic patient:

1. Has an onset of symptoms or change in dyspeptic symptoms after age 45 years.
2. Tests positive for *H. pylori* or is taking NSAIDs before age 45 years.
3. Has had dyspepsia for more than 1 year.
4. Has anorexia, weight loss, anemia, or blood in the stools and colonic pathology has been excluded.
5. Is immunocompromised.

Patients, especially young patients, with unexplained dyspepsia and no alarming symptoms should be tested and treated for *H. pylori* rather than undergo endoscopy.

Esophageal reflux can be observed on upper GI radiographs. Esophagitis can be detected by esophagoscopy, and its symptoms can be produced by instillation of dilute hydrochloric acid in the distal esophagus (Bernstein test). Esophageal pH monitoring is the most sensitive test.

Gastritis is best diagnosed by gastroscopy, at which time tests for *H. pylori* should be performed. Gallbladder disease can be diagnosed with sonography, cholecystography, and isotopic studies.

LESS COMMON DIAGNOSTIC CONSIDERATIONS

When the patient finds that abdominal discomfort is intensified by bending over or wearing a tight garment, *gas entrapment* (e.g., hepatic or splenic flexure syndrome) should be suspected. Sometimes this discomfort is relieved by the passage of flatus. Gas entrapment can be confirmed if flexion of the right or left thigh on the abdomen replicates the pain or if an abdominal radiograph shows a large bubble of trapped gas in the hepatic or splenic flexure. The pain of gas entrapment in the hepatic or splenic flexure is often referred to the chest, and the patient may complain of chest pain.

Differential Diagnosis of Heartburn, Indigestion, and Dyspepsia

CAUSE	NATURE OF PATIENT	NATURE OF SYMPTOMS	ASSOCIATED SYMPTOMS	PRECIPITATING AND AGGRAVATING FACTORS	AMELIORATING FACTORS	PHYSICAL FINDINGS	DIAGNOSTIC STUDIES
Reflux esophagitis	Adults More common in pregnant women in later months	Severe heartburn Water brash with and without recumbency Recurrent pain radiates to back (40%), arms, or neck (5%)	Chest pain Dysphagia Belching (from aerophagia) Cough Asthma, especially nocturnal	Recumbency Straining or lifting Drinking alcoholic, caffeinated, or carbonated beverages Eating heavy meals or fatty, spicy, or acidic foods Smoking Pregnancy Exercise	Raising head of bed Antacids, proton-pump inhibitors Small, frequent, low-fat meals Avoidance of tight garments		Pain often relieved by viscous lidocaine Esophagoscopy Upper GI radiograph Esophageal pH monitoring
Gastritis	Especially alcoholics	Abdominal pain Vague indigestion Heartburn	Decreased appetite Sense of fullness Nausea and vomiting	Alcohol Meals Drugs (aspirin, NSAIDs, corticosteroids, antibiotics, antiasthma agents)	Bile gastritis may be relieved by vomiting Proton-pump inhibitors	Tenderness on abdominal palpation or epigastric percussion	Endoscopy Upper GI radiograph Gastric biopsy
Active, chronic gastritis	Especially older adults	Indigestion	Indigestion		Bismuth compounds (Pepto-Bismol) Proton-pump inhibitors Antimicrobials		Gastric mucosal biopsy Urea breath test Serologic test for *H. pylori*
Nonulcer dyspepsia		Diffuse abdominal pain or discomfort	Nocturnal pain uncommon		Pain not usually relieved by antacids Occasional relief of symptoms after treatment for *H. pylori*		Endoscopy

Continued

Differential Diagnosis of Heartburn, Indigestion, and Dyspepsia—cont'd

CAUSE	NATURE OF PATIENT	NATURE OF SYMPTOMS	ASSOCIATED SYMPTOMS	PRECIPITATING AND AGGRAVATING FACTORS	AMELIORATING FACTORS	PHYSICAL FINDINGS	DIAGNOSTIC STUDIES
Functional GI disorder	Children and adults	Distention Awareness of peristalsis and gurgling Intermittent symptoms Vague, nonspecific symptoms No weight loss Continuous pain	Significant emotional investment Other anxiety symptoms Belching (from aerophagia)	Social/environmental stresses	Reduction in stress	No signs of systemic disease	Study findings normal
Excessive intestinal gas	Common in elderly	Vague feelings of indigestion	Abdominal bloating Belching Passing flatus	Increased ingestion of flatulogenic foods (e.g., bagels, legumes, high-fiber foods) GI stasis Gut hypomotility Bacterial change Constipation Lack of exercise	Belching Passing flatus		
Gas entrapment (hepatic or splenic flexure syndrome)		Abdominal discomfort Pain often referred to chest	Chest pain	Bending over Wearing tight garments	Passing flatus	Flexion of thigh on abdomen replicates symptoms	Abdominal radiograph shows trapped gas in hepatic or splenic flexure
Gallbladder disease		Vague abdominal discomfort Occasional distention Indigestion	Nausea Pain in right shoulder	Fatty foods		Pain and tenderness on palpation in RUQ	Cholecystograms Sonograms

GI, Gastrointestinal; *NSAIDs,* nonsteroidal anti-inflammatory drugs; *RUQ,* right upper quadrant.

Heartburn may be caused by viral *esophagitis* and *esophageal candidiasis*. *Disseminated sclerosis* that invades the esophagus may also cause severe heartburn. Indigestion may be the presenting symptom in *uremia, pulmonary tuberculosis, migraine, gastric dilatation, glaucoma, hypercalcemia, diabetes,* and *CAD*. Although they are often asymptomatic, *Barrett's esophagus* and *gastric cancer* may cause symptoms of indigestion.

Selected References

Bazaldua OV, Schneider FD: Evaluation and management of dyspepsia, *Am Fam Physician* 60: 1773-1788, 1999.

Conroy RT, Siddiqi B: Dyspepsia, *Prim Care* 34:99-108, 2007.

Crane SJ, Talley NJ: Chronic gastrointestinal symptoms in the elderly, *Clin Geriatr Med* 23: 721-734, 2007.

Dent J: Definitions of reflux disease and its separation from dyspepsia, *Gut* 50(Suppl 4):17-20, 2002.

De Luca VA: Gastroduodenal dyspepsia: a personal view integrating clinical, endoscopic, histological, and management criteria, *Dig Dis* 14:27-42, 1996.

Geeraerts B, Tack J: Functional dyspepsia: past, present, and future, *J Gastroenterol* 43:251-255, 2008.

Gremse DA, Sacks AI: Evaluation of dyspepsia, *Pediatr Ann* 26:251-259, 1997.

Jones MP: Evaluation and treatment of dyspepsia, *Postgrad Med J* 79:225-229, 2003.

McOmber MA, Shulman RJ: Pediatric functional gastrointestinal disorders, *Nutr Clin Pract* 23: 268-274, 2008.

Pound SE, Heading RC: Diagnosis and treatment of dyspepsia in the elderly, *Drugs Aging* 7: 347-354, 1995.

Richard LG: Nonulcer dyspepsia, *Mayo Clin Proc* 10:1011-1015, 1999.

Richter JE: Dyspepsia: organic causes and differential characteristics from functional dyspepsia, *Scand J Gastroenterol* 26(Suppl 182):11-16, 1991.

Smucny J: Evaluation of the patient with dyspepsia, *J Fam Pract* 50:538-543, 2001.

Talley NJ, Seon Choung R: Functional (non-ulcer) dyspepsia and gastroparesis-differentiating these conditions and practical management approaches, *Rev Gastroenterol Disord* 9:E48-E53, 2009.

Talley NJ, Silverstein MD, Agreus L, et al: AGA technical review: evaluation of dyspepsia, *Gastroenterology* 114:582-595, 1998.

Insomnia

19

Patients usually describe insomnia as poor quality or quantity of sleep despite adequate time for sleep, resulting in daytime fatigue, irritability, and decreased concentration.

Of all the sleep problems, disorders of initiating and maintaining sleep (insomnia) are the most common. Studies have shown that hypnotics are used regularly by about 25% of the adult population. Insomnia includes the following problems: delay in falling asleep, poor quality of sleep (deficiency of deep and rapid eye movement [REM] sleep), frequent awakening, and early-morning wakefulness. *Because patients with insomnia may present complaining of trouble with sleeping, daytime sleepiness, or fatigue, the physician must be alert to all of these presenting complaints.*

Comorbid insomnias are those associated with medical, psychiatric, or specific sleep disorders, and substance abuse. **Idiopathic insomnia is a diagnosis of exclusion.**

Insomnia may be chronic or transient. Chronic insomnia can be caused by *physical disorders* (e.g., congestive heart failure, pregnancy, hyperthyroidism, nocturnal asthma, nocturnal seizures), *painful* or *uncomfortable syndromes* (e.g., toothache, arthritis, restless legs syndrome), *psychiatric illnesses* (e.g., depression, anxiety, schizophrenia, mania), use or withdrawal of *drugs* (e.g., caffeine, alcohol, antidepressants, sympathomimetics, beta blockers, hypnotics), and *situational stressors*. **The most common causes of chronic insomnia are ingestion of caffeine, alcohol consumption, sleep apnea, medical disorders, nocturia, anxiety, and depression.** Transient insomnia is usually caused by stressful events, time zone shifts, and short-term pain-producing events.

NATURE OF PATIENT

Nocturnal enuresis (bed-wetting), *sleepwalking, talking while asleep,* and *night terrors* are thought to be arousal disorders because they usually occur with emergence from deep non-REM sleep. Children who experience nocturnal enuresis and sleepwalking often have difficulty sleeping. Bed-wetting is the most common sleep-arousal disorder in children between ages 3 and 15 years. It is more prevalent in males than females. When no obvious organic or psychological cause exists, bed-wetting usually occurs in the first part of the night as the child emerges from delta sleep and before the first REM sleep. The change of sleep state is often accompanied by body movements and increased muscle tone; urination occurs during this period. Although most of these problems have a psychological cause, many investigators believe that such disorders have a psychophysiologic rather than strictly psychological basis.

Insomnia occurs more frequently in children with attention deficit hyperactivity disorder (ADHD) and bipolar disorders.

Nightmares and night terrors often disturb sleep. In both children and adults, nightmares occur during REM sleep. Night terrors, characterized by sudden screams and arousal, occur during deep sleep. **Insomnia in children is most often caused by psychological stress but occasionally results from organic disease** (e.g., hip disorder).

Sleep-disordered breathing is more common in men, but sleep-disordered breathing and insomnia are more common in women.

Some patients who snore have *sleep-induced apnea,* which causes nocturnal wakefulness and daytime drowsiness. These patients are typically obese and/or snorers. They may have as many as 100 episodes of sleep apnea each night; many episodes lead to brief arousal.

Too often, complaints of insomnia by the elderly are ignored as being part of the usual aging process. Sleep patterns often change with aging. Although some elderly people require less sleep than they did in their younger years, many complain of trouble sleeping. Elderly patients often complain of both a delay in falling asleep and poor sleep quality. They are more likely to awaken from environmental stimuli such as noise and temperature and often have associated medical or painful conditions that interfere with the quality of sleep.

Many patients who ingest products that contain *caffeine* (e.g., coffee, tea, cola) complain of insomnia. Even those patients who had previously tolerated caffeine well may experience sleeping problems. Because the half-life of caffeine may range from 2 to more than 6 hours in different people, the ingestion of caffeine, especially after 6 PM, may contribute significantly to insomnia. Patients may or may not be aware that caffeine is the cause of their insomnia. People who drink *alcohol,* even in moderate amounts (i.e., two drinks at night), as well as recovering alcoholics often experience poor sleep quality with frequent awakening.

Poor sleep at night may be related to napping or dozing during the day, which is more common in elderly people. Elderly patients with *dementia* are often restless and wakeful at night. *Depression,* a common cause of sleep disturbances, is frequently undiagnosed in elderly patients.

Patients of all ages with depression (unipolar affective disorder) frequently experience insomnia characterized by delayed sleep onset (prolonged latency), frequent awakening, and *classic early-morning wakefulness.* Young adults without apparent depression who have insomnia have a higher incidence of depression in later life. Patients with *bipolar affective disorder* may experience marked insomnia, especially just before and during the manic phase. Patients who suffer from *anxiety* may have trouble falling asleep but seldom experience early-morning wakefulness.

NATURE OF SYMPTOMS

Patients usually describe insomnia rather loosely as "trouble sleeping." The physician must determine whether they have difficulty with falling asleep (prolonged sleep latency), staying asleep (poor quality), early-morning wakefulness, or a combination of these problems. Because a patient may have one or more types of insomnia, the physician must question him or her specifically for each type of insomnia to diagnose the cause correctly and provide effective, specific therapy. *Short-term* (less than 3 weeks) insomnia is most often caused by a life stress such as emotion, noise, pain, stimulation, grief, anxiety, jet lag, or a change in working hours. *Chronic* insomnia may result from psychiatric disorders (e.g., depression, dysthymic disorder), conditioned insomnia, drugs, caffeine, or alcohol.

Asking patients what they are thinking about before they fall asleep and when they awaken often provides significant clues to the cause of their insomnia. It is also important to interview the sleep partner of an insomniac about snoring, apnea, leg twitches, seizures, and unusual sleep postures. Bedside tape recorders may also help to document snoring.

Prolonged sleep latency (the time from turning the lights out until stage 1 sleep) is most common in anxious patients, caffeine and alcohol users, and elderly patients, especially those who sleep during the day. Most patients overestimate the latency period. Some complain of poor-quality sleep when they do not feel rested despite adequate sleep; this is usually caused by a deficiency of deep-REM sleep and is particularly common in patients with painful syndromes, pregnant women, people who consume alcohol, and recovering alcoholics.

Some patients, particularly alcoholics, complain of frequent awakening; this usually accompanies stage 2 sleep. Early-morning awakening from which a patient cannot return to sleep is most common and particularly characteristic of depressed patients. Some studies show depressed patients to have prolonged sleep latency, decreased total sleep, increased intermittent awakening, and less deep sleep than other patients.

ASSOCIATED SYMPTOMS

Many patients present complaining of fatigue when they really have daytime sleepiness caused by sleep disorders. *Painful* and *uncomfortable conditions* such as pleurisy, peptic esophagitis, toothaches, hip disorders, pregnancy, and even severe itching can interfere with normal sleep. *Restless legs* while awake, especially in the evenings, may be associated with *periodic limb movements* while asleep, thus disturbing sleep or even causing full awakening. Paroxysmal nocturnal dyspnea, nocturnal asthma, hyperthyroidism, alcoholism, use of caffeine or other drugs, recent cessation of hypnotic or antidepressant therapy, and severe snoring may also contribute to sleep problems. **Sleep-disordered breathing, especially obstructive sleep apnea, is often associated with insomnia. It is important to make this diagnosis as it is usually correctable.**

Although anxiety and depression often cause insomnia, patients with these conditions usually have additional symptoms. *Anxious patients* often have somatic complaints such as headaches, chest pain, palpitations, dizziness, gastrointestinal distress, nervousness, and feelings of foreboding. *Depressed patients* frequently complain of decreased appetite, weight loss, lack of energy, lack of interest in activities, decreased libido, constipation, and vague aches and pains. Patients with fibrositis *(fibromyalgia)* and insomnia (which some investigators attribute to depression) may obtain excellent relief of their aches, pains, and insomnia with antidepressant medication.

The daytime consequences of insomnia may provide diagnostic clues. Fatigue, poor performance, impaired concentration, and irritability are common in both insomnia and depressive disorders. Automobile accidents are more common in patients with insomnia and may be a clue to sleep problems.

PRECIPITATING AND AGGRAVATING FACTORS

Patients who complain of insomnia should be questioned about whether certain situations (e.g., a death in the family, financial concerns, family crises, school examinations, changes in life patterns, alterations in work schedules, changes in drug habits) coincided with the onset of insomnia. *Rebound insomnia* often occurs with cessation of benzodiazepine drugs, especially at higher dosage levels. Paradoxically, these drugs may have originally been used as hypnotics. The patient should also be questioned about prior episodes of insomnia and what may have precipitated them. Transient insomnia may occur in anticipation of a joyous event or during periods of excitement.

According to one study of patients referred to a sleep center, the most common cause of insomnia is ingestion of *caffeine* in any form. Many of these patients had previously tolerated caffeine well. The second most common cause is *alcohol.* Although small amounts of alcohol may facilitate sleep onset for some patients, it may also cause early awakening or nightmares, a finding that is contrary to common belief. These patients often note poor quality of sleep and frequent awakening.

Medications that may contribute to insomnia include beta blockers, thyroid hormones, calcium channel blockers, decongestants, bronchodilators, anticholinergics, stimulating antidepressants, and nicotine.

In evaluating sleep disturbances, physicians should have patients keep a sleep diary for 1 week. They should note the time they retire, their latency period, the number of awakenings, the time of last awakening, any sleep events (e.g., dreams, nightmares, need to urinate), and any comments made by the sleep partner. **Sleep partners should be questioned as to snoring and apneic periods.** It is particularly important for patients to note their thoughts during latency and on awakening, because these ideas may help establish the cause of their insomnia.

Other precipitating and aggravating factors in insomnia include fear of illness and even pruritus. Although these factors may be tolerated during the day when the patient is active, they may be distracting enough to cause insomnia when the patient is at rest.

AMELIORATING FACTORS

Hypnotics, including over-the-counter preparations, are occasionally helpful for short periods of insomnia. However, their continued use (for more than 1 week) may exacerbate insomnia, particularly if REM sleep has been suppressed. Hypnotics are *rarely* indicated to treat the symptoms of insomnia. **Insomnia is treated by dealing with its cause.**

Daytime naps or pain can be identified as the probable cause of insomnia if cessation of the former or relief of the latter results in improved sleep. If avoidance of caffeine (in all forms) after noon permits the return of normal sleep patterns, caffeine was probably responsible for the insomnia. When changes in work shifts are associated with insomnia, patients should be advised to try to return to their original sleep schedule to determine whether doing so eliminates their insomnia. Avoidance of noisy or extremely warm environments and strenuous exercise at night may also facilitate a return to normal sleep patterns.

PHYSICAL FINDINGS

The physical examination is usually not helpful in determining the cause of insomnia. Medical conditions that contribute to insomnia may occasionally yield abnormal physical findings, including hyperthyroidism, congestive heart failure, peptic esophagitis, pulmonary disease, ulcer disease, seizure disorders, and prostatism. Any condition that causes frequent nocturia may interfere with normal sleep patterns.

DIAGNOSTIC STUDIES

When the cause of insomnia cannot be determined and the patients cannot find relief, they should be referred to a sleep center for polysomnographic studies.

LESS COMMON DIAGNOSTIC CONSIDERATIONS

Insomnia-causing conditions that occur less frequently include nocturnal *myoclonus*, painful erections, central *sleep apnea*, and *restless legs syndrome*. The last two conditions are more common in elderly people. Sleep apnea is often exacerbated by hypnotics and alcohol.

Physicians have been increasingly recognizing *primary* sleep disorders rather than assuming that insomnia is a symptom of other disorders.

Differential Diagnosis of Insomnia

CAUSE	NATURE OF PATIENT	NATURE OF SYMPTOMS	ASSOCIATED SYMPTOMS	PRECIPITATING AND AGGRAVATING FACTORS
Bed-wetting (nocturnal enuresis)	Children (especially ages 3-15 yr) More common in males	Arousal after deep sleep	Sleepwalking	
Nightmares and night terrors	More common in children	Arousal during rapid eye movement sleep		Environmental or psychological stresses and fears
Painful or uncomfortable conditions	Any age	Delayed latency Poor sleep quality	Symptoms related to physical disorder or painful or uncomfortable conditions	Toothache Pleurisy Arthritis
Physical disorders				Pregnancy Esophagitis Nocturnal asthma or seizures Congenital hip lesions Hyperthyroidism Nocturia
Change in sleep habits	Elderly people	Delayed sleep latency Poor sleep quality	Daytime naps or dozing	
Unipolar depression	Depressed	Delayed sleep latency Early-morning wakefulness	Anorexia Fatigue Lack of interest in activities Decreased libido Constipation Vague aches and pains	Conditions, medications, and situations that produce depression
Bipolar depression	Manic Manic-depressive	May not sleep at all during manic phases	Agitation Hyperactivity Flight of ideas	Worse just before and during manic phase

Continued

Differential Diagnosis of Backache—cont'd

CAUSE	NATURE OF PATIENT	NATURE OF SYMPTOMS	ASSOCIATED SYMPTOMS	PRECIPITATING AND AGGRAVATING FACTORS
Anxiety	Any age	Delayed sleep latency	Somatic complaints Headaches Chest pain Palpitations Dizziness Gastrointestinal symptoms Nervousness Feelings of foreboding	Situations that produce anxiety
Sleep apnea	Adults Often obese males	Frequent awakening Poor sleep quality	Snoring Excess daytime sleepiness	Sleep apnea Obstruction Central apnea
Caffeine	Any age	Delayed sleep latency Poor sleep quality	May have previously tolerated caffeine well	Use of caffeine (especially after 6 PM)
Alcohol	Teenagers Adults Elderly	Delayed sleep latency Frequent awakening	Nervousness Signs of alcoholism	Alcohol Alcoholic withdrawal Recovering alcoholics
Withdrawal of antidepressants or hypnotics	Any age	Similar to prior symptoms	May redevelop symptoms of anxiety and/or depression	
Medications and drugs	Any age	Poor sleep quality Prolonged sleep latency	Depends on drug responsible	Psychotropics Beta blockers Bronchodilators Sympathomimetics Diuretics Hypnotics Appetite suppressants Amphetamines Cocaine

Selected References

Attarian HP: Helping patients who say they cannot sleep: practical ways to evaluate and treat insomnia, *Postgrad Med* 107:127-130, 133-137, 140-142, 2000.

Billiard M, Bentley A: Is insomnia best categorized as a symptom or a disease? *Sleep Med* 5(Suppl 1):835-840, 2004.

Bonnet MH, Arand DL: Diagnosis and treatment of insomnia, *Respir Care Clin North Am* 5:333-348, 1999.

Caples SM, Gami AS, Somers VK: Obstructive sleep apnea, *Ann Intern Med* 142:187-198, 2005.

Eddy M, Walbroehl GS: Insomnia, *Am Fam Physician* 59:1911-1916, 1918,1999.

Folks DG, Fuller WC: Anxiety disorders and insomnia in geriatric patients, *Psychiatr Clin North Am* 20:137-164, 1997.

Krell SB, Kapur VK: Insomnia complaints in patients evaluated for obstructive sleep apnea, *Sleep Breath* 9:104-110, 2005.

Krishnan P, Hawranik P: Diagnosis and management of geriatric insomnia: a guide for nurse practitioners, *J Am Acad Nurse Pract* 20:590-599, 2008.

Lavie P: Insomnia and sleep-disordered breathing, *Sleep Med* 8(Suppl 4):S21-S25, 2007.

Lieberman JA 3rd, Neubauer DN: Understanding insomnia: diagnosis and management of a common sleep disorder, *J Fam Pract* 56(Suppl A):35A-49A, 2007.

Pallesen S, Bjorvatn B, Nordhus IH, et al: A new scale for measuring insomnia: The Bergen Insomnia Scale, *Percept Mot Skills* 107:691-706, 2008.

Passarella S, Duong MT: Diagnosis and treatment of insomnia, *Am J Health Syst Pharm* 65:927-934, 2008.

Pring PN, Vitiello MV, Raskind MH, Thorpy MJ: Geriatrics: sleep disorders and aging, *N Engl J Med* 323:520-526, 1990.

Spielman AJ, Nunes J, Glovinsky PB: Insomnia, *Neurol Clin* 14:513-543, 1996.

Yousaf F, Sedgwick P: Sleep disorders, *Br J Hosp Med* 55:353-358, 1996.

Menstrual Irregularities

20

ABNORMAL BLEEDING

Menstrual irregularity is especially common in the perimenarchal and perimeno-pausal years. Bleeding from the vagina is considered *abnormal* when it occurs at an unexpected time of life (before menarche or after menopause) or varies from the norm in amount or pattern. *Spontaneous abortions, pregnancy complications,* and *bleeding from polyps* or other pathologic processes account for approximately 25% of the cases of abnormal vaginal bleeding.

Dysfunctional uterine bleeding is a confusing, nonspecific diagnostic term. It has been defined as abnormal uterine bleeding not due to structural or systemic disease. Therefore, this diagnosis may be reached only by a process of exclusion. It is almost always associated with anovulatory cycles. With advances in the understanding of the neuroendocrinologic basis of the menstrual cycle, diagnosis and therapy have become more specific (see Selected References).

To understand and diagnose the various causes of menstrual irregularities, the examiner must have a thorough knowledge of normal physiology (Fig. 20-1). **Although the history is important, it is seldom diagnostic and serves only as a guide to the origin of the bleeding. In most patients, hormonal or cytologic studies are necessary to establish the correct diagnosis.**

Anovulatory Bleeding

Hormonal mechanisms of endometrial bleeding include estrogen-withdrawal bleeding, estrogen-breakthrough bleeding, progesterone-withdrawal bleeding, and progesterone-breakthrough bleeding. **Anovulatory, hormone-related bleeding is most common.** This form of dysfunctional uterine bleeding is caused by estrogen-withdrawal or estrogen-breakthrough bleeding in polycystic ovary syndrome (PCOS).

Estrogen-Withdrawal Bleeding. In estrogen-withdrawal bleeding, the endometrium proliferates and remains stable as long as the estrogen level remains above the threshold. When the estrogen falls below the threshold, bleeding occurs. In the absence of progesterone, the endometrium is not in the

THE MENSTRUAL CYCLE

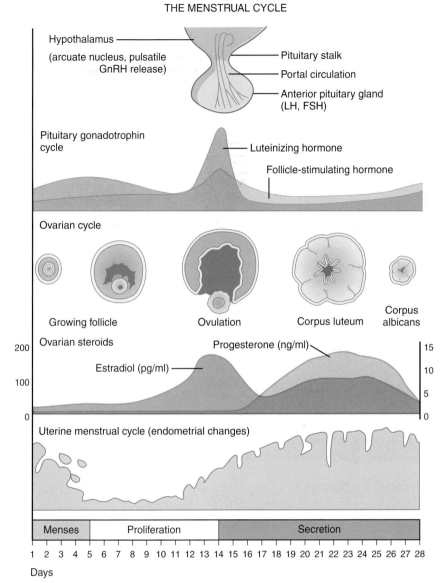

Figure 20-1. Normal menstrual cycle, with pituitary anatomy and levels of gonadotropins, ovarian activity and levels of ovarian steroids, and changes in endometrium. *GnRH, gonadotropin-releasing hormone.* (From Braverman PK, Sondheimer SJ: Menstrual disorders. Pediatr Rev 18:18, 1997. Illustration by Marcia Smith.)

secretory phase, and bleeding is often prolonged and profuse. This type of bleeding often occurs during adolescence and the climacteric.

Estrogen-Breakthrough Bleeding. Estrogen-breakthrough bleeding has been divided into two categories. The first is associated with low but constant levels of estrogen (near the threshold), which cause portions of the endometrium to degenerate and results in spotting. **This type of threshold-breakthrough bleeding occurs with the use of low-dose oral contraceptives and in PCOS.**

The second type of estrogen-breakthrough bleeding occurs when estrogen levels are initially well above the threshold, causing the endometrium to proliferate and become hyperplastic. Areas of endometrium outgrow their bloodborne hormone supply, resulting in degeneration and irregular, prolonged bleeding.

Progesterone-Withdrawal Bleeding. As in PCOS, progesterone-withdrawal bleeding occurs only with an estrogen-primed endometrium. When estrogen therapy is continued as progesterone is withdrawn, this type of bleeding occurs. It is also observed when intramuscular progesterone or oral medroxyprogesterone acetate (Provera) is administered as a test for the presence of endogenous estrogen.

Progesterone-Breakthrough Bleeding. Progesterone-breakthrough bleeding occurs when a high dose of a progestational drug is given.

Dysfunctional Ovulatory Bleeding

Dysfunctional ovulatory bleeding may be suspected from the history and confirmed with simple investigations (Table 20-1). Ovulatory bleeding is usually associated with a regular cycle length, occasional ovulation pain (mittelschmerz), premenstrual symptoms (e.g., breast soreness, bloating, weight gain, mood changes), and a biphasic basal body temperature. *Anovulatory bleeding* causes an irregular cycle in which bleeding is not preceded by or associated with subjective symptoms. The basal body temperature pattern is monophasic.

Bleeding Patterns

Recognition of particular bleeding patterns is another way of considering cases of abnormal vaginal bleeding (Table 20-2). *Menorrhagia,* or *hypermenorrhea* (excessive menstrual bleeding, >60-80 mL), is often caused by local gynecologic disease (e.g., polyps, cancer, salpingitis, uterine fibroids). It also occurs in association with intrauterine contraceptive devices (IUDs).

Metrorrhagia (intermenstrual spotting between otherwise normal periods) is also often caused by local disease. It is frequently associated with exogenous estrogen therapy. *Menometrorrhagia* is bleeding that is unpredictable with regard to amount and frequency. It can be caused by local lesions, complications of early gestation, or endocrine dysfunction (e.g., dysfunctional bleeding).

Polymenorrhagia is excessive cyclic hemorrhage occurring at intervals of 21 days or less. This type of bleeding is most often the result of anovulatory cycles.

TABLE 20-1. Differentiation of Ovulatory and Anovulatory Bleeding

CRITERIA	OVULATORY BLEEDING	ANOVULATORY BLEEDING
History	Regular cycle length Ovulation pain (mittelschmerz) Premenstrual molimina (breast soreness, bloating, weight gain, mood change) Dysmenorrhea (cramps up to 12 hr before flow and/or for first 2 days of flow)	Irregular cycles in which bleeding is not preceded by or associated with subjective symptoms
Basal body temperature record	Biphasic pattern	Monophasic pattern
Cervical mucus	Preovulatory: thin, clear, watery mucus with stretchability (spinnbarkeit) and ferning	Always dominated by estrogen
Maturation index	Preovulatory: dominated by superficial cells Postovulatory: shift to high percentage of intermediate cells	Always a marked right shift due to high estrogen level
Premenstrual endometrial biopsy	Secretory endometrium	Proliferative and possibly hyperplastic changes
Serum progesterone level	Preovulatory: <1 ng/mL Postovulatory: >5 ng/mL	Never exceeds 5 ng/mL; usually preovulatory values

From Strickler RC: Dysfunctional uterine bleeding: diagnosis and treatment. Postgrad Med 66:135-146, 1979.

TABLE 20-2. Nomenclature to Describe Menstrual Disturbances

TERM	BLEEDING PATTERN
Menorrhagia	Excessive flow (amount and/or duration) with normal cycle (21-35 days)
Polymenorrhea	Normal flow with cycle shorter than 21 days
Polymenorrhagia	Excessive flow with cycle shorter than 21 days
Metrorrhagia	Excessive flow that is acyclic
Metrostaxis	Continuous bleeding
Ovulatory bleeding (pseudopolymenorrhea)	Spotting or light flow at time of midcycle estrogen nadir
Premenstrual staining	Spotting or light flow up to 7 days before menstruation in ovulatory cycle

From Strickler RC: Dysfunctional uterine bleeding: diagnosis and treatment. Postgrad Med 66:135-146, 1979.

NATURE OF PATIENT

Before menarche, a characteristic sequence of events begins at about age 8 years (Fig. 20-2). Breast buds develop, pubic hairs appear, breasts enlarge, axillary hairs appear, and finally a height spurt occurs. Menstrual function usually begins after the height spurt. About 6 months before menarche, physiologic leukorrhea

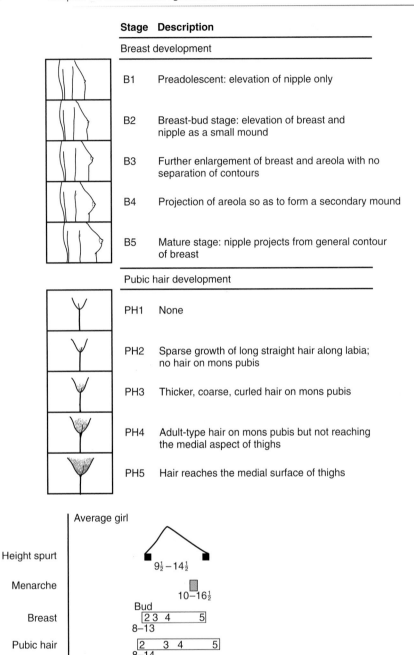

Stage	Description
Breast development	
B1	Preadolescent: elevation of nipple only
B2	Breast-bud stage: elevation of breast and nipple as a small mound
B3	Further enlargement of breast and areola with no separation of contours
B4	Projection of areola so as to form a secondary mound
B5	Mature stage: nipple projects from general contour of breast
Pubic hair development	
PH1	None
PH2	Sparse growth of long straight hair along labia; no hair on mons pubis
PH3	Thicker, coarse, curled hair on mons pubis
PH4	Adult-type hair on mons pubis but not reaching the medial aspect of thighs
PH5	Hair reaches the medial surface of thighs

Figure 20-2. Relationship of pubertal events in adolescent girls. (From Lopez RI: Menstrual irregularities in teenage girls. Drug Ther April:49, 1981.)

occurs. In the first year after menarche, 55% of menses are anovulatory, with a sharp decline to about 7% by 8 years after menarche. Usually, 15 months is required for completion of the first 10 menstrual cycles. This means that when menses begin, it is unusual for them to occur at regular monthly intervals.

The average age at which girls begin to menstruate is 12 years. Table 20-3 shows the characteristics of normal menstruation. Bleeding that occurs before 9 to 10 years of age is abnormal, and local pathology as well as adrenal and ovarian tumors must be suspected. Because some teenage girls are reluctant to volunteer information about their menstrual periods, it is essential that physicians routinely ask a series of questions, as follows:

1. When did your menses begin?
2. How often do your menstrual periods occur?
3. On what date did your last period occur?
4. Is there any pain associated with menstruation?
5. Are you sexually active?
6. Are you practicing any form of birth control?

These questions must be asked in a nonthreatening way so that the patient feels at ease and understands that the physician is willing to listen. Likewise, when asking questions about sexual activities, the physician must remain non-judgmental. The teenager should be reassured that any discussion of this nature will remain a private matter between patient and physician.

The adolescent typically has cycles of variable length. Anovulation may be associated with both short and long cycles together with short follicular and luteal cycles. Menarche may be delayed in underweight adolescents as well as in some teenage girls who are on strict diets to remain fashionably thin and in athletes with normal body weight but low body fat. Menarche often has a familial pattern; girls often start menstruating at about the same age as their mothers and older sisters did.

Several significant age-associated conditions can cause abnormal vaginal bleeding. In children, insertion of *foreign bodies* into the vagina may cause bleeding.

In adolescence, amenorrhea, dysmenorrhea and abnormal uterine bleeding are common, affecting about 75% of adolescents. Both primary and secondary amenorrhea can occur. When pelvic anatomy and ovarian function are normal, dysmenorrhea is considered *primary. Secondary dysmenorrhea* occurs when dysmenorrhea is associated with pelvic or hormonal pathology. In adolescents,

TABLE 20-3. Characteristics of Menstruation*

CHARACTERISTICS	RANGE	AVERAGE
Menarche (age of onset)	9-17 yr	12.5 yr
Cycle length (interval)	21-35 days	28 days
Duration of flow	1-8 days	3-5 days
Amount of flow	10-80 mL	35 mL
Onset of menopause	45-55 yr	47-50 yr

*Range and averages for American women.
From Hamilton C: Vaginal bleeding: evaluation and management. Res Staff Physician Nov:62-64, 1981.

anovulation causes virtually all instances of dysfunctional uterine bleeding and 90% of all instances of abnormal uterine bleeding.

During the reproductive years, *dysfunctional uterine bleeding* and bleeding from *pregnancy complications, tumors,* or *fibroids* may occur (Table 20-4). **A menstruating woman of any age can bleed from complications of pregnancy.** Anovulatory *estrogen-withdrawal bleeding* is the most common cause of irregular menses during the reproductive and perimenopausal years, accounting for 40% of menstrual disturbances in the perimenopausal years.

Other, less common causes of abnormal vaginal bleeding in perimenopausal women are *organic lesions* (neoplasm or inflammatory diseases of the cervix, vagina, and endometrium), *constitutional diseases* (hypothyroidism, hyperthyroidism, Cushing's disease, cirrhosis, thrombocytopenia), and certain *drugs* (Table 20-5). In postmenopausal women, bleeding may result from *endometrial* and *cervical cancers.*

NATURE OF SYMPTOMS

Prolonged irregular and profuse bleeding may occur with either estrogen-breakthrough or estrogen-withdrawal bleeding. The bleeding may be spotty (threshold-breakthrough bleeding). Anovulatory bleeding is usually unexpected and painless. Anovulatory cycles may result in *polymenorrhagia*. With ovulatory menstrual abnormalities there may be a short luteal phase, in which case menstrual cycles may be variable in length with excessive flow. Patients with these problems may also complain of premenstrual bleeding or staining. When *menorrhagia* is present, *tumors, fibroids, cancer, polyps, salpingitis,* or *IUDs* may be the cause. *Endometriosis* (see Chapter 21), *salpingitis,* and *cancer* may also cause minimal bleeding and should be suspected if purulent discharge is present.

During the reproductive years, abnormal vaginal bleeding often represents *pregnancy complications.* The patient may have a history of sexual activity without adequate contraceptive measures. In addition, symptoms of pregnancy, such as missed periods, morning sickness, and breast tenderness, may be present. In these patients the uterine bleeding initially results from endometrial sloughing; therefore, spotting rather than amenorrhea may occur before gross hemorrhage.

Gross hemorrhage may be concealed or visible. *Ectopic pregnancy* is strongly suggested by an adnexal or cul-de-sac mass in a pregnant woman who has a normal or only slightly enlarged uterus. Concealed pelvic hemorrhage from a ruptured ectopic pregnancy can occur either with or without vaginal bleeding. This diagnosis should be suspected when the patient has amenorrhea, pelvic or abdominal fullness, abdominal pain (particularly if unilateral or referred to the shoulder), tenesmus, and urinary frequency or urgency. Fever, signs of peritoneal irritation, purulent vaginal discharge, and pain can be seen in patients with ectopic pregnancy or salpingitis.

Copious vaginal bleeding most often results from pregnancy complications and less often from local gynecologic disease or dysfunctional bleeding. Bright-red hemorrhage with clots suggests a brisk nonmenstrual flow. A darker tint

TABLE 20-4.   Causes of Vaginal Bleeding in the Reproductive Years

Menstruation and variations:

Ovulatory spotting (midcycle)

Pregnancy complications:

Early (<20 wk):

Implantation bleeding

Abortion

Ectopic pregnancy

Trophoblastic disease

Late (>20 wk):

Placenta previa, vasa praevia, other

Postpartum:

Uterine atony

Retained products

Normal delivery

Disorders of central nervous system—hypothalamic-ovarian-pituitary axis

Dysfunctional uterine bleeding:

Anovulatory (80%-90%)

Ovulatory

Functioning ovarian cysts or tumors

Emotional stress

Anticholinergic drugs

Exogenous hormones:

Estrogen

Estrogen-progestin oral contraceptives

Trauma

Anticoagulant drugs

Organic gynecologic disease:

Pelvic infections

Neoplastic diseases:

Benign

Malignant

Adenomyosis

Systemic disease

Generalized bleeding disorders

Thyroid disease

From Hamilton C: Vaginal bleeding: evaluation and management. Res Staff Physician Nov:62-64, 1981

TABLE 20-5.   Common Drugs That May Alter Menstrual Bleeding

GROUP AND GENERIC NAMES	TRADE AND COMMON NAMES
Amphetamines	Desoxyn, Obetrol*
Anticoagulants	Coumadin, heparin
Benzodiazepines:	
Diazepam, oxazepam	Valium, Serax*
Benzamide derivatives:	
Procainamide, procarbazine	Pronestyl, Matulane
Butyrophenones	Haldol, Inapsine*
Cannabis	Marijuana
Chlordiazepoxide	Librium
Cimetidine	Tagamet
Ethyl alcohol	Whiskey, wine, beer
Isoniazid	Isonicotinic acid hydrazide*
Methyldopa	Aldomet*
Monoamine oxidase inhibitors	Eutonyl, Nardil
Opiates*	Morphine, heroin, methadone*
Phenothiazines*	Compazine, Thorazine, Phenergan*
Prostaglandin inhibitors	Motrin, Indocin
Rauwolfia	Raudixin
Reserpine*	Serpasil*
Spironolactone*	Aldactone*
Steroids	
Estrogens*	Premarin, oral contraceptives*
Progesterones*	Provera, oral contraceptives*
Testosterone*	Android*
Thyroid hormones	Synthroid, Cytomel
Thioxanthenes*	Navane*
Tricyclic antidepressants*	Elavil*

*May also produce galactorrhea.
Modified from Murata JN: Abnormal genital bleeding and secondary amenorrhea: common gynecological problems. J Obstet Gynecol Neonatal Nurs 19:26-36, 1990.

of blood implies slower hemorrhage acted on by cervical or vaginal secretions. Irregular bleeding during pregnancy may result from separation of the placenta or the embryo from its attachment, but malignant cervical erosions, polyps, and local vaginal lesions must be excluded.

Menorrhagia during puberty is usually caused by anovulation. This gradually abates within several months of the onset of menarche. If menstrual irregularity continues for 2 to 3 years after menarche, PCOS should be considered.

Menorrhagia during the reproductive years can also result from anovulation, as can *polymenorrhagia*. Menorrhagia that occurs during the reproductive years may be caused by *fibromyomas*. **The chief characteristic of a uterine fibroid is an asymmetrically enlarged uterus.** More than one fibroid may be present in the uterus, and the shape can be extremely irregular. As a rule, the consistency of the fibroid is hard and unyielding. Usually, the cervix and uterine fibroid move together.

It may be difficult for the physician to distinguish a fibromyoma from an *ovarian cyst*. **A helpful point in the differentiation of fibroids from ovarian cysts is that ovarian cysts almost never cause menorrhagia.** Ovarian tumors usually create no menstrual disturbances. *Adenomyoma* of the uterus usually causes symmetrical uterine enlargement, but absolute differentiation must be accomplished by pathologic examination.

Chronic salpingo-oophoritis (hydrosalpinx, tubo-ovarian abscess, or *chronic salpingitis)* and *ovarian endometriosis* can cause menorrhagia, and congestive (premenstrual) dysmenorrhea is usually present as a prominent symptom. Menorrhagia can also be caused by IUDs, thrombocytopenia, and other coagulation defects.

Irregular menstrual bleeding may be divided into three groups:

- **Irregular bleeding during menstrual life**
- **Bleeding before puberty and after menopause**
- **Bleeding during pregnancy**

Irregular Bleeding During Menstrual Life

Metrorrhagia. The most common cause of bleeding or spotting between regular menses is breakthrough bleeding associated with oral contraceptives, but complications of pregnancy must always be considered. The lesions of the reproductive organs that cause metrorrhagia include *cervical carcinoma, benign* and *malignant uterine tumors, endometritis,* and (rarely) *tuberculous endometritis.* *Fibromyomas* usually cause menorrhagia but can occasionally cause metrorrhagia. Fibroids tend to produce irregular bleeding when they are submucosal or in the process of extrusion. A carcinoma can develop in a patient known to have uterine fibroids, and a fibroid can occasionally undergo sarcomatous degeneration. Rapid enlargement of the uterus associated with irregular bleeding is very suggestive of a *sarcoma*. However, several fibroids can be present in the same uterus and are a common cause of rapid uterine enlargement. *Choriocarcinoma* is a rare cause of uterine enlargement that follows a *hydatidiform mole* in about 50% of the recorded cases. It should be suspected during early pregnancy, when abortion is a threat and the uterus is extremely enlarged. Choriocarcinoma is also likely in women who have persistent uterine enlargement.

Cervical erosions do not usually bleed. If irregular bleeding occurs from the erosion or the cervix bleeds during an examination, cancer should be excluded.

Menorrhagia. *Polyps* and *fibroids* are common causes of menorrhagia, which has been defined as blood loss of more than 80 mL per period or menses lasting longer than 7 days. Typical menstrual blood loss is 30 to 40 mL.

Dysfunctional uterine bleeding can occur at any age. Half of the cases occur in women between ages 40 and 50 years, about 10% develop at puberty, and the remaining 40% occur between puberty and age 40 years. Dysfunctional uterine bleeding, most frequently due to an anovulatory cycle, is usually in the form of menorrhagia, although the interval between periods may be shortened.

Women using *estrogen preparations* to control menstrual symptoms or prevent conception may experience menorrhagia while the drugs are being taken or after their withdrawal. The menorrhagia is often related to the dosage of estrogen.

Coagulopathy and hypothyroidism may manifest as menorrhagia.

Bleeding associated with *ovulation* is uncommon; when it occurs, it is midway between the periods (at approximately the time of ovulation). Mid–menstrual cycle bleeding accompanied by lower abdominal pain is termed *mittelschmerz*.

Bleeding Before Puberty and After Menopause

Vaginal bleeding in neonates is usually caused by a temporarily *high fetal estrogen concentration*. Postmenopausal bleeding may result from *malignant growths, polyps, senile endometritis,* or *cervicitis. Carcinoma of the uterine body* seldom causes much uterine enlargement, and any increase in size usually occurs slowly. Because the postmenopausal uterus shrinks considerably, a uterine size that would be regarded as normal in a younger woman indicates abnormal enlargement in a postmenopausal woman.

Bleeding During Pregnancy

It is important for the physician to differentiate the uterine hemorrhage of extrauterine gestation from that due to threatened abortion. Bleeding can be caused by *placenta previa* and *abruptio placentae.*

Associated Symptoms

Ovulatory irregular bleeding is often associated with midcycle ovulation pain (mittelschmerz), premenstrual symptoms, and dysmenorrhea. Fever, purulent vaginal discharge, and pain may be clues to *pregnancy complications,* including spontaneous and induced *abortion.* These same signs and symptoms may be observed in cases of *ectopic pregnancy* and *salpingitis.* Irregular menses associated with galactorrhea suggests a *prolactinoma.* Anovulatory irregular bleeding associated with hirsutism and occasionally hypertension, obesity, acne, and diabetes suggests *PCOS.*

Precipitating and Aggravating Factors

Anovulatory irregular menstrual bleeding often occurs during the first 12 to 18 months after menarche. It is seen most often in obese patients; in women who have adrenal disease, pituitary tumors, PCOS, Cushing's disease, diabetes, malnutrition, chronic illness, or hypothyroidism; and in patients who use phenothiazines or opiates (Table 20-5).

Physical Findings

Physical examination should include thorough pelvic, vaginal, and abdominal evaluations. It should be directed at detection of systemic diseases such as *endocrinopathies*, including adult-onset adrenal hyperplasia, Cushing's disease, thyroid dysfunction, polycystic ovaries, and obesity. Persistent acne and hirsutism support a diagnosis of PCOS.

Diagnostic Studies

Diagnostic tests useful in the differential diagnosis of patients with abnormal vaginal bleeding include a complete blood count, reticulocyte count, platelet count, and coagulation studies; pregnancy tests; thyroid-stimulating hormone, follicle-stimulating hormone, and luteinizing hormone tests; plasma glucose measurement; and urinalysis. A free testosterone level greater than 50 ng/dL as well as a luteinizing hormone–to–follicle-stimulating hormone (LH/FSH) ratio greater than 2 is suggestive of polycystic ovarian syndrome. Other diagnostic tests that help the physician evaluate the cause of abnormal vaginal bleeding include uterine curettage; endometrial, vaginal, and cervical biopsies; a Papanicolaou test for detection of cancer; and Gram stain and culture for determination of infections. Transvaginal ultrasonography is used to measure the thickness of the endometrium when endometrial cancer is suspected. It is usually accompanied by endometrial biopsy (an office procedure). Infusing a small amount of sterile saline into the uterine cavity prior to ultrasonography (called *sonohysterography*) improves sensitivity of the imaging for uterine fibroids and endometrial polyps.

Pelvic ultrasonography helps the physician diagnose ectopic pregnancies, ovarian cysts, and tumors. **Because most patients of reproductive age who have severe uterine bleeding are pregnant, human chorionic gonadotropin (HCG) levels should be determined.** HCG is produced during intrauterine or ectopic pregnancy, development of hydatidiform moles, and formation of choriocarcinoma. The most sensitive test for detecting early pregnancy is the quantitative serum test for the beta unit of HCG. This test often allows the physician to detect pregnancy as early as 1 week after fertilization. Newer urine pregnancy tests have been reported to be 90% sensitive one day after the missed period and 97% after one week. Although with the increased sensitivity of newer urine tests, a negative office urine pregnancy test result is reassuring, women in whom an ectopic pregnancy is suspected should undergo a serum quantitative HCG determination, particularly since this information is used to determine when a pregnancy should be able to be reliably visualized on ultrasonography. A negative serum HCG test result almost always excludes an ectopic pregnancy.

Although ectopic pregnancy accounts for only 0.5% of all pregnancies, it is the cause of 10% to 15% of maternal deaths. More than 90% of ectopic pregnancies are caused by tubal implants that rupture during the first trimester. Major risk factors for ectopic pregnancy include a history of a previous ectopic pregnancy, salpingitis, a previous tubal procedure, and pregnancy that occurs while an IUD is in place.

Catastrophic ruptures usually manifest as hemodynamic instability; however, some ectopic pregnancies leak slowly over several days, so they may go unrecognized until the patient's second or third visit. Ultrasonography helps rule out an ectopic pregnancy by confirming the presence of a uterine gestational sac with an intrauterine pregnancy. Unruptured ectopic pregnancies are diagnosed by transvaginal ultrasonography in conjunction with serial serum quantitative HCG measurements. Ruptured ectopic pregnancies are addressed surgically in an emergency manner. Unruptured ectopic pregnancies may be managed medically or surgically, depending on their size and location.

Less Common Diagnostic Considerations

Patients with *endometriosis* may have abnormal vaginal bleeding but usually have dull backaches and dyspareunia associated with congestive dysmenorrhea. *Cervical erosions* can be detected on physical examination. *Bleeding disorders,* including idiopathic thrombocytopenic purpura, may manifest as menometrorrhagia. *Thrombocytopenia* is often seen in patients with disseminated lupus.

Because *clear cell adenocarcinoma* of the vagina or cervix can be fatal, the possibility of this tumor must always be considered. It is most common in the daughters of the 2 to 3 million women who took diethylstilbestrol (DES) as a fertility drug. These *DES daughters* may also have congenital abnormalities of the cervix, uterus, and upper vagina. In addition, they demonstrate an increased risk of pregnancy complications (e.g., threatened, spontaneous, or induced, incomplete abortion and ectopic gestation).

Abnormal vaginal bleeding may also be a sign of a *coagulation defect,* especially platelet deficiency, von Willebrand's disease, or leukemia.

AMENORRHEA

The average age at menarche in the United States is 12.7 years, and the age range for menarche is 11 to 15 years (99% of females reach menarche by 16 years). *Primary amenorrhea* refers to the condition in women who fail to menstruate at all. Most young patients simply have delayed menarche. **Failure to menstruate by age 15 years in the presence of normal secondary sexual development should be investigated.** Because weight loss, excessive exercise training, and eating disorders can result in delayed menarche, it is particularly important for the physician to determine the patient's diet and level of physical activity. In addition, substances such as amphetamines, cannabis, estrogens, and phenothiazines may interfere with the onset of menstruation (Table 20-6).

Primary amenorrhea is rare. It is usually associated with an endocrine imbalance or congenital abnormalities. In patients with this condition, the physician must rule out chromosomal aberrations and genital malformations. In cases in which gonadal failure is suspected, chromatin analysis of a buccal smear should be performed.

Short stature and a webbed neck should suggest *Turner's syndrome.* Age is a significant factor in the diagnosis. For example, a 15-year-old girl who has not yet

TABLE 20-6.   Common Drugs That May Cause Amenorrhea

GENERIC NAME	TRADE AND COMMON NAMES
Amphetamines	Desoxyn, Obetrol
Benzodiazepines:	
Diazepam, oxazepam	Valium, Serax
Benzamide derivatives	Pronestyl, Matulane
Butyrophenones	Haldol, Inapsine
Calcium channel blockers:	
Nifedipine, verapamil, diltiazem	Adalat, Cardizem, Calan
Cannabis	Marijuana
Chemotherapeutics	Cytoxan, Myleran, Leukeran, Platinol
Cimetidine	Tagamet
Isoniazid	Isonicotinic acid hydrazide
Methyldopa	Aldomet
Monoamine oxidase inhibitors	Eutonyl, Nardil
Opiates	Morphine, heroin
Phenothiazines	Compazine, Thorazine, Phenergan
Rauwolfia	Harmonyl, Raudixin
Reserpine	Serpasil
Spironolactone	Aldactone
Steroids:	
Gonadal	Ingredients of oral contraceptives
Estrogens	
Progesterones	
Thyroid hormones	Synthroid, Cytomel
Thioxanthenes	Navane
Tricyclic antidepressants	Elavil

Modified from Murata JN: Primary amenorrhea. Pediatr Nurs 15:125-129, 1989.

menstruated usually has a delayed menarche, whereas a 17-year-old girl who has not begun to menstruate is considered to have primary amenorrhea (Fig. 20-3).

Patients with *secondary amenorrhea* have menstruated but then stop. **During the reproductive years the most common cause of secondary amenorrhea is pregnancy.** An endocrine imbalance may be an associated factor, but tumors seldom cause secondary amenorrhea. When pregnancy, lactation, and menopause have been ruled out, the most common causes are PCOS, ovarian failure, hyperprolactinemia, and hypothalamic amenorrhea. A vaginal smear and evaluation of the cervical mucus will help determine whether there is ovarian estrogen production. Various endocrinologic tests help determine whether ovarian progesterone production is normal and levels of ovarian androgen are normal

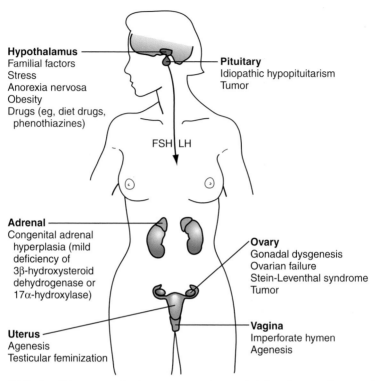

Hypothalamus
Familial factors
Stress
Anorexia nervosa
Obesity
Drugs (eg, diet drugs,
  phenothiazines)

Pituitary
Idiopathic hypopituitarism
Tumor

FSH LH

Adrenal
Congenital adrenal
  hyperplasia (mild
  deficiency of
  3β-hydroxysteroid
  dehydrogenase or
  17α-hydroxylase)

Ovary
Gonadal dysgenesis
Ovarian failure
Stein-Leventhal syndrome
Tumor

Uterus
Agenesis
Testicular feminization

Vagina
Imperforate hymen
Agenesis

Figure 20-3. Possible causes of primary amenorrhea and delayed menarche. *FSH,* follicle-stimulating hormone; *LH,* luteinizing hormone. (From Lopez RI: Menstrual irregularities in young girls. Drug Ther April:42, 1981.)

or elevated. If a patient with secondary amenorrhea has galactorrhea, a *prolactinoma* is probable. Table 20-7 lists the various causes of secondary amenorrhea.

Diagnostic studies that are useful in the evaluation of amenorrhea include, blood and urine hormone estimation (follicle-stimulating hormone, thyroid-stimulating hormone, luteinizing hormone, prolactin), chromosome analysis, basal body temperature, vaginal smear, magnetic resonance imaging (MRI) or computed tomography (CT) of the pituitary fossa (to investigate elevated prolactin value), and a progesterone withdrawal test for determination of whether estrogen is being manufactured. A pelvic examination can reveal structural abnormalities, such as an imperforate hymen and transverse vaginal septum. Pelvic ultrasonography can detect gonadal dysgenesis or polycystic ovaries.

Less common causes of amenorrhea include *nutritional disorders* and strict *dieting; systemic disorders* such as tuberculosis, diabetes, prolactinoma, hypothyroidism, and hyperthyroidism; and *psychogenic disturbances,* including severe stress and anorexia nervosa.

Hyperandrogenic chronic anovulation, which includes PCOS, should be suspected in young obese women who have normal sexual development, hypertension, and hirsutism. They may have secondary amenorrhea or oligomenorrhea.

TABLE 20-7. Possible Causes of Secondary Amenorrhea

| | Ovarian Hormone Production | | |
NORMAL (CYCLE)	DECREASED (ACYCLIC)		INCREASED (ACYCLIC)
	HIGH GONADOTROPIN LEVELS	LOW OR NORMAL GONADOTROPIN LEVELS	
Asherman's syndrome Endometrial destruction Infective tuberculosis, schistosomiasis Iatrogenic (curettage, irradiation)	Premature ovarian failure Castration (surgical or radiation)	Functional aberrations of hypothalamic-pituitary axis Psychogenic factors Nutritional factors Nongonadal endocrine disorders(thyroid, adrenals, pancreas) Systemic infections and chronic diseases Pharmacologic factors (psychotropic drugs, postpill oversuppression, drug addiction) Central nervous system disease (tumor or trauma)	Polycystic ovary syndrome Virilizing ovarian tumors (arrheno-blastoma, hilus cell tumor) Feminizing ovarian tumors (granulose cell, thecal cell)

From Lehmann F: Diagnostic approach to ovarian dysfunction. Hormone Res 9:319-338, 1978.

Early PCOS may include severe dysfunctional bleeding and elevated serum gonadotropin levels. The patient may also have severe acne. *Congenital adrenal hyperplasia* (virilizing tumor) is also manifested by hirsutism and severe acne.

Secondary amenorrhea has been reported in female marathon runners, a finding that is probably related to the marked decrease in total body fat in these women. It has also been reported in competitive swimmers and ballet dancers for the same reason.

Asherman's syndrome is amenorrhea resulting from destruction of the basal layer of the endometrium and adhesions following *overenthusiastic* uterine curettage.

Differential Diagnosis of Menstrual Irregularities

CAUSE	NATURE OF PATIENT	NATURE OF SYMPTOMS	ASSOCIATED SYMPTOMS	PRECIPITATING AND AGGRAVATING FACTORS	PHYSICAL FINDINGS	DIAGNOSTIC STUDIES
Dysfunctional uterine bleeding (hormonal causes):	Can occur at any age 10% of cases occur at puberty 50% of cases occur between ages 40 and 50 yr	Usually due to anovulatory cycles Menorrhagia Interval between periods may be decreased				Diagnosis only by process of exclusion
Anovulatory cycles	Normal occurrence in 55% of girls within first year of menarche	Irregular cycle length Polymenorrhagia Bleeding not preceded by or associated with subjective symptoms		Obesity Adrenal or pituitary disease Polycystic ovaries Diabetes Malnutrition Chronic illness Hypothyroidism Phenothiazines or opiates	Obesity, hypertension, hirsutism, acne, and sometimes diabetes suggest PCOS	Monophasic basal body temperature Serum progesterone level never exceeds 5 ng/mL
Estrogen-withdrawal bleeding	Most common cause of irregular menses in reproductive years, especially in adolescence and climacteric	Prolonged, irregular, profuse bleeding	Painless			Endometrial biopsy Serum FSH and LH Pregnancy test
Estrogen-breakthrough bleeding	Women on oral contraceptives, women with PCOS	Spotty bleeding	Painless			Serum FSH/LH/Estrogen, pregnancy test
Threshold bleeding		Spotty bleeding		Low-dose oral contraceptives		

With estrogen levels above threshold	Prolonged, irregular, profuse bleeding				
Progesterone-breakthrough bleeding					
Progesterone-withdrawal bleeding				High-dose progestational drugs	
				Intramuscular progesterone or oral medroxyprogesterone acetate (Provera) as test for endogenous estrogen	
Ovulatory cycles	Cycle length is usually regular, Premenstrual staining or bleeding, Dysmenorrhea	Mittelschmerz, PMS			Biphasic basal body temperature, Serum progesterone level >3 ng/mL
Complications of pregnancy:	Spotting precedes gross hemorrhage (visible or concealed)	Missed periods, Morning sickness, Breast tenderness	Reproductive age		Serum HCG
Ectopic pregnancy	Amenorrhea, Pelvic or abdominal fullness, Abdominal pain (usually unilateral), May refer to shoulder, May or may not be vaginal bleeding, Purulent vaginal discharge	Tenesmus, Increased urinary frequency or urgency	Increased risk with previous ectopic pregnancy, salpingitis, previous tubal procedure, or pregnancy with IUD	Adnexal or cul-de-sac mass, Normal or slightly enlarged uterus, Peritoneal irritation	

Continued

Differential Diagnosis of Menstrual Irregularities—cont'd

CAUSE	NATURE OF PATIENT	NATURE OF SYMPTOMS	ASSOCIATED SYMPTOMS	PRECIPITATING AND AGGRAVATING FACTORS	PHYSICAL FINDINGS	DIAGNOSTIC STUDIES
During uterine pregnancy		Irregular bleeding due to separation of placenta or embryo from its attachment				
Spontaneous abortion		Hemorrhage (sometimes with clots)	Fever Purulent vaginal discharge or pain			
Endometriosis (see Chapter 21)		Slight bleeding	Dysmenorrhea Purulent vaginal discharge Dull backache		Implants may be palpable	Pelvic ultraso- nography
Endometrial and cervical cancer	Postmenopausal women	Extent of bleeding may vary	Purulent vaginal discharge			Dilatation and curettage Biopsy Papanicolaou smear
Fibroids	Women of reproductive age	Menorrhagia and occasionally metrorrhagia Irregular bleeding			Uterus is asym- metrically enlarged Fibroids are hard and unyielding Cervix and fibroids usually move together	Pelvic sonogram
IUD		Menorrhagia	Cervical discharge		IUD	

Salpingitis	Usually occurs in reproductive years	Menorrhagia or slight bleeding	Purulent discharge Fever Abdominal pain Dysmenorrhea		Signs of peritoneal irritation	
Insertion of foreign body into vagina	Most common cause of abnormal vaginal bleeding in children				Foreign body	
Amenorrhea:						
Primary	In girls up to age 17 yr; delayed menarche most common cause Girls 18 yr or older who have not yet menstruated (rare)			Severe malnutrition Weight loss Vigorous exercise Amphetamines Phenothiazines Cannabis Endocrine and congenital abnormalities Chromosomal aberrations	Abnormal pubertal development Abnormal external or internal genitalia Short stature	Chromatin analysis
Secondary	Patients have menstruated and then stopped menstruating			Pregnancy Endocrine imbalance Tumors Breast-feeding Oral contraceptives Postpill amenorrhea		Vaginal smear and evaluation of cervical mucus to determine ovarian estrogen production and other hormone levels Serum HCG
Prolactinoma			Galactorrhea			Serum prolactin levels CT scan of sella

CT, Computed tomography; *FSH,* follicle-stimulating hormone; *HCG,* human chorionic gonadotropin; *IUD,* intrauterine device; *LH,* luteinizing hormone; *PCOS,* polycystic ovarian syndrome; *PMS,* premenstrual syndrome.

Selected References

ACOG Committee on Practice Bulletins–Gynecology: ACOG Practice Bulletin No. 108: Polycystic ovary syndrome, *Obstet Gynecol* 114:936-949, 2009.

American College of Obstetricians and Gynecologists: ACOG Practice Bulletin No. 94: Medical management of ectopic pregnancy, *Obstet Gynecol* 111:1479-1485, 2008.

American College of Obstetricians and Gynecologists: ACOG Committee Opinion No. 426: The role of transvaginal ultrasonography in the evaluation of postmenopausal bleeding, *Obstet Gynecol* 113:462-464, 2009.

Barnhart KT: Clinical practice: Ectopic pregnancy, *N Engl J Med* 361:379-387, 2009.

Creatsas G, Deligeoroglou E: Polycystic ovarian syndrome in adolescents, *Curr Opin Obstet Gynecol* 19:420-426, 2007.

Hart R: Polycystic ovarian syndrome—prognosis and treatment outcomes, *Curr Opin Obstet Gynecol* 19:529-535, 2007.

Heiman DL: Amenorrhea, *Prim Care* 36:1-17, 2009.

Hill D: Abnormal uterine bleeding: avoid the rush to hysterectomy, *J Fam Pract* 58:136-142, 2009.

Hurskainen R, Grenman S, Komi I, et al: Diagnosis and treatment of menorrhagia, *Acta Obstet Gynecol Scand* 86:749-757, 2007.

Practice Committee of American Society for Reproductive Medicine: Current evaluation of amenorrhea, *Fertil Steril* 90(Suppl):S219-S225, 2008.

Slap GB: Menstrual disorders in adolescence: best practice and research, *Clin Obstet Gynecol* 17:75-92, 2003.

Menstrual Pain

21

Dysmenorrhea means painful menstruation. It may begin shortly before menstruation. Approximately 60% of postpubescent women experience dysmenorrhea; 10% of these women are incapacitated by pain for 1 to 3 days per month. It is the major cause of lost working hours and school days among young women and is associated with substantial economic losses to the entire community as well as to the patient. In some patients, anticipatory fear of the next menstrual period can cause anxiety during the intermenstrual period.

In evaluating a patient with pelvic pain at menstruation, the physician must first decide whether the patient has premenstrual syndrome (PMS) or dysmenorrhea. PMS usually begins 2 to 12 days before the menstrual period and subsides at the onset or early in the course of menstruation. The major symptoms of PMS are a diffuse, dull pelvic ache; mood changes (irritability, nervousness, headaches, depression); swelling of the breasts and extremities; occasional weight gain; and a sensation of abdominal bloating. PMS is quite common and causes minor mood changes, whereas premenstrual dysphoric disorder (PMDD) affects only 3% to 8% of women and is characterized by severe irritability, tension, dysphoria, and lability of mood that seriously interfere with lifestyle. *Diagnostic and Statistical Manual of Mental Disorders,* 4th edition (DSM IV) diagnostic criteria for PMDD are presented in Table 21-1. The American College of Obstetrics and Gynecology also recommends charting symptoms for at least one menstrual cycle prior to making the diagnosis of PMS. Women with presumed *PMS* or *PMDD* should be evaluated for conditions such as depression, anxiety disorder, and hypothyroidism, symptoms of which can be similar. Patients should also be screened for domestic violence as well as substance abuse.

Dysmenorrhea is classified as primary or secondary. *Primary dysmenorrhea* is the most common menstrual disorder, occurring in 30% to 50% of young women. Its prevalence decreases with age, with the highest prevalence being in those 20 to 24 years old. Dysmenorrhea is classified as primary (intrinsic, essential, or idiopathic) if it occurs in a woman who has no pelvic abnormality.

245

TABLE 21-1.   Clinical Criteria for Premenstrual Dysphoric Disorder

In most menstrual cycles, at least five of the following symptoms should be present for most of the last week of the luteal phase, remitted within a few days after onset of menses, and remain absent in the week after menses. At least one symptom must be *1, 2, 3,* or *4.*

1. Depressed mood or dysphoria
2. Anxiety or tension
3. Affect lability
4. Irritability
5. Decreased interest in usual activities
6. Concentration difficulties
7. Marked lack of energy
8. Marked changed in appetite, overeating, or food cravings
9. Hypersomnia or insomnia
10. Feeling overwhelmed
11. Other physical symptoms, e.g., breast tenderness, bloating
    • Symptoms markedly interfere with work, school, social activities, or relationships.
    • Symptoms are not just an exacerbation of another disorder.

The first three criteria must be confirmed by prospective daily ratings for at least two consecutive menstrual cycles.

Adapted from Yonkers KA, O'Brien PM, Eriksson E: Premenstrual syndrome. Lancet 371(9619):1201, 2008.

About 95% of female adolescents have primary dysmenorrhea, and this problem is a major cause of school absenteeism. Primary dysmenorrhea is thought to be caused by the increased secretion of prostanoid and eicosanoid (hence, nonsteroidal anti-inflammatory drugs [NSAIDs] often provide relief), which in turn cause abnormal uterine contractions and uterine hypoxia,

Secondary dysmenorrhea (extrinsic or acquired) results from organic pelvic diseases such as *endometriosis, fibroids, adenomyosis, bacterial infections,* and infections caused by *intrauterine contraceptive devices* (IUDs). Because effective therapy is now available for primary and secondary dysmenorrhea, it is not sufficient to merely diagnose *dysmenorrhea*. The physician must distinguish among PMS, primary dysmenorrhea, and secondary dysmenorrhea.

Some women will not initiate a discussion of dysmenorrhea with their physician. They may have been taught that it is normal or that relief cannot be obtained. It is therefore essential that the practitioner ask the patient whether dysmenorrhea is a problem.

NATURE OF PATIENT

Primary dysmenorrhea is common in adolescent girls and young women, with the greatest incidence in the late teens and early 20s. **When dysmenorrhea begins within the first 2 to 3 years of menarche, primary dysmenorrhea is the most likely diagnosis.** Primary dysmenorrhea usually occurs with ovulatory cycles, which normally begin 3 to 12 months after menarche, when ovulation occurs regularly. Primary dysmenorrhea usually begins within 6 months of menarche and becomes progressively more severe.

If a patient has gradually increasing monthly pain without menstruation, a *congenital abnormality* obstructing menstrual flow must be considered. These rare abnormalities may lead to hematocolpos, hematometra, and eventually intraperitoneal bleeding.

Secondary dysmenorrhea usually begins many years after menarche. Dysmenorrhea that develops after age 20 years is usually of the secondary type. A history of pelvic infection, menorrhagia, or intermenstrual bleeding suggests underlying pelvic pathology. Dysmenorrhea can often be caused by an *IUD*. If dysmenorrhea develops after cervical conization, cautery, or radiation, *acquired cervical stenosis* or *cervical occlusion* may be the cause. Dysmenorrhea after uterine curettage may be due to *intrauterine synechiae* (Asherman's syndrome). Secondary dysmenorrhea due to *endometriosis* is usually late in onset (beginning when the patient is in her 30s) and worsens with age. Endometriosis is uncommon in teenagers. *Adenomyosis* may be a cause of secondary dysmenorrhea, particularly in parous women older than 40 years and if menorrhagia is present.

NATURE OF SYMPTOMS

Pain that begins with menstrual flow or a few hours before flow commences and lasts for 6 hours to 2 days is most characteristic of *primary dysmenorrhea*. The pain is usually crampy but may be a dull ache. It is normally located in the midline of the lower abdomen just above the symphysis. It occasionally radiates down the anterior aspect of the thighs or to the lower back.

In teenagers, endometriosis may mimic the pain of primary dysmenorrhea in that the pain may be limited to the first day of menstruation. Likewise, endometriosis should be suspected if pelvic pain occurs at times other than menstruation, such as that occurring with defecation, during intercourse, or in midcycle.

The pain of *secondary dysmenorrhea* often begins several hours or even a few days before menses and is often relieved by the menstrual flow. This pain is usually a dull, continuous, diffuse lower abdominal pain but may be crampy. Like the pain of primary dysmenorrhea, it can radiate down the thighs and into the back. *Secondary dysmenorrhea should be suspected if pain occurs during the first few cycles after menarche; pain begins after age 25; and/or there are pelvic abnormalities, infertility, and no response to nonsteroidal anti-inflammatory drugs and/or oral contraceptives.*

When *pelvic inflammatory disease* causes dysmenorrhea, the pain is greatest premenstrually and is relieved with the onset of vaginal bleeding. A common cause of secondary dysmenorrhea is *endometriosis*. The symptoms in patients with this disorder become progressively more severe with each cycle; the pain usually begins (and increases in severity) 2 to 3 days premenstrually and persists for more than 2 days after the onset of flow. It is most severe on the first and second days of bleeding. The usual drop in basal body temperature, which normally occurs 24 to 36 hours after menses, is delayed until the second or third menstrual day.

Despite the differences between primary and secondary dysmenorrhea, their symptoms can overlap and vary greatly in intensity and do not necessarily occur with every menstrual period. The physician must recognize that patients with primary dysmenorrhea may also have pelvic pathology and so have additional superimposed symptoms of secondary dysmenorrhea. These patients can have constant crampy pain beginning 1 to 2 days before menstrual flow and continuing for 2 to 3 days after menstrual flow.

ASSOCIATED SYMPTOMS

Systemic symptoms such as nausea, vomiting, diarrhea, headache, fatigue, nervousness, and dizziness are more characteristic of *primary dysmenorrhea* than secondary dysmenorrhea. If menorrhagia and colicky pain are associated with menstruation, *uterine fibroids* should be suspected, although fibroids are seldom responsible for menstrual pain. If a nonpregnant patient with an enlarged, soft uterus complains of menorrhagia and dysmenorrhea, *adenomyosis* should be suspected. Bleeding from glandular tissue located deep within the myometrium has been implicated as the cause of the pain.

The pain of *endometriosis* may continue into the intermenstrual period. Rectal pain on defecation during the menstrual period also suggests endometriosis as a cause of dysmenorrhea. When dysmenorrhea is associated with dyspareunia, rectal pain, tenesmus, backache, and urgent micturition, endometriosis should be suspected.

PRECIPITATING AND AGGRAVATING FACTORS

Primary dysmenorrhea is often associated with and aggravated by *PMS. IUDs* may cause secondary dysmenorrhea and, in some patients, may aggravate pre-existing primary dysmenorrhea. Early menarche, smoking, *menstrual flow* that continues longer than 8 days, and *emotional stress* also appear to intensify dysmenorrhea. By itself, retroversion does not cause dysmenorrhea; however, some conditions that cause retroversion also cause dysmenorrhea.

AMELIORATING FACTORS

Dysmenorrhea is not consistently alleviated by any known physical measure. Some patients may state that lying on the floor in the knee-chest position gives some relief. Dysmenorrhea that occurs soon after the onset of menarche frequently disappears as the menstrual cycles become more regular. Pregnancy often relieves primary dysmenorrhea and secondary dysmenorrhea due to endometriosis. The pain may be alleviated for several months or, on occasion, permanently.

Differential Diagnosis of Menstrual Pain

CAUSE	NATURE OF PATIENT	NATURE OF SYMPTOMS	ASSOCIATED SYMPTOMS	PRECIPITATING AND AGGRAVATING FACTORS	AMELIORAT-ING FACTORS	PHYSICAL FINDINGS	DIAGNOSTIC STUDIES
PMS		Begins 2-12 days before menses and subsides at onset or during first days of period Diffuse, dull pelvic ache May coexist with dysmenorrhea	Irritability Nervousness Headache Swelling of breasts and extremities Bloating and weight gain Breast tenderness	Emotional stress Dysmenorrhea	Menses	Breasts tender on palpation	
Primary dysmenorrhea	30%-50% of young women 95% of adolescents	Most common menstrual disorder, especially in adolescents Begins within 3-12 mo of menarche with ovulatory cycles Becomes more severe with age Pain: Just precedes or begins with menstrual flow Lasts for 6 hr to 2 days Is crampy or a dull ache Is usually in midline of lower abdomen May radiate down thighs and to lower back	Nausea and vomiting Diarrhea Headache Fatigue Nervousness Dizziness	PMS IUD Emotional stress	Pain may lessen as menstrual cycles become regular Pregnancy Oral contraceptives NSAIDs	None	

Continued

Differential Diagnosis of Menstrual Pain—cont'd

CAUSE	NATURE OF PATIENT	NATURE OF SYMPTOMS	ASSOCIATED SYMPTOMS	PRECIPITATING AND AGGRAVATING FACTORS	AMELIORATING FACTORS	PHYSICAL FINDINGS	DIAGNOSTIC STUDIES
Secondary dysmenorrhea	Older than 25 yr Often a history of recurrent pelvic inflammatory disease	Secondary to organic disease Begins years after menarche; may occur with anovulatory cycles Pain: Begins several hours before menses Is a dull, continuous, diffuse lower abdominal pain May be crampy Can radiate down thighs and to back		Cervical stenosis secondary to cervical conization or radiation IUD Pelvic abnormalities Vaginitis	Menses	Depends on cause of secondary dysmenorrhea	Papanicolaou test Tests for gonorrhea and chlamydia Laparoscopy Ultrasonography for myomas and ovarian cysts HCG Wet mounts for Candida, clue cells, and Trichomonas
Endometriosis	Usually older than 30 yr Teenagers uncommonly affected	Symptoms worsen with each cycle Pain: Begins 2-3 days before menses and persists for 2 days after May continue into intermenstrual period	Rectal pain with defecation Dyspareunia Tenesmus Backache Urgent micturition		Pregnancy Oral contraceptives	Pelvic examination best done in late luteal phase Nodularity felt in uterosacral ligaments or other sites of endometrial implants	Fern test Basal body temperature Laparoscopy Ultrasonography
Fibroids		Uncommon cause of dysmenorrhea	Menorrhagia			Uterine mass	Ultrasonography
Pelvic inflammatory disease		Pain is greatest premenstrually	Menorrhagia	Onset at menses		Cervical discharge Chandelier sign	Gonorrhea culture Leukocytosis Chlamydial culture

HCG, Human chorionic gonadotropin; IUD, intrauterine device; NSAIDs, nonsteroidal anti-inflammatory drugs; PMS, premenstrual syndrome.

Nonsteroidal anti-inflammatory drugs and oral contraceptives usually alleviate the pain of primary dysmenorrhea and endometriosis. Spontaneous alleviation of dysmenorrhea may occur with advancing age, but this is not usually the case.

PHYSICAL FINDINGS

In patients who have primary dysmenorrhea, no physical abnormalities are usually found. In patients with secondary dysmenorrhea, physical findings depend on the specific cause. When primary dysmenorrhea is considered likely, the pelvic examination should be performed while the patient is experiencing pain.

The practitioner must perform a careful physical examination to check for pelvic infection, endometriosis, pelvic mass, uterine enlargement, and other pelvic disease. When evidence of endometriosis is being sought, the pelvic examination should ideally be performed in the late luteal phase immediately before menstruation, when the endometrial implants (often in the uterosacral ligaments) are the largest and therefore most palpable. Using a laxative to promote bowel evacuation facilitates pelvic examination for endometrial implants. Special attention should focus on genital development; vaginal discharge; stigmata of pelvic infection; the appearance of the cervix; and the size, shape, consistency, and position of the uterus.

DIAGNOSTIC STUDIES

A Papanicolaou test as well as human chorionic gonadotropin, chlamydial, and gonococcal tests should be performed in all patients with secondary dysmenorrhea. Enzyme immunoassay, direct-smear immunofluorescent antibody, and DNA probe tests offer greater sensitivity and specificity. Wet-mount preparations of vaginal secretions for *Candida*, clue cells, and *Trichomonas* help diagnose vaginitis (although commercial immunoassays are currently available), which may contribute to menstrual pain. Abdominal and transvaginal ultrasonography, laparoscopy, and hysteroscopy are often useful diagnostic tools.

LESS COMMON DIAGNOSTIC CONSIDERATIONS

Less common causes of dysmenorrhea include *congenital malformations, uterine hypoplasia,* and true *cervical stenosis* or *obstruction* that results from cauterization, conization, or radiation therapy. Endometrial *carcinoma* and *tuberculosis* are rare causes of secondary dysmenorrhea. A *foreign body* (e.g., an IUD or any object inserted into the vagina) can cause dysmenorrhea.

Selected References

American College of Obstetricians and GynecologistsAmerican College of Obstetricians and Gynecologists: ACOG practice bulletin: premenstrual syndrome, *Int J Gynecol Obstet* 73:183-191, 2001.

Baines PA, Allen GM: Pelvic pain and menstrual related illnesses, *Emerg Med Clin North Am* 19:763-780, 2001.

Bulun SE: *Endometriosis. N Engl J Med* 360:268-279, 2009.

Coco AS: Primary dysmenorrhea, *Am Fam Physician* 60:489-496, 1999.

Dawood MY: Primary dysmenorrhea: advances in pathogenesis and management, *Obstet Gynecol* 108:428-441, 2006.

French L: Dysmenorrhea, *Am Fam Physician* 71:285-291, 2005.

Morrow C, Naumburg EH: Dysmenorrhea, *Prim Care* 36:19-32, 2009.

Pearlstein T, Steiner M: Premenstrual dysphoric disorder: burden of illness and treatment update, *J Psychiatry Neurosci* 33:291-301, 2008.

Rapkin AJ, Mikacich JA: Premenstrual syndrome and premenstrual dysphoric disorder in adolescents, *Curr Opin Obstet Gynecol* 20:455-463, 2008.

Ross LE, Steiner M: A biopsychosocial approach to premenstrual dysphoric disorder, *Psychiatr Clin North Am* 26:529-546, 2003.

Sanfilippo J, Erb T: Evaluation and management of dysmenorrhea in adolescents, *Clin Obstet Gynecol* 51(2):257-267, 2008.

Steiner M: Premenstrual syndromes, *Annu Rev Med* 48:447-455, 1997.

Yonkers KA, O'Brien PM, Eriksson E: Premenstrual syndrome, *Lancet* 371(9619):1200-1210, 2008.

Nausea and/or Vomiting Without Abdominal Pain

22

Chronic nausea and vomiting are not uncommon in primary care practice. Approximately 3% of the population has reported nausea once a week, and 2% reported vomiting at least once a month. The cost of acute gastrointestinal infections in the United States is thought to exceed $3.4 billion per year. *Nausea* is a vague, unpleasant sensation; it may herald the onset of vomiting or occur without vomiting. *Vomiting* is the forceful expulsion of gastric contents through the mouth and must be differentiated from *regurgitation*. The latter is an effortless backflow of small amounts of ingested food or liquid during or between meals or feedings. Dribbling of milk from a child's mouth is an example of regurgitation. When a patient complains of vomiting, it is helpful for the physician to distinguish acute from chronic and cyclic vomiting.

The most common cause of acute nausea and vomiting in adults and children is *gastroenteritis*. Other common causes are *gastritis, migraine, excessive alcohol ingestion,* certain *drugs, motion sickness,* and (in children) *otitis media*. Common causes of chronic nausea and sometimes vomiting include *pregnancy, gastritis, drugs* (especially narcotics, codeine, digitalis glycosides, antiarrhythmics, salicylates, nonsteroidal anti-inflammatory drugs [NSAIDs], theophylline, chemotherapeutic agents, and antibiotics), *uremia,* and *hepatic failure.* Recurrent nausea that occurs without vomiting is often a reaction to *environmental* or *emotional stresses.* This form of nausea is temporally related to the stressful period and usually disappears when the stress is removed.

NATURE OF PATIENT

In children (as well as adults) it is important to get a complete history that should include when vomiting started and any associated symptom or precipitating factors, the nature of emesis, the characteristics of vomitus, the frequency and forcefulness of vomiting, hydration status, ingestion of medications or poisons, and family history of gastrointestinal (GI) disease. In neonates, vomiting with the first feeding suggests *esophageal or intestinal atresia* or some other congenital GI anomaly (e.g., malrotation, Hirschsprung's disease). Abnormalities of the oropharynx, sepsis, metabolic disorders, and necrotizing enterocolitis can cause vomiting in the newborn. The most common causes of vomiting in the first year are *gastroesophageal reflux, GI infection, urinary tract infection* (UTI), *dietary protein intolerance* or *allergies,* and *septicemia.* When projectile vomiting occurs in infants younger than 3 months (usually ages 2 to 3 weeks), *pyloric stenosis* must be considered. Although it is uncommon, recurrent vomiting of bile-stained material in neonates may indicate *intestinal obstruction* due to atresia, stenosis, or volvulus of the small bowel.

The most common causes of vomiting in children are *viral* and *bacterial infections, high fevers* of any cause, and *otitis media.* Otitis media has its highest incidence in young children and may manifest as unexplained vomiting and fever. **Cyclic vomiting, with or without typical migraine symptoms, may be caused by abdominal migraine, which is more common in children.** Cyclic vomiting syndrome is itself an entity characterized by periods of intense vomiting lasting less than a week (three or more episodes per year) with symptom-free intervals in between. It is thought to be related to a mitochondrial DNA mutation and has several triggers, including infection, stress, motion sickness, lack of sleep, menstruation, exhaustion, and certain foods, such as monosodium glutamate, cheese, and chocolate.

In adults the common causes of acute nausea or vomiting are *gastritis* (alcohol or drug induced), *viral gastroenteritis, psychogenic conditions,* and, occasionally, *labyrinthine disorders.* Common viral pathogens include *rotavirus, adenovirus,* and *norovirus.* Nausea and vomiting can also be the presenting symptoms in patients with *hepatitis, myocardial infarction,* and *diabetic ketoacidosis.* Chronic vomiting in adults usually results from *gastritis, mechanical obstruction, gut motility disorders* (including *diabetic gastroparesis*), *achalasia, drugs, labyrinthine disorders,* and *uremia.* Hyperemesis gravidarum may cause chronic vomiting during pregnancy. Both *food contamination* and *chemical poisoning* must be considered as causes of vomiting, particularly if several people are affected at the same time; in cases of food poisoning, more than one person is usually experiencing symptoms. Toxins from *Staphylococccus aureus* or *Bacillus cereus* are often implicated in gastroenteritis from poorly prepared or stored foods. Nausea and vomiting of *pregnancy* must be considered in women of reproductive age; some pregnant women experience morning sickness in the first trimester of pregnancy, often before they are aware of their pregnancy.

Self-induced vomiting should be suspected in patients with anxiety, depression, or eating disorders, such as anorexia and bulimia. If these patients are questioned carefully, they may admit to a feeling of nausea, which they attempt to relieve by gagging themselves to produce vomiting. If an elderly patient presents with persistent vomiting, gastric or intestinal obstruction secondary to *neoplasm* should be suspected.

NATURE OF SYMPTOMS

When vomiting is painless or has preceded abdominal pain by a considerable period, a surgical lesion is unlikely. Repeated episodes of unexplained vomiting and nausea may indicate *pancreatitis,* which is not always associated with abdominal pain. Persistent vomiting without any bile staining is an indication of *pyloric obstruction.* In children this may be caused by *pyloric stenosis,* and in adults, by ulcer scarring or tumor. Vomiting or regurgitation of undigested food indicates *esophageal obstruction.* Vomiting secondary to *increased intracranial pressure* (ICP) is often projectile and not preceded by nausea.

Nausea and vomiting are frequent manifestations of *digitalis toxicity.* These symptoms are not necessarily from high serum levels of the digitalis glycoside; a GI adverse effect of the drug may occur at normal serum levels. Although many patients with *gastritis* have abdominal pain, some patients experience unexplained nausea or vomiting without pain. *Substance abuse* (alcohol, caffeine, and drugs) may also be associated with unexplained nausea or vomiting. Prolonged use of marijuana can cause chronic nausea, which is often relieved with a hot shower.

When children vomit more than four times per hour, cyclic vomiting due to abdominal migraine is probable. It usually occurs a few times a month. Chronic vomiting once or twice an hour that occurs around 30 times a month is usually caused by peptic or infectious GI disorders.

The timing of vomiting may be of diagnostic importance. Patients with *uremia, pregnant* women, and *chronic alcoholics* often experience early-morning nausea and vomiting. Vomiting immediately before food is ingested may be a manifestation of *anxiety, depression, or an eating disorder,* whereas vomiting shortly after eating may be a consequence of *gastric outlet obstruction* caused by a pyloric channel ulcer, adenocarcinoma, or other infiltrative lesions.

Postprandial vomiting may also be of *functional origin,* although organic gastric disease should be suspected. The Rome III criteria define three separate entities of functional nausea and vomiting: chronic idiopathic nausea, cyclic vomiting syndrome, and functional vomiting. Criteria for these entities are presented in the table "Differential Diagnosis Nausea and/or Vomiting without Abdominal Pain" at the end of the chapter. Vomiting soon after eating occurs frequently in patients with *gastritis* and those with *digitalis toxicity.* Vomiting that begins 20 to 40 minutes after meals suggests *gastric atony* associated with diabetes, prior gastric surgery, or peritonitis. If vomiting begins 1 to 2 hours after a meal, disease of the biliary tract or pancreas may be the cause. In these latter instances, pain is usually not relieved by vomiting. Recurrent vomiting that occurs 1 to 4 hours after eating may be due to gastric or duodenal lesions causing *gastric outlet obstruction.* Vomiting that follows and relieves an episode of epigastric pain is usually caused by an *intragastric lesion* or *pyloric spasm.*

The odor of vomitus may also provide a clue to the cause. If the vomitus lacks the pungent odor of gastric acid, a *dilated esophagus* (possibly from a stricture or achalasia) may be the cause. Patients with this condition frequently vomit in the morning and vomit or regurgitate undigested food. If vomitus has a fecal odor, *intestinal obstruction* or a *gastrocolic fistula* should be suspected.

ASSOCIATED SYMPTOMS

If headache (especially a unilateral one) is associated with nausea or vomiting, *migraine* should be suspected. Occasionally, recurrent or cyclic nausea and vomiting may be the only manifestations of migraine; acephalic migraine is more common in children and adolescents. If vertigo and tinnitus are associated with nausea and vomiting, *Ménière's syndrome or disease* or other middle ear disturbances should be considered. If symptoms of depression are present with little or no weight loss despite a history of long-standing emesis, psychogenic vomiting is probable. Anxiety, and to a lesser degree depression, may cause chronic or recurrent nausea. As with *anorexia nervosa,* women experience psychogenic vomiting more often than men.

If chest pain or other symptoms of myocardial infarction (MI) are associated with vomiting, the vomiting may be caused by myocardial infarction. Nausea and vomiting often precede the development of chest pain. Chest pain and vomiting are rarely caused by a strangulated diaphragmatic hernia. In these instances, electrocardiographic (ECG) abnormalities may erroneously suggest posterior infarction.

Acute nausea and vomiting associated with diarrhea and occasionally with abdominal pain are most often caused by *gastroenteritis.* When vertigo accompanies vomiting, *labyrinthine disorders* should be suspected. When vomiting without vertigo is induced by a recumbent posture, a *posterior fossa lesion* should be suspected. Vomiting may be the initial manifestation of *diabetic ketoacidosis.* It is a particularly common presentation in patients with juvenile diabetes.

PRECIPITATING AND AGGRAVATING FACTORS

Nausea and vomiting are frequently precipitated by *medications* such as digitalis, theophylline, quinidine, potassium preparations, chemotherapeutic agents, antibiotics, narcotics, hormone preparations, and antihypertensives. Iron preparations, salicylates, and nonsteroidal anti-inflammatory drugs s also cause nausea and occasionally vomiting. *Nicotine* poisoning and excessive use of nicotine patches and gum may cause vomiting. *Radiation therapy* may also cause nausea and vomiting.

Anticipatory nausea and vomiting may occur before radiation therapy or chemotherapy, especially in anxious patients. *Postoperative nausea and vomiting,* no longer attributed to anesthetic agents, occurs often and is usually caused by central mechanisms and perioperative medications. If vomiting is preceded by a cough, it may be the primary manifestation of *asthma* when wheezing is trivial or not present.

AMELIORATING FACTORS

Vomiting usually relieves the symptoms of fullness and pain caused by pyloric obstruction. Vomiting relieves nausea if it is being caused by nauseating substances in the stomach. It does not usually alleviate nausea caused by gastroenteritis, gastritis, uremia, or drugs that cause nausea through a central effect.

PHYSICAL FINDINGS

The presence of fever in a vomiting patient suggests that *infection* is causative. The presence of hypotension, dehydration, abdominal mass, or weight loss suggests more serious etiologies. In children, physical findings of *otitis media* suggest that it may be the probable cause of the vomiting. A walnut-size mass may be palpable in the epigastrium of infants with *hypertrophic pyloric stenosis*. A cloudy sensorium, focal neurologic deficits, or papilledema suggests an *intracranial lesion*, whereas nystagmus suggests a labyrinthine cause. Jaundice or hepatomegaly suggests *hepatitis* or *cirrhosis* as the cause. A distended abdomen accompanying nausea and vomiting may indicate *paralytic ileus* or *mechanical obstruction* of the intestine. Abdominal tenderness, distention, and occasionally visible peristalsis suggest *GI obstruction*. A succussion splash suggests *diabetic gastroparesis*. The location of abdominal pain may provide clues about which organ is responsible for the symptoms.

Chronic vomiting results in weight loss. If a patient's weight is maintained despite a history of chronic nausea and vomiting, the origin of symptoms is probably *psychogenic*. When an infant has chronic post-feeding *non-bilious* vomiting that is *not* projectile *and* continues to thrive, this latter observation is reassuring, and watchful waiting may be appropriate. Decreased skin turgor suggests that the vomiting has caused significant fluid loss. Physical findings consistent with congestive heart failure (e.g., tachycardia, gallop, peripheral edema) suggest that nausea may be from *hepatic capsule distention* and *mesenteric congestion*.

DIAGNOSTIC STUDIES

Initial studies to investigate nausea and vomiting that is not self-limited usually include a complete blood cell count and a complete metabolic profile. Serum amylase and lipase measurements should be included if pancreatitis is suspected. Urine and blood cultures may help determine whether a systemic infection is involved. A urine or serum pregnancy test should be performed in all women of child-bearing age. Plain films of the abdomen may be ordered if an obstruction is suspected. Further studies are guided by the clinical presentation and may include an upper GI series, endoscopy, and abdominal computed tomography (CT) with intravenous and oral contrast material. Ultrasonography is the diagnostic procedure of choice for the diagnosis of *infantile hypertrophic pyloric stenosis* as well as *cholecystitis*. Detailed neurologic studies, including spinal tap and brain magnetic resonance imaging (MRI) or CT, should be performed only if an intracranial process is suspected. A metabolic cause may be suspected if laboratory test results include abnormal serum levels of substances such as urea nitrogen, creatinine, glucose, bilirubin, and calcium. Digitalis excess may be diagnosed on the basis of elevated serum digitalis values. Toxicology screening may detect toxins and drugs that cause vomiting.

Differential Diagnosis of Nausea and/or Vomiting Without Abdominal Pain

CAUSE	NATURE OF PATIENT	NATURE OF SYMPTOMS	ASSOCIATED SYMPTOMS	PRECIPITATING AND AGGRAVATING FACTORS	PHYSICAL FINDINGS	DIAGNOSTIC STUDIES
Gastroenteritis	Most common cause at any age	Acute nausea and vomiting	Diarrhea Fever Abdominal pain		Hyperactive peristalsis	
Gastritis		Acute or chronic nausea and vomiting occur postprandially	Abdominal pain	Viral infection Alcohol or drug induced		Endoscopy
Viral or bacterial infection	Common cause of vomiting in children	Acute nausea and vomiting	Fever		High temperature	
Drugs		Acute or chronic nausea and vomiting		Chemotherapeutic agents Codeine Digitalis glycosides Quinidine Salicylates Theophylline Antihypertensives Antibiotics		Serum drug level measurements
		Postprandial vomiting		Iron preparations Proton pump blockers Nonsteroidal anti-inflammatory drugs Nicotine (also patches, gum)		
Otitis media	Children	Acute nausea and vomiting	Fever Earache		Inflamed tympanic membrane	
Excessive alcohol ingestion	Alcoholics Social drinkers	Early-morning vomiting				Gastroscopy

Condition	Nature of Patient	Nature of Symptoms	Associated Symptoms	Predisposing Factors	Physical Findings	Diagnostic Studies
Uremia		Chronic nausea and vomiting Usually in early morning				Elevated blood urea nitrogen and serum creatinine measurements
Morning sickness	Pregnant females	Early-morning nausea and vomiting Usually in first trimester				Serum human chorionic gonadotropin measurement
Environmental or emotional stresses		Episodic nausea usually without vomiting				
Diabetic gastroparesis	Diabetics				Succussion splash	Radiograph of abdomen
Pyloric obstruction	In infants aged <3 mo, may be due to pyloric stenosis In adults, may be secondary to ulcer scarring or tumor	Projectile vomiting	Abdominal pain		Palpable mass Succussion splash	Ultrasonography
Esophageal obstruction and achalasia		Vomiting or regurgitation of undigested food Odorless vomitus Usually occurs in early morning or after large meals				Esophageal radiograph Endoscopy
Increased intracranial pressure		Projectile vomiting not preceded by nausea			Papilledema	Neurologic examination Spinal fluid analysis, CT
Pancreatitis	Alcoholics	Repeated episodes of unexplained nausea and vomiting	Abdominal pain	Excessive alcohol intake		Elevated serum amylase value CT scan of pancreas

More sophisticated tests include radioisotope studies of liquid and solid gastric emptying as well as esophageal pH and motility studies. Enteroclysis or capsule endoscopy may be used to investigate the small bowel. Psychiatric assessment, including the Minnesota Multiphasic Personality Inventory, may also be helpful.

LESS COMMON DIAGNOSTIC CONSIDERATIONS

Several writers have categorized the causes of vomiting as follows: allergies, cerebromedullary factors, toxins, visceral problems, deficiency states, and motion sickness. *GI allergies* should be considered if sudden nausea or vomiting consistently follows ingestion of specific food. The less common *cerebromedullary causes* include increased intracranial pressure, trauma, cerebral tumors, abscesses, hydrocephalus, intracranial hemorrhage, and acephalic migraine. *Hepatic coma* and *Addison's disease* are less common causes of nausea and vomiting. *GI disorders,* such as the cyclic vomiting syndrome, gastroparesis, ulcers, obstructive tumors (particularly those of the stomach and proximal small bowel), adhesive bands, volvulus, eosinophilic esophagitis, eosinophilic gastroenteritis, *Helicobacter pylori* infection, and Crohn's disease, may also cause nausea and vomiting. *Blood* in the GI tract is another cause.

Patients with *pyelonephritis* and *pelvic inflammatory disease* may present with a chief complaint of vomiting, particularly if they also have reflex ileus. Patients with *anorexia nervosa,* particularly in the early stages, may induce the vomiting. However, because anorectic patients seldom complain of this symptom, it may be difficult for the physician to diagnose the condition before pronounced weight loss has occurred. Vomiting may also be caused by conditions that alter neural control of gut motility.

Selected References

Acker ME: Vomiting in children, *Adv Nurse Pract* 10:51-56, 2002:68.

American Gastroenterology Association Medical Position Statement: Nausea and vomiting, *Gastroenterology* 120:261-262, 2001.

Camilleri M: Gastrointestinal problems in diabetes, *Endocrinol Metab Clin North Am* 25:361-378, 1996.

Chandran L, Chitkara M: Vomiting in children: reassurance, red flag, or referral? *Pediatrics in Review* 29:183-192, 2008.

Haug TT, Mykletum A, Dahl AA: The prevalence of nausea in the community: psychological, social, and somatic factors, *Gen Hosp Psychiatry* 24:81-86, 2002.

Khan S, Di Lorenzo C: Chronic vomiting in children: new insights into diagnosis, *Curr Gastroenterol Rep* 3:248-256, 2001.

Li BU, Lefevre F, Chelimsky GG, et al: North American Society for Pediatric Gastroenterology, Hepatology, and Nutrition consensus statement on the diagnosis and management of cyclic vomiting syndrome, *J Pediatr Gastroenterol Nutr* 47:379-393, 2008.

Metz A, Hebbard G: Nausea and vomiting in adults—a diagnostic approach, *Austral Fam Physician* 36:688-692, 2007.

Olden KW, Chepyala P: Functional nausea and vomiting, *Nature Clin Pract Gastroenterol Hepatol* 5:202-208, 2008.

Pareek N, Fleisher DR, Abell T: Cyclic vomiting syndrome: what a gastroenterologist needs to know, *Am J Gastroenterol* 102:2832-2840, 2007.

Quigley EMM, Hasler WH, Parkman HP: AGA technical review on nausea and vomiting, *Gastroenterology* 120:263-286, 2001.

Quinlan JD, Hill DA: Nausea and vomiting of pregnancy, *Am Fam Physician* 68:121-128, 2003.

Rollins MD, Shields MD, Quinn RJM, et al: Value of ultrasound in differentiating causes of persistent vomiting in infants, *Gut* 32:612-614, 1991.

Scorza K, Williams A: Evaluation of nausea and vomiting, *Am Fam Physician* 76:76-84, 2007.

Pain in the Foot

23

Foot pain is usually caused by inappropriate footwear, local disease, or an abnormality but occasionally results from referred pain. Therefore, examination of the foot should begin with the spine and proceed distally. Foot pain is often caused by *muscular* or *ligamentous strain* associated with *trauma,* unaccustomed or strenuous *physical activity,* and *sports.* Women frequently experience foot pain from new shoes or a change in shoe heel height. Other common causes are *gout; rheumatoid arthritis,* which usually affects the forefoot and midfoot; *plantar warts; callosity;* and *metatarsal stress fracture (march fracture).* Isolated pain in the heel can result from *plantar fasciitis, subcalcaneal syndrome, arterial insufficiency, Achilles tendinitis* or *bursitis,* and *jogger's trauma.* In adolescents, pain in the heel may be caused by *calcaneal apophysitis.*

NATURE OF PATIENT

Foot pain in children is rare. When it does occur, it usually results from acute bone and ligament injuries or bone-tendon disorders such as traction apophysitis (Sever's disease), which causes pain at the posterior and superior tip of the calcaneus. Overuse syndrome, especially Achilles tendinitis, often occurs in teenagers. It is caused only rarely by tumors, infections, or juvenile arthritis.

Because foot pain usually results from *muscular* or *ligamentous strain,* it is more likely to occur in people who are physically active, particularly those who are unaccustomed to physical exercise and muscular strain in their feet, such as unconditioned athletes and "weekend athletes." The gradual development of forefoot pain in a new military recruit suggests a *metatarsal stress fracture,* which is most common in the second metatarsal, followed by the third and fourth metatarsals. Joggers and runners may experience *Achilles tendinitis, tarsal tunnel syndrome,* or *plantar fasciitis.* Ankle sprains and repetitive injuries are common in ballet dancers and athletes. Ankle pain can occur in rheumatoid arthritis and Lyme disease.

Gout is more common in men older than 40 years but does occur in women, especially those who are postmenopausal. The patient may present with a history of previous attacks of painful joints or urolithiasis. Often a family history of gout may be elicited.

Pain in the heel caused by *plantar fasciitis* and its associated soft tissue irritation is most common in obese patients older than 40 years. When adolescents complain of pain in the heel, it most likely is caused by *calcaneal apophysitis*. *Achilles tendinitis,* which also causes heel pain, is usually caused by trauma (e.g., injury from jogging), although the trauma may not be recalled by the patient. Achilles tendinitis is more common in patients with Reiter's syndrome and ankylosing spondylitis who are positive for human leukocyte antigen (HLA) B27, even without a history of trauma. The physician should ask about recent use of fluoroquinolone antibiotics because this class of medications is known to increase risk of both Achilles tendinitis and tendon rupture. In patients with *rheumatoid arthritis,* foot pain is second in frequency only to knee pain, which is most common. In a diabetic patient, pain in an otherwise insensate foot may indicate Charcot's foot, a form of neuroarthropathy. However, this condition manifests as erythema, warmth, and swelling of the foot, so osteomyelitis, arterial insufficiency, and deep vein thrombosis need to be considered.

NATURE OF SYMPTOMS

As with other types of pain, a careful history of the location (forefoot, midfoot, or hindfoot) and quality of the pain (how it began, what intensifies it) is most helpful in determining its cause.

Forefoot pain, generally referred to as *metatarsalgia,* has many causes. They include metatarsal stress fracture, interdigital neuroma, Freiberg's infraction, gout, sesamoiditis, synovitis or dislocation of the metatarsophalangeal (MTP) joint, plantar warts, and atrophy of the plantar fat pad. *Midfoot pain* is an infrequent complaint but usually results from tendinitis or acquired flatfoot. *Inferior heel pain* is often used to describe *hindfoot pain*. This common complaint is most commonly caused by plantar fasciitis. Other common causes are calcaneal apophysitis, heel pad fat atrophy, nerve entrapment, tarsal tunnel syndrome, and arterial insufficiency. *Posterior heel pain* is usually due to Achilles tendinitis or rupture.

Foot pain described as a dull ache is probably caused by *foot strain*. This is more likely to occur in older adults, overweight people, people wearing new shoes, and those who are on their feet for much of the day. It is critical that the physician establish the precise location of the ache because this fact determines which ligaments, tendons, or fascia is involved (torn or under strain). For example, pain below the ankle on the inner aspect of the heel suggests a tear or strain of the ligamentous fibers attached to the internal malleolus. Symptoms such as burning, tingling, or numbness suggest *neuropathy*.

Plantar warts and *callosity* can cause severe pain, particularly with weight bearing. These conditions are typically located on the plantar surface of the foot in the metatarsal region. Pain from a *calcaneal spur* or *plantar fasciitis* is usually continuous, although it may worsen with weight bearing. The spur is usually located in the center of the undersurface of the heel, about 2.25 cm from the back of the foot; however, the pain may be more toward the back of the heel. The condition called *jogger's foot* or *tarsal tunnel syndrome* may produce the complaint of a burning pain in the heel, aching in the arch, or diminished sensation in the sole behind the large toe.

Patients with entrapment of the tibial nerve (tarsal tunnel syndrome) may report poorly localized burning pain around the medial malleolus that radiates to the plantar surface of the foot and toes.

The pain of *Achilles tendinitis* is usually over the Achilles tendon and may be associated with tenderness on palpation and swelling.

With *gout* the pain is usually acute, frequently recurrent, and often agonizing, although atypical cases of gout may cause less severe symptoms. The attacks usually have a sudden onset and characteristically start during the early hours of the day, while the patient is still in bed. Before gout is diagnosed, the patient may attribute the bouts of pain to minor trauma such as "stubbing the toe" or "spraining" the involved joint. Once the diagnosis of gout has been established, the patient usually recognizes subsequent attacks. Although the MTP joint of the big toe is classically affected, one or more other joints, including the ankle, may also be affected.

In general, systemic causes of foot pain, such as gout, rheumatoid arthritis, and diabetes occur at rest, whereas biomechanical causes of foot pain, such as sprains and calcaneal spurs, occur with ambulation and decrease with rest.

PRECIPITATING AND AGGRAVATING FACTORS

Most foot pain is precipitated by *trauma*, unaccustomed or strenuous *physical activity*, and *athletics*. A change in occupation or work that involves constant jarring of the foot or walking or standing on concrete floors may lead to foot strain. Constant vibration or jarring frequently leads to heel pain that may result from calcaneal periostitis. Likewise, new shoes or a change in heel size can lead to foot strain.

Gouty pain in the foot may have no particular precipitating factors, although several reports have indicated that a gouty diathesis may be caused by minor trauma to the involved joint.

PHYSICAL FINDINGS

The foot should be examined with the patient bearing weight and not bearing weight on it. The gait should be observed, as should be the knees and hips during walking. In addition to careful examination of the foot for local discoloration, coldness, hair loss, swelling, and areas tender on palpation, a careful examination of the lower back and legs should be performed in patients who complain of foot pain, because foot pain may result from referred pain. A painful, discolored (red) foot with pallor on elevation suggests ischemia.

Pain with medial to lateral compression of the calcaneus suggests a stress fracture. When pain is caused by *foot strain*, the forefoot may flatten on weight bearing, and there may be calluses under the metatarsal heads. With *metatarsal stress fracture*, the head of the involved metatarsal is tender on palpation. With *interdigital neuroma*, the examiner can reproduce pain often radiating to the toe by performing interdigital palpation with one hand and application of side-to-side pressure with the other. When the pain is from *gout*, there is usually a warm, violaceous, tender, swollen joint, typically the MTP joint of the big toe or the ankle. Tophi may be present in the foot, other joints, or the ear lobe.

When the pain is from a *calcaneal spur* or *plantar fasciitis*, there may be spot tenderness with deep palpation, particularly on the undersurface of the heel. If this finding is associated with radiographic evidence of a calcaneal spur, the diagnosis is obvious. In cases with radiographic confirmation of a calcaneal spur, the pain may be caused by plantar fasciitis.

Although the diagnosis of *ankle sprain* is usually obvious from the history, patients may not remember the traumatic incident. Sprained ankles most often result from an inversion injury and have tenderness and swelling over the anterior talofibular ligament. Likewise, *fractures* are usually associated with a history of significant trauma. A radiograph is usually necessary to diagnose small fractures of the ankle. In patients with a history suggesting a sprained ankle, the Ottawa ankle and foot rules can be applied to determine the need for a radiograph. An ankle radiograph is required if there is pain in the malleolar area along with one of the following findings: tenderness at the posterior edge of the lateral or medial malleolus and the inability to bear weight (walk 4 steps) immediately and at evaluation. A foot radiograph is required if there is pain in the midfoot along with one of the following: bony tenderness at the base of the fifth metatarsal or at the navicular and inability to walk 4 steps at the time of the injury and at evaluation. These rules have been found to be 97% sensitive and 31% specific for fractures of the ankle and foot.

Bunions can also cause foot pain, particularly at the MTP joint. This pain is usually worse with extension of the big toe. *Heel fasciitis*, also called *calcaneal periostitis*, may produce chronic pain in the bottom of the foot. Patients with this condition usually have pain and tenderness localized to the insertion of the long plantar tendon into the base of the calcaneus. When *peripheral ischemia* gives rise to isolated heel pain without other evidence of peripheral vascular disease, there is often cornification of the heel skin and coolness in this area.

DIAGNOSTIC STUDIES

Doppler ultrasonography studies help the physician detect arterial insufficiency. Radiographs may demonstrate calcaneal spurs and fractures, including small stress fractures, although magnetic resonance imaging (MRI) is often required to detect stress fractures. Arthropathies, including Charcot foot, can be detected on plain radiographs. Quantitative scintigraphs help the physician identify abnormal weight distribution and its associated fasciitis. MRI is often helpful in diagnosing midfoot and forefoot problems in some patients as well as nerve entrapment, such as tarsal tunnel syndrome. Occasionally, a computed tomography (CT) scan or arthroscopic examination is helpful. Ultrasonography is helpful in the diagnosis of plantar fasciitis. Bone scans may detect avascular necrosis, stress fracture, osteomyelitis, or (rarely) metastatic carcinoma.

In children, less common causes of heel pain include enthesopathy (inflammation of the cartilaginous attachment of ligaments and tendons to bone), juvenile arthritis, fractures, and tumors.

LESS COMMON DIAGNOSTIC CONSIDERATIONS

Metatarsalgia is not a cause but a symptom of pain in the forefoot (Table 23-1). *Primary metatarsalgia* is pain in the forefoot due to a chronic disorder of weight distribution across the MTP joints. Pain in the metatarsal region can result from other local processes (e.g., plantar warts, tarsal tunnel syndrome, plantar fasciitis) or systemic disease (e.g., rheumatoid arthritis, sesamoiditis, gout). *Neuralgia* and *polyneuritis* from alcohol ingestion, lead poisoning, or diabetes may produce pain in one or both feet. In addition, affected patients frequently complain of burning sensations or paresthesias of the soles. Decreased tactile and vibratory sensations may be observed on physical examination.

If foot pain is precisely located on the plantar surface between a pair of metatarsal heads, *Morton's neuroma* should be suspected (Fig. 23-1). This relatively rare condition is more common in women than men. The usual history is foot pain for 2 or more years that is relieved by shoe removal and unchanged by conservative measures. This pain is often described as *burning, shooting, needles, daggers*, or *like walking on a stone*. It may radiate to the toes. Patients may complain of numbness and tingling. Physical findings include pain with compression of the toes, a palpable click after the release of pressure in the affected area, occasional swelling, and some sensory changes. The pain is precipitated by walking and is aggravated by compression of the toes and weight bearing.

In addition to having tingling and numbness, patients with *Raynaud's disease* may present with pain in the toes that is often associated with pain in the fingers. These pains may be precipitated by exposure to cold, emotional stress, beta blockers, and cigarette smoking. Patients with *Fabry's disease*,

TABLE 23-1.   Forefoot Pain: 23 Diagnoses in 98 Patients

DIAGNOSIS	NUMBER
Primary Metatarsalgia	
Static disorders	12
Iatrogenic (postoperative)	12
Secondary to hallux valgus	9
Hallux rigidus	3
Morton's foot (neuroma)	3
Congenital	3
Long first ray	2
Freiberg's disease	1
Total	45
Secondary Metatarsalgia	
Rheumatoid arthritis	11
Sesamoiditis	10
Post-traumatic	4
Neurogenic	3
Stress fractures	2
Gout	1
Short ipsilateral lower limb	2
Total	33
Pain under Forepart of Foot	
Morton's neuroma	5
Plantar fasciitis	3
Causalgia	2
Tarsal tunnel syndrome	2
Tumors	2
Intermittent claudication	1
Buerger's disease	1
Plantar verrucae (warts)	4
Total	20

Modified from Scranton PE: Metatarsalgia: diagnosis and treatment. J Bone Joint Surg 62:723-732, 1980.

a recessively inherited disorder linked to the X chromosome, may present with disabling crises of burning pain in the feet and hands. Some patients with *rheumatoid arthritis* have marked prominence of the metatarsal heads with pain in this region. Bilateral ankle pain may occur in patients with acute sarcoid arthritis, which may be associated with a reddish-bluish dislocation around the ankle.

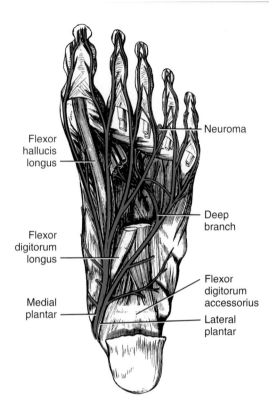

Neuroma

Flexor
hallucis
longus

Deep
branch

Flexor
digitorum
longus

Flexor
digitorum
accessorius

Medial
plantar

Lateral
plantar

Figure 23-1. Anatomy of Morton's neuroma. (From Morris MA: Morton's metatarsalgia. Clin Orthop Rel Res 127:203-207, 1977.)

Foot ulcerations, which are not necessarily associated with significant pain, can occur in patients with diabetes mellitus, tabes dorsalis, leprosy, paraplegia, Raynaud's disease, and thromboangiitis obliterans (Buerger's disease). These conditions should be suspected whenever an ulcer exists without much pain. They may all cause some degree of neuropathy that interferes with pain perception.

Erythromelalgia is painful dilatation of the superficial vessels of the foot. The pain is burning in quality and may be severe. It may be seen in patients with lead poisoning, polycythemia, or syringomyelia and in some psychologically disturbed patients.

Differential Diagnosis of Foot Pain

CAUSE	NATURE OF PATIENT	NATURE OF SYMPTOMS	PRECIPITATING AND AGGRAVATING FACTORS	PHYSICAL FINDINGS	DIAGNOSTIC STUDIES
Muscular and ligamentous strain	Physically active, especially those unaccustomed to exercise	Pain in region of strained muscles or ligaments	Trauma Unaccustomed or strenuous physical activity	Localized tenderness on palpation	
Tarsal tunnel syndrome	Nonspecific	Poorly localized numbness and burning, medial malleolus	Exercise, night pain	Presence of Tinel's sign, pain with dorsiflexion	MRI or nerve conduction study may be needed
Charcot foot	Diabetic	Diffuse pain in otherwise insensate foot	Worse with walking	Warmth, erythema, edema Vascular or infectious process may need to be ruled out	Radiography, CT
Foot strain	Older adults Overweight patients	Dull ache in foot, especially forefoot	New shoes Change in heel size Prolonged standing	Forefoot may splay with weight bearing	
Plantar warts and callosity		Pain on plantar surface in metatarsal region	Weight bearing	Plantar callosity	
Jogger's foot	Joggers	Burning in heel Aching in arch			
Fractures	Patients with history of trauma Joggers		Trauma	Decreased sensation behind big toe	Radiography or MRI may be needed to diagnose small fractures of ankle and march fractures of metatarsals

Continued

Differential Diagnosis of Foot Pain—cont'd

CAUSE	NATURE OF PATIENT	NATURE OF SYMPTOMS	PRECIPITATING AND AGGRAVATING FACTORS	PHYSICAL FINDINGS	DIAGNOSTIC STUDIES
Calcaneal spur or plantar fasciitis		Pain on undersurface of heel Continuous 2.25 cm (1 inch) from back of heel	Worse with weight bearing	Worse with dorsiflexion of toes	Radiography may show calcaneal spur Ultrasonography
Achilles tendinitis or bursitis	Joggers	Heel pain over Achilles tendon	Trauma Running	Swelling and tenderness over Achilles tendon	
Calcaneal apophysitis	Adolescents	Pain in back of heel	Running and jumping	Pain on palpation of Achilles tendon insertion	
Arterial insufficiency	Older adults Diabetics	Rest pain in heel or toes		Coolness Decreased pulses Cornification of heel skin	Arteriography
Gout	Males, especially >40 yr old Postmenopausal females	Acute, severe pain in big toe metatarsophalangeal joint and occasionally other toes or ankle	Trauma	Warm, violaceous, tender, swollen joints	Uric acid Radiography

CT, Computed tomography; *MRI,* magnetic resonance imaging.

Selected References

Aldrige T: Diagnosing heel pain in adults, *Am Fam Physician* 70:332-338, 2004.

Ashman CJ, Klecker RJ, Yu JS: Forefoot pain involving the metatarsal region: differential diagnosis with MR imaging, *Radiographics* 21:1425-1440, 2001.

Balint GP, Korda J, Hangody L, et al: Foot and ankle disorders, *Best Pract Res Clin Rheumatol* 17:887-911, 2003.

Barrett SL, O'Malley R: Plantar fasciitis and other causes of heel pain, *Am Fam Physician* 59: 2200-2206, 1999.

Becker MA, Ruoff GE: What do I need to know about gout? *J Fam Pract* 59(Suppl):S1-S8, 2010.

Bessen T, Clark R, Shakib S, et al: A multifaceted strategy for implementation of the Ottawa ankle rules in two emergency departments, *BMJ* 339:b3056, 2009.

Buchbinder R: Plantar fasciitis, *N Engl J Med* 350:2159-2166, 2004.

Buttke J: Identifying the Charcot foot, *Adv Skin Wound Care* 19:189-190, 2006.

Clemow C, Pope B, Woodall HE: Tools to speed your heel pain diagnosis, *J Fam Pract* 57:714-723, 2008.

Dalinka MK, Alazraki N, Berquist TH, et al: Imaging evaluation of suspected ankle fractures. American College of Radiology. ACR Appropriateness Criteria, *Radiology* 215(Suppl):239-241, 2000.

Di Marcangelo MT, Yu TC: Diagnostic imaging of heel pain and plantar fasciitis, *Clin Podiatr Med Surg* 14:281-301, 1997.

Frykberg RG, Zgonis T, Armstrong DG, et al: Diabetic foot disorders: a clinical practice guideline (2006 revision). [Update of J Foot Ankle Surg. 2000;39(Suppl):S1–S60; PMID: 17280936]. J Foot Ankle Surg 45(Suppl):S1-S66, 2006.

Gibbon WW, Cassar-Pullicino VN: Heel pain, *Ann Rheum Dis* 53:344-348, 1994.

Joong MA, El-Khoury GY: Radiologic evaluation of chronic foot pain, *Am Fam Physician* 76: 975-983, 2007.

Markinson BC: Three-step approach to in-office assessment of the geriatric foot, *Geriatrics* 56: 48-52, 2001.

Richette P, Bardin T: Gout. *Lancet* 375(9711):318-328, 2010.

Stern SH: Ankle and foot pain, *Prim Care* 15:809-826, 1988.

Van Wyngarden TM: The painful foot, part I: common forefoot deformities, *Am Fam Physician* 55:1866-1876, 1997.

West SG, Woodburn J: Pain in the foot, *Br Med J* 310:860-864, 1995.

24 Pain in the Lower Extremity in Adults

To diagnose pain in the lower extremity accurately, the physician must determine whether the pain is *articular* (hip, knee, or ankle) or *nonarticular* (muscular, vascular, or neurologic). In addition, the examiner should note whether the pain is present at rest or is primarily associated with exercise. The most likely causes of pain in a child's leg are different from those in an adult. Therefore, lower extremity pain in adults and lower extremity pain and a limp in children are reviewed in separate chapters.

In adults the most common causes of leg pain are *muscular* and *ligamentous strains; degenerative joint disease* (DJD), particularly of the hip and knee; *intermittent claudication* due to arterial insufficiency; *spinal stenosis; sciatica; night cramps; varicose veins; thrombophlebitis; gout;* and *trauma.* **The major clues to diagnoses are as follows:**
1. The location of the pain
2. The age of the patient, and
3. Whether the pain is related to exertion

NATURE OF PATIENT

Knee pain in children and adolescents is usually due to patellar subluxation, patellar tendinitis, tibial apophysitis, or musculoligamentous strain.

The most common cause of leg pain in adults is *muscular or ligamentous strain,* seen more frequently in "weekend athletes." Questioning usually reveals a history of unusual or strenuous exercise. The usual causes of leg pain in joggers and runners are *shin splints, stress fractures,* and *compartment syndromes.* The most common is shin splints, a musculotendinous inflammation of the anterior tibia that occasionally involves the periosteum. The pain is usually on the anterior aspect of the tibia, particularly the distal third along the medial crest, but it can occur on the lateral aspect of the tibia as well. Shin splints are most common in less well-conditioned athletes and are most frequently reported early in the running season. Skiers often experience anterior knee pain due to *patellofemoral problems.*

272

Anterior knee pain due to abnormal patellar tracking is more common in women and adolescents. Patellar problems are more common in young women, often beginning in adolescence. During pregnancy the common causes of painful legs include *venous insufficiency, postphlebitic syndrome, thrombophlebitis, muscle cramps,* and *trauma.* Patients who kneel frequently (carpet installers and floor washers) often have prepatellar bursitis.

DJD is uncommon in patients younger than 40 years unless it has been facilitated by unequal leg length (causing DJD of the hip) or prior trauma, such as athletic injuries of the knee. After age 40, pain in the hip or knee is typically caused by DJD. Sports injuries, including trauma, ligamentous sprains and tears, meniscal tears, and overuse syndromes, are also more common in adults older than 40 years. Inflammatory arthritis includes rheumatoid arthritis, septic arthritis, and gout. Osteoarthritis and Baker's cyst occur more frequently in older adults.

In patients age 50 or older, calf pain precipitated by walking or exercise that abates with rest is most likely from *peripheral arterial insufficiency (peripheral artery disease).* **Pain in the hip from intermittent claudication is seen in patients with aortoiliac disease.** When exercise-induced calf pain occurs in younger adults, frequently with a history of phlebitis, *venous claudication* is probable. *Gout* is most common in older men but can occur in women, particularly those who have had early menopause (natural or surgically induced). Patients with gout may or may not have a family history of the condition. Often a history of a prior attack can be elicited. Classic gouty pain occurs in the big toe, but it may occur in other toes or the ankles or knees; it is rare in the hip.

NATURE OF SYMPTOMS

Anterior knee pain is most often caused by *patellar tendinitis, patellofemoral malalignment,* or *chondromalacia patellae* (also known as *anterior knee pain syndrome*). Pain due to patellofemoral malalignment is usually aching in quality, has a gradual onset, and is located in the peripatellar region. It is often bilateral and is worse with activity such as stair climbing, hill climbing, skiing, and squatting and after prolonged sitting. Sharp pain in the knee, particularly the medial aspect, suggests *synovial impingement* or structural difficulties such as loose bodies. Aching joint pain is usually seen in inflammatory conditions with diffuse involvement of the synovium, such as those found in *rheumatoid arthritis.*

Degenerative Joint Disease
When the knee or hip joints are painful and stiff in the morning, improve during the day, and worsen toward the end of the day, DJD is probable. Osteoarthritis (DJD) usually occurs in older patients but may occur earlier under special circumstances. These pains may be exacerbated by certain activities (e.g., descending stairs). Patients with osteoarthritis of the hip may present with pain in the groin or the knee. Therefore, the diagnosis of DJD of the hip must be considered

in patients who present with knee or groin pain when no pathology is noted in these areas. With DJD of the hip, hip motion is usually restricted and radiographic findings are abnormal. *Obturator nerve involvement* can also cause pain in the groin and medial aspect of the thigh and knee. A hernia may be suspected because of groin pain; if no hernia is found, obturator involvement should be considered.

Osteoarthritis of the hip may also manifest as pain in the buttock; therefore, the causes of buttock pain must be considered in the differential diagnosis. Buttock pain caused by *lumbar disk disease* is worse with extension of the spine and relieved by rest in the fetal position. Buttock pain caused by osteoarthritis of the hip is not usually exacerbated by spinal extension or relieved by rest in the fetal position. Likewise, no evidence of nerve root compression is usually seen with osteoarthritis of the hip.

Sciatica
Typical sciatica causes pain in the buttock that radiates down the posterolateral aspect of the leg. It may radiate into the dorsum of the foot and tends to follow standard dermatome patterns. Sciatic pain may be sharp or burning. It is frequently made worse by coughing, straining at stool (if sciatica is caused by a herniated disc), or walking down steps; it may be precipitated by sudden strenuous movements. The patient may present with pain initiated by an attempt to lift a heavy object or by vigorous turning or twisting with the back flexed (e.g., pulling the rope on a lawn mower or outboard engine).

Effects of Exercise and Rest on Pain
Leg pain that develops during walking occurs in patients with arterial insufficiency, venous insufficiency, spinal stenosis, and thrombophlebitis.

Arterial Insufficiency (Peripheral Artery Disease). The pain of arterial insufficiency *(intermittent claudication)* is usually described as soreness, a cramp, or a burning sensation in the calf. The discomfort may also be described as tightness, heaviness, tiredness, or achiness rather than pain. The discomfort is usually precipitated by walking and relieved by rest. It rarely occurs while the patient is at home. It usually develops after the patient has walked a predictable (by the patient) distance and is relieved by rest in a standing position after a predictable (by the patient) time. After resting, the patient can resume walking a similar distance before the pain starts again; relief is achieved again after resting.

A common mistake is the diagnosis of osteoarthritis of the hip when gluteal claudication is the problem. This error is more likely if buttock pain is not associated with pain in the calf. Some patients with vascular disease of the iliac artery complain only of the symptoms of gluteal claudication, which are usually felt when the patient walks outside.

Rest pain (often nocturnal) in the toes or heel is almost pathognomonic of arterial insufficiency. The leg of a patient with arterial insufficiency may have pallor on elevation, rubor on dependency, and loss of hair on the toes. Some men with aortoiliac disease may present with pain in the upper leg or the buttock and an inability to develop or sustain an erection. Pain from intermittent claudication is usually unilateral but can be bilateral. When the pain is present bilaterally, it seldom occurs in both legs simultaneously. The onset of pain in one leg may prevent the patient from walking enough to produce symptoms in the other leg. Physical examination for evidence of arterial insufficiency must therefore be performed on both legs. Comparing the blood pressure of the ankle and the arm provides the ankle-brachial index (ABI). An ABI less that 0.9 is abnormal. An ABI less than 0.4 is suggestive of severe peripheral artery disease.

Venous Insufficiency. Venous claudication is difficult to distinguish from claudication due to arterial insufficiency. In both conditions, walking causes calf pain that may be severe enough for the patient to stop walking. Patients with venous claudication usually have no physical signs of arterial insufficiency.

Spinal Stenosis. Spinal stenosis is another cause of leg pain that is exacerbated by exercise. The pain (*pseudoclaudication*) is similar to that associated with arterial insufficiency; it also occurs more frequently in older men. The first clue that the pain in the leg is not caused by arterial insufficiency is the presence of normal pedal pulses. **Although both begin with exercise, the pain of spinal stenosis is less often relieved by rest than the pain of arterial insufficiency** (Table 24-1). The pain of intermittent claudication is relieved within a few minutes, whereas the pain of spinal stenosis requires 10 to 30 minutes to subside. Some patients with calf pain from spinal stenosis state that they must sit or lie down with the thighs flexed to relieve the discomfort.

The pain of spinal stenosis is caused by localized narrowing of the spinal canal due to a structural abnormality that results in *cauda equina compression.* Patients occasionally complain of backache or buttock pain as well as numbness and tingling in the feet with walking. Walking uphill is easier than walking downhill for these patients. They have no problem riding a bicycle, probably because the stooped position assumed during this activity reduces the amount of cauda equina compression. The examiner must remember that vascular claudication and spinal stenosis can coexist.

Thrombophlebitis. Unilateral pain and swelling in the calf are usually caused by thrombophlebitis. The pain is usually present at rest and is seldom worsened by exercise. In a patient with thrombophlebitis who experiences calf pain while walking, acute exacerbation of the calf pain occurs immediately after the foot is placed on the ground. Although the history and physical examination of thrombophlebitis are well known to most physicians (i.e., pain, swelling, tenderness on palpation, occasionally a history of prior trauma or previous bouts of phlebitis), this relatively common cause of leg pain is often misdiagnosed. Several studies have suggested that venous ultrasonography should be used to confirm the clinical diagnosis because thrombophlebitis has often been incorrectly diagnosed in the absence of ultrasonographic evidence.

TABLE **24-1.**   Comparison of Symptoms and Signs in Vascular and Spinal (Neurogenic) Claudication

	VASCULAR CLAUDICATION	NEUROGENIC CLAUDICATION
Backache	Uncommon; occurs in aortoiliac occlusion	Common but need not be present
Leg symptoms	Quantitatively related to effort	May be brought on by effort; directly related to posture of extension of spine
Quality	Cramplike, tight feeling; intense fatigue; discomfort; pain may be absent	Numbness, cramplike, burning, paresthetic; sensation of cold or swelling; pain may be absent
Relief	Rest of affected muscle group	Rest not enough; postural altera-tion of spine to allow flexion is necessary in most
Onset	Simultaneous onset in all parts affected	Characteristic march up or down legs
Urinary incontinence	Does not occur	Very rare
Impotence	Common in aortoiliac disease (failure to sustain erection)	Very rare (failure to achieve erection)
Wasting of legs	Global in aortoiliac disease	Cauda equina distribution in severe cases
Trophic changes	May be present; absent in aortoiliac disease	Absent but may be present in combined disease
Sensory loss	Absent	Not uncommon; common after exercise
Ankle jerks	Often absent in patients > 60 yr old	Common, particularly after exercise
Straight-leg raising	Full	Often full

From DeVilliers JC: Combined neurogenic and vascular claudication. SA Med J 57:650-654, 1980.

Other Conditions

Other causes of painful swelling of the calf are *traumatic rupture* of the plan-taris tendon or the medial head of the gastrocnemius, *muscle trauma*, and *muscle stiffness* after unaccustomed exercise. *Popliteal (Baker's) cyst,* called the "pseudothrombophlebitis syndrome," causes painful swelling of the calf, thus mimicking thrombophlebitis. Therefore, all patients with painful calf swelling should be examined for a popliteal cyst. In one large series, most patients with painful popliteal cysts also had inflammatory joint disease of the knee, usually rheumatoid arthritis (Table 24-2).

Diffuse aching in one or both calves with no relation to exercise sug-gests *varicose veins.* Patients with this condition frequently complain of night cramps and that their legs hurt when they go to bed at night. The pain of venous insufficiency is vague, nonspecific, and unrelated to any specific

TABLE 24-2.   Disease Entities Associated with
Pseudothrombophlebitis Syndrome

Rheumatoid arthritis
Psoriatic arthritis
Osteoarthritis
Juvenile rheumatoid arthritis
Reiter's syndrome
Gonococcal arthritis
Gouty arthritis
Traumatic arthritis
Meniscal injury
Osteochondritis dissecans
Villonodular synovitis
Systemic lupus erythematosus
Ankylosing spondylitis
Mixed connective tissue disease

From Katerndahl DA: Calf pain mimicking thrombophlebitis. Postgrad Med 68:107-115, 1980.

muscle groups. Superficial varicosity may suggest the diagnosis, but deep venous insufficiency may be present without noticeable superficial serpiginous varicosity.

A first attack of *gouty arthritis* of the knee or (rarely) of the hip may be difficult to diagnose unless the patient has a warm, swollen joint in the big toe (podagra) and a prior history of gout. When the first attack is a warm, swollen, painful knee, the diagnosis is less apparent and may be confused with *pyogenic arthritis*. Patients with gout do not usually have as many systemic signs and symptoms (rash, malaise, fever) as those with pyogenic arthritis. Patients with gouty arthritis often have a hot, red, tender, swollen joint. The involved joint is sensitive to external pressure; some patients cannot even tolerate the weight of a sheet or blanket on the joint.

ASSOCIATED SYMPTOMS

Patients with *DJD* often have pain and stiffness in other joints. A limp may be present in cases of DJD of the hip. Patients with *sciatica* may have numbness, paresthesia, weakness, and sensory deficits as well as abnormal knee or ankle jerks (hyperactive early; diminished to absent later). Patients with *intermittent claudication* may complain of numbness in the foot, which may erroneously suggest *peripheral neuropathy*. If men with claudication also report *impotence*, an *aortoiliac lesion* is probable.

Night cramps, edema of the legs, and stasis abnormalities suggest *chronic venous insufficiency.*

PRECIPITATING AND AGGRAVATING FACTORS

Pain during activity is usually seen with structural abnormalities, whereas pain at rest or after activity suggests inflammatory processes. Bone pain occurs at rest and increases with weight bearing. The pain of *DJD* worsens with exercise and prolonged weight bearing. *Sciatic* pain is aggravated by coughing, straining at stools, sneezing, walking, stooping, lifting, and spinal extension. As mentioned earlier, both the pain of *intermittent claudication* and that of *spinal stenosis* are brought on by walking and exercise. Pain in the knee after sitting for a while suggests patellofemoral disorders.

AMELIORATING FACTORS

Patients with *DJD* report that their morning stiffness, aches, and pain often abate during the day as they move the joint. *Sciatic* pain is often alleviated by recumbency in the fetal position. The pain of *intermittent claudication* abates within a few minutes after cessation of walking; the pain of *spinal stenosis* is relieved more slowly and by spinal flexion. The pain of *varicose veins* is alleviated somewhat by elevation of the involved limb; the resting (nocturnal) pain of *arterial insufficiency* is often relieved by lowering the involved limb. **Relief of symptoms with an adequate dose of colchicine is pathognomonic of gout.**

PHYSICAL FINDINGS AND DIAGNOSTIC STUDIES

A careful history and physical examination are essential in all patients who complain of pain in the extremities. The physician should especially note any history of previous joint disease, precipitating events, previous diagnoses, and medications, particularly oral contraceptives, that are associated with a higher incidence of thrombophlebitis.

Physical examination should include observation of gait, neurologic evaluation (Fig. 24-1), attempts to reproduce the pain by palpation or maneuver, determination of range of motion of all joints, measurement of both calves and both thighs, and inspection and palpation for arterial insufficiency. Examination of the knee and popliteal space should be performed in both the supine and erect positions. Joint effusions are more readily detected in the supine position, whereas Baker's cysts are more prominent when the patient is erect. The absence of any abnormal physical finding essentially rules out a meniscal tear, whereas a positive McMurray test result strongly suggests a meniscal tear.

L3 Root	Lateral Femoral Cutaneous Nerve	Common Peroneal Nerve	Deep Peroneal Nerve
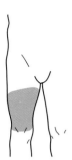	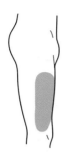	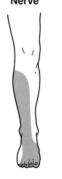	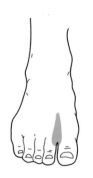
Weakness: Hip flexion Hip adduction Knee extension	Weakness: None	Weakness: Foot eversion while plantarflexed Foot dorsiflexion Toe dorsiflexion	Weakness: Toe dorsiflexion

A

L4 Root	L5 Root	S1 Root
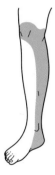	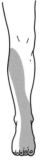	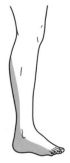
Weakness: Hip adduction Hip abduction Knee extension Knee flexion Foot dorsiflexion Toe dorsiflexion	Weakness: Hip abduction Knee flexion Foot plantarflexion Foot inversion and eversion while plantarflexed Toe dorsiflexion	Weakness: Knee flexion Foot plantarflexion Foot inversion and eversion while plantarflexed
Reflex: Patellar		Reflex: Achilles

B

Figure 24-1. Common root and peripheral nerve syndromes (lower extremity). Syndromes are usually incomplete. Dermatomes and innervations can vary in some patients. (From Birnbaum JS: The Musculoskeletal Manual, 2nd ed. Philadelphia, WB Saunders, 1986.)

Muscular and Ligamentous Strains and Tears

When a patient complains of pain in the knee, the joint should be palpated (Figs. 24-2 and 24-3). Tenderness at the joint line suggests damage to the medial or collateral ligaments, the capsular ligament, or the meniscus. Radiographs, magnetic resonance imaging (MRI), and arthroscopic examination may be needed for an accurate diagnosis. The stability of the knee ligaments should be determined by careful physical examination (Figs. 24-4 and 24-5). Tenderness above or below the joint line suggests a muscle pull or strain (Fig. 24-6). With acute muscle tears there is usually local tenderness, bruising, and possibly a gap in the muscle.

With *acute, gouty arthritis* the joint is usually warm, red, tender, and swollen. Although pain can be as severe as that seen in pyogenic arthritis, patients with gouty arthritis do not have comparable systemic symptoms. The serum uric acid value is usually elevated, and uric acid crystals may be seen in the joint aspirate.

Useful diagnostic studies in the evaluation of leg pain include plain radiographs, MRI, computed tomography (CT), Doppler ultrasonography studies, venograms, arthroscopy, arthrograms, and measurement of patellofemoral congruency.

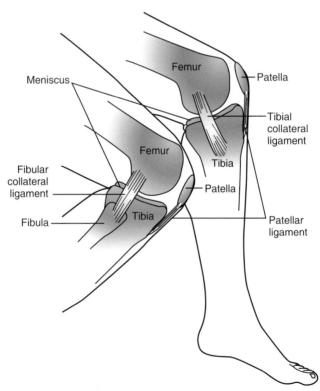

Figure 24-2. Major landmarks in examination of the knee. (From Smith JB: Knee problems in children. Pediatr Clin North Am 24:4, 1977.)

Degenerative Joint Disease

Pain in the hip is frequently caused by DJD but may also result from other common conditions (Fig. 24-7). The major physical findings that suggest DJD of the knee include joint crepitus, limitation of joint movement, and elicitation of presenting symptoms at extremes of joint movement. Patients with advanced disease may have fixed flexion contractures, joint effusions, and radiographic evidence of arthritis. Patients with DJD are often in the same age group as those

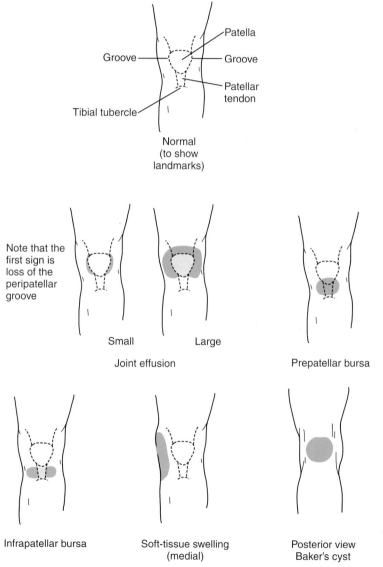

Figure 24-3. Knee swelling. (From Birnbaum JS: The Musculoskeletal Manual, 2nd ed. Philadelphia, WB Saunders, 1986.)

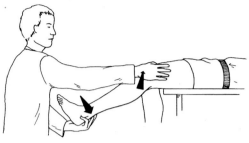

Medial Collateral Ligament

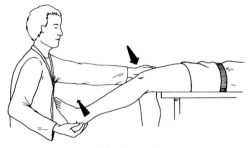

Lateral Collateral Ligament

Good muscular relaxation is essential
Don't allow the thigh or leg to rotate while performing the test
Always compare to the uninvolved knee

Figure 24-4. Tests for collateral ligament stability. (From Birnbaum JS: The Musculoskeletal Manual, 2nd ed. Philadelphia, WB Saunders, 1986.)

with vascular insufficiency, in whom the symptoms are referable to soft tissue. The physician must remember that the two conditions can coexist. If a careful examination reveals no swelling of the joint, there is probably no serious problem inside the joint.

Sciatica

Some common physical findings in sciatica include restriction of spinal movement (hyperextension often reproduces sciatic pain), limitation of straight-leg raising, and spasm over the sacrospinal muscles (which may be tender on palpation). Changes in reflex activity may occur as well as sensory or motor loss over the involved segments (see Fig. 24-1). Myelography, CT, and MRI are rarely necessary for diagnosis; they are used to determine the extent of the spinal cord compression.

Intermittent Claudication

Physical findings in intermittent claudication include pallor on elevation, rubor on dependency (most noticeable in the toes and sole), loss of hair on the toes, and diminished arterial pulsations. The presence of normal pedal pulses at rest

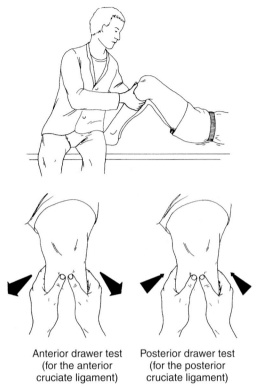

Anterior drawer test   Posterior drawer test
(for the anterior   (for the posterior
cruciate ligament)   cruciate ligament)

Figure 24-5. Drawer tests to evaluate cruciate ligament stability. (From Birnbaum JS: The Musculoskeletal Manual, 2nd ed. Philadelphia, WB Saunders, 1986.)

and after walking virtually rules out arterial insufficiency. An ABI less that 0.9 is abnormal. An ABI less than 0.4 is suggestive of severe peripheral artery disease.

Patients with *venous claudication* usually have varicose veins. Occasionally they can identify a tender point in the calf, but examination is not revealing. These patients should exercise to the point of discomfort, at which time a group of varices may be noted. Venography may be required for diagnosis.

Thrombophlebitis
The classic findings in patients with thrombophlebitis are swelling and a measurable increase in calf circumference in comparison with the opposite side. The clinician can often palpate a tender cordlike vein between the heads of the gastrocnemius muscle. The patient may have dilatation of other veins, edema, erythema, and Homans's sign. These findings are variable and not always reliable for the diagnosis of thrombophlebitis. Inflation of a sphygmomanometer around each calf until pain is produced is a sensitive test. The most important tests are venography and duplex Doppler ultrasonography.

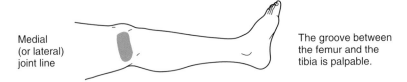

Medial (or lateral) joint line

The groove between the femur and the tibia is palpable.

Tenderness here can be in the ligament, in the meniscus or can indicate degenerative arthritis.
The point of maximal tenderness will usually move posteriorly a bit when the knee is flexed if a painful *MENISCUS* is responsible (called Steinman's test.)
Tenderness may extend a bit above and below the joint line if it arises from the *LIGAMENT*.
Joint-line tenderness due to *DEGENERATIVE ARTHRITIS* is usually fairly diffuse.

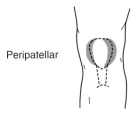

Peripatellar

Tenderness here can be found in *CHONDROMALACIA PATELLAE* or *DEGENERATIVE ARTHRITIS* of the patello-femoral joint, but the patellar compression test is more specific.

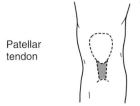

Patellar tendon

Tenderness anywhere here indicates *PATELLAR TENDONITIS*

A

Figure 24-6. Sites of tenderness around the knee. (From Birnbaum JS: The Musculoskeletal Manual, 2nd ed. Philadelphia, WB Saunders, 1986.)

Because cellulitis of the calf can mimic thrombophlebitis, the two conditions must be differentiated. In *cellulitis*, the pain is described as being on the surface, no palpable cord is present, and Homans's sign is absent. Careful examination reveals that pain is induced by light palpation rather than deep palpation over the course of the vein. Likewise, the area of erythema is more clearly demarcated, occasionally with an associated open wound. An inflated sphygmomanometer requires high pressure to reproduce the pain of cellulitis, and often there is no difference in pressure between the two calves. These findings contrast

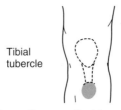

Tibial
tubercle

Tenderness (and sometimes swelling) here in a
teenager implies *OSGOOD-SCHLATTER'S DISEASE*

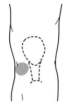

The bony prominence where
the anserine tendons insert
is easily palpable inferior
to the joint line on the
antero-medial tibia.

Tenderness here indicates *ANSERINE TENDONITIS*

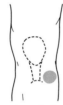

Gerdy's tubercle
on the anterolateral tibia

Tenderness here indicates *ILIOTIBIAL BAND TENDONITIS*
B

Figure 24-6, cont'd.

with those reported in patients with thrombophlebitis. **Because thrombophlebitis may coexist with a popliteal (Baker's) cyst, venous Doppler ultrasonography should be performed in all patients with popliteal cysts.**

Other Conditions

The diagnosis of *joint sprain* is made by demonstrating instability of the joint. Tears of joint ligaments can often be demonstrated by the use of stress-view radiographs of the joint involved. With suspected *fractures*, a radiograph that includes the joints at both ends of the fractured bone should always be performed. Instability of joints suggests ligamentous tears. Angulation in valgus or varus with the knee slightly flexed suggests either medial or lateral ligament instability. Abnormal forward or backward shift of the tibia on the femur indicates anterior cruciate or posterior cruciate ligament instability, respectively (see Fig. 24-5). Occasionally, abnormal rotations may be present; these suggest a complicated combination injury of the knee.

If the diagnosis is still unclear after a complete physical examination is conducted with special attention to the musculoskeletal, vascular, and nervous

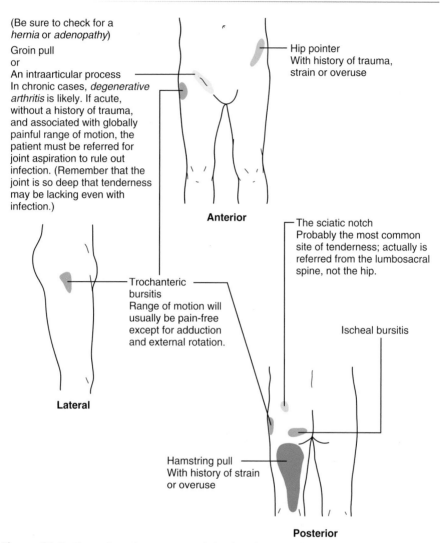

(Be sure to check for a
hernia or *adenopathy*)

Groin pull
or
An intraarticular process
In chronic cases, *degenerative
arthritis* is likely. If acute,
without a history of trauma,
and associated with globally
painful range of motion, the
patient must be referred for
joint aspiration to rule out
infection. (Remember that the
joint is so deep that tenderness
may be lacking even with
infection.)

Hip pointer
With history of trauma,
strain or overuse

Anterior

The sciatic notch
Probably the most common
site of tenderness; actually is
referred from the lumbosacral
spine, not the hip.

Trochanteric
bursitis
Range of motion will
usually be pain-free
except for adduction
and external rotation.

Ischeal bursitis

Lateral

Hamstring pull
With history of strain
or overuse

Posterior

Figure 24-7. Sites of tenderness around the hip. (From Birnbaum JS: The Musculoskeletal
Manual, 2nd ed. Philadelphia, WB Saunders, 1986.)

systems, noninvasive and invasive studies of the vascular system, electromyography, CT, MRI, and occasionally myelography may be helpful.

LESS COMMON DIAGNOSTIC CONSIDERATIONS

Sudden onset of pain in the leg, especially the lower leg and sometimes associated with paralysis, paresthesia, pallor, or absence of arterial pulsation, suggests acute arterial *embolism*. The likelihood of this diagnosis is increased by

the presence of atrial fibrillation. Vague arthralgias and muscle aches are often seen with viral and flulike *infections*, but no joint abnormality can be detected on physical examination in these cases. Primary bone *tumors* are rare in adults; however, pain from metastatic bone disease is frequently seen in patients with breast, lung, and prostatic tumors.

Chondromalacia patellae, though more common in adolescents than adults, may be seen in patients in their 40s and 50s. These patients characteristically have pain, stiffness, grating, or locking of the knee. The pain is worse when the knee is weight bearing in flexion. Crepitation and pain with manipulation of the patella over the femoral condyle are characteristic. Pain is exacerbated when the patient tenses the quadriceps with the knee in free extension while the examiner is depressing the upper pole of the patella.

Meralgia paresthetica, which is slightly more common in men than women, is caused by entrapment of the lateral femoral cutaneous nerve by the tensor fasciae latae. The patient complains of pain, burning, or tingling over the lateral aspect of the thigh that is occasionally worse at night or after exercise. It is alleviated by rest, particularly in the sitting position.

Peripheral neuropathy is more common in diabetic patients but may be seen in others. Patients complain of burning, tingling, and numbness, particularly in the feet. They may have a sensation of coldness, but no decrease in vascular pulsations is noted in those with pure peripheral neuropathy. Diabetic patients with peripheral neuropathy often have associated vascular insufficiency. Physical findings include sensory loss (often symmetrical), muscle wasting, weakness, decreased tendon reflexes, and signs of arterial insufficiency.

Obturator hernias, an uncommon cause of pain, occur more frequently in elderly debilitated women than in other patients. The female-to-male ratio is 6:1. Patients usually present with pain along the anteromedial aspect of the thigh. This pain is increased by adduction of the thigh. Pain may also be felt in the hip or knee. The pain may be associated with intermittent bouts of nausea, vomiting, abdominal pain, and distention, all signs of small bowel obstruction. **Obturator hernias should be given particular consideration in elderly women who complain of pain in the hip or knee with no objective evidence of DJD or other common causes.**

Iliopsoas bursitis, a rare condition, should be suspected if the patient has gradual onset of groin pain that is exacerbated by flexion or internal rotation of the hip.

Half of the patients with *pseudothrombophlebitis* due to a popliteal (Baker's) cyst have rheumatoid arthritis. In one study of patients with a confirmed popliteal cyst, only 50% had palpable masses and 12% had masses below the popliteal space. **Baker's cyst should be suspected in all patients with thrombophlebitis and rheumatoid arthritis and in all patients with suspected thrombophlebitis but no venographic evidence of phlebitis.** An arthrogram is essential to the diagnosis of a popliteal cyst. Ultrasonography may help the physician diagnose an intact cyst, but it is often not useful in the diagnosis of a ruptured popliteal cyst.

Rheumatoid arthritis is a relatively uncommon cause of pain in the lower extremity. The joint pain usually lasts for a few weeks, with characteristic morning stiffness, joint tenderness, and pain with motion. The patient frequently has joint effusion, soft tissue swelling, and synovial thickening. Pseudothrombophlebitis should be suspected when calf pain occurs in any patient with rheumatoid arthritis, especially if active inflammation of the knee is present.

Spinal stenosis (neurogenic claudication, cauda equina claudication) is often difficult to differentiate from intermittent claudication due to arterial insufficiency. The patient's history is particularly important because the two conditions affect the same age group. Patients with calf pain due to spinal stenosis state that the pain starts insidiously, is exacerbated by walking, and is particularly related to extension of the spine. They may have associated backache or buttock pain, which is relatively uncommon in patients with intermittent claudication. A paresthetic quality to the pain suggests a neurogenic origin. Patients with spinal stenosis do not experience prompt relief of pain with cessation of exercise (as do those with arterial insufficiency); they feel greater relief when they lie or sit down with their thighs flexed; they also do not have pain while riding a bicycle because the spine is in a flexed position. In any patient who has signs of intermittent claudication and rides a bicycle without difficulty, spinal stenosis should be suspected.

Musculotendinous rupture of the gastrocnemius or plantaris muscle, particularly during athletic activities such as jogging, running, and tennis, is characterized by a sudden onset of pain in the leg ("it felt like I got a shot in the leg"). Frequently, the physician can palpate the retracted end of the plantaris muscle.

Trochanteric bursitis, a relatively uncommon cause of leg pain, usually manifests as pain over the greater trochanter, in the buttock, and in the lateral thigh along the distribution of the second lumbar dermatome. On physical examination, the patient may be found to limp and usually to have marked point tenderness over the greater trochanter. The differential diagnosis consists of arthritis of the hip or lumbar spine problems. The major factors in differential diagnosis include pain on palpation over the trochanteric bursa and the absence of sensory loss, which would be seen with lumbar disc disease. The pain is not exacerbated by coughing and sneezing but is by squatting, climbing stairs, and sitting with the painful leg crossed over the other one. It is alleviated by infiltration of the trochanteric bursa with local anesthetics, steroids, or both.

Cyclic hip pain that coincides with menstruation suggests *endometriosis*. The pain is usually unilateral. Other uncommon causes of knee pain are meniscal cysts, bipartite patella, fat pad irritation (Hoffa's syndrome), and neuromas.

THE LEG AND SPORTS MEDICINE

The most common causes of chronic leg pain in runners include *shin splints, stress fractures,* and *compartment syndromes* (Fig. 24-8). Shin splints represent musculotendinous inflammation from overuse and probably subclinical

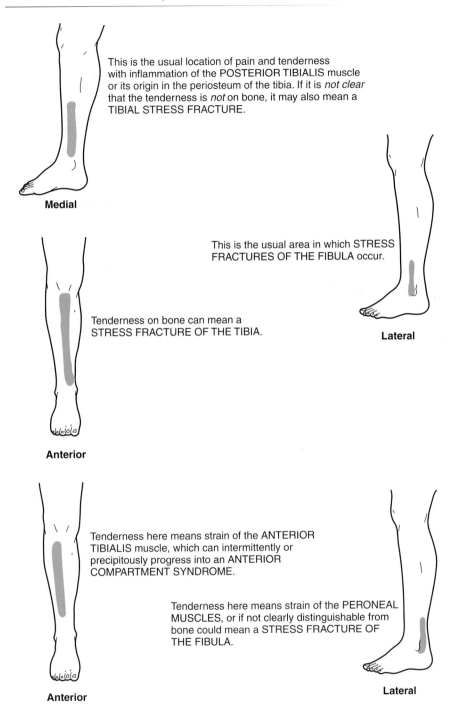

This is the usual location of pain and tenderness with inflammation of the POSTERIOR TIBIALIS muscle or its origin in the periosteum of the tibia. If it is *not clear* that the tenderness is *not* on bone, it may also mean a TIBIAL STRESS FRACTURE.

Medial

This is the usual area in which STRESS FRACTURES OF THE FIBULA occur.

Tenderness on bone can mean a STRESS FRACTURE OF THE TIBIA.

Lateral

Anterior

Tenderness here means strain of the ANTERIOR TIBIALIS muscle, which can intermittently or precipitously progress into an ANTERIOR COMPARTMENT SYNDROME.

Tenderness here means strain of the PERONEAL MUSCLES, or if not clearly distinguishable from bone could mean a STRESS FRACTURE OF THE FIBULA.

Lateral

Anterior

Figure 24-8. Pain in the shin, often seen in runners.

periosteal reaction. The pain is either anterolateral or posteromedial along the distal tibia. The painful areas are tender on palpation.

With stress fractures there is usually point tenderness over the involved bone, and the diagnosis may be confirmed radiographically. Stress fractures are more common in experienced long-distance runners, particularly those who attempt to run more than 20 to 30 miles per week. These fractures may occur in the tibia, fibula, or metatarsus. Lateral knee pain in long-distance runners suggests *iliotibial band friction syndrome.*

Compartment syndromes occur when the fascial compartment is too small to accommodate the approximately 20% increase in muscle size that occurs with strenuous exercise. This results in limited venous outflow and tends to produce ischemic pain of the involved tissue. Patients with compartment syndromes usually present with a gradual onset (over 1 or more years) of bilateral pain that is progressive, dull, aching, and particularly worse after long runs. Paresthesias may also be present. The anterior compartment of the leg is usually affected; the next most likely affected is the posterior compartment, followed by the posterior superficial compartment. Physical findings include tenderness in the muscle mass itself but not as much in the bone and tendons. Elevated compartment pressures are diagnostic.

Differential Diagnosis of Lower Extremity Pain in Adults

CAUSE	NATURE OF PATIENT	NATURE OF SYMPTOMS	ASSOCIATED SYMPTOMS	PRECIPITATING AND AGGRAVATING FACTORS	AMELIORATING FACTORS	PHYSICAL FINDINGS	DIAGNOSTIC STUDIES
Muscular or ligamentous strain	Weekend athletes Those with trauma Often older than 40 yr	Pain Swelling of joint Sudden onset		Unaccustomed or strenuous activity		With ligamentous injury of joint, possible tenderness at joint line and swelling of joint Local tenderness Positive McMurray test result suggests meniscal tear	MRI for injury of knee, especially meniscal and ligamentous
Degenerative joint disease	Older than 40 yr (except those with prior trauma)	Knee or hip pain Morning stiffness Gradual onset	Pain and stiffness in other joints Occasional limp	Standing and weight bearing Descending stairs	Movement	Buttock pain not worse with hyperextension No evidence of nerve root compression Crepitation of joint Limitation of joint movement, effusion	Radiographs Arthroscopy of knee MRI
Lumbar disc disease (sciatica)	More common in men older than 40 yr	Pain in buttock and postero-lateral aspect of leg Acute onset Lancinating or like toothache Less severe previous episodes	Paresthesias Dysesthesias Weakness	Lifting Turning Twisting Spinal extension Coughing Straining	Fetal position	Spasm of hamstrings Abnormal straight or flexed leg raising Neurologic abnormalities in lower leg Reversal of lordotic curve Pain of sciatic distribution with spinal hyperextension Asymmetrical limitation of motion	CT Electromyography MRI

Continued

Differential Diagnosis of Lower Extremity Pain in Adults—cont'd

CAUSE	NATURE OF PATIENT	NATURE OF SYMPTOMS	ASSOCIATED SYMPTOMS	PRECIPITATING AND AGGRAVATING FACTORS	AMELIORATING FACTORS	PHYSICAL FINDINGS	DIAGNOSTIC STUDIES
Anterior compartment syndrome (shin splint)	Runners	Achy Tightness Claudication type of pain	Occasional muscle weakness or sensory symptoms	Exercise	Rest	Tenderness on palpation over medial border of shin	Isotopic bone scan
Varicose veins		Diffuse aching of one or both calves Worse at night	Edema and stasis abnormalities		Elevation of limb	Varicose veins may or may not be apparent	Venography Duplex Doppler ultrasonography studies
Thrombophlebitis	History of phlebitis Use of oral contraceptives	Unilateral Pain at rest	Swelling	Placing foot on ground		No evidence of arterial insufficiency Swelling of calf with tenderness and warmth Palpable cord	Venography Duplex Doppler studies
Arterial insufficiency	Older than 50 yr, but diabetic patients younger	Pain in calf with walking Intermittent claudication of hip with aortoiliac disease Rest pain in calf, toes, or heel suggests severe arterial insufficiency Usually unilateral	Impotence with aortoiliac disease	Walking	Rest Dependency of involved limb	Decreased pulses Pallor on elevation, rubor on dependency Cool Loss of hair on toes ABI <0.9	Arteriography Doppler ultrasonography studies MRI

Spinal stenosis	Older patients More common in men	Calf pain induced by walking and leg exercise	Paresthesias Backache Buttock pain	Exercise Not precipitated by exercise with spine flexed (bicycling)	Not quickly relieved by rest Spinal flexion	Good pedal pulses Transient neurologic deficit	Electromyography CTMRI
Gout	More common in men	Acute onset Toe and knee pain Rare in hip		Occasionally precipitated by trauma		Joint warm, swollen, exquisitely tender	Serum uric acid test Uric acid crystals found in joint aspirate

ABI, Ankle-brachial index; *CT*, computed tomography; *MRI*, magnetic resonance imaging.

Selected References

Balint GP, Korda J, Hangody L, et al: Foot and ankle disorders, *Best Pract Res Clin Rheumatol* 17:87-111, 2003.

Bennett DL, Daffner RH, Weissman BN, et al: *Expert Panel on Musculoskeletal Imaging: ACR Appropriateness Criteria: Nontraumatic knee pain*, Reston, VA, 2008, American College of Radiology, Available at http://www.acr.org/SecondaryMainMenuCategories/quality_safety/app_criteria/pdf/ExpertPanelonMusculoskeletalImaging/NonTraumaticKneePainDoc15.aspx.

Bussières AE, Taylor JA, Peterson C: Diagnostic imaging practice guidelines for musculoskeletal complaints in adults-an evidence-based approach, part 1: lower extremity disorders, *J Manipulative Physiol Ther* 30:684-717, 2007.

Calmbach WL, Hutchens M: Evaluation of patients presenting with knee pain, part 1: history, physical examination, radiographs, and laboratory tests, *Am Fam Physician* 68:907-912, 2003.

Calmbach WL, Hutchens M: Evaluation of patients presenting with knee pain, part 2: differential diagnosis, *Am Fam Physician* 68:917-922, 2003.

Choksi P, Thomas R, Simmons D: Charcot arthropathy: an often overlooked complication of diabetes mellitus, *J Ark Med Soc* 103:229-231, 2007.

Ebell MH: Diagnosis lumbar spinal stenosis, *Am Fam Physician* 80:1145-1147, 2009.

Hirsch AT, Haskal ZJ, Hertzer NR: ACC/AHA 2005 guidelines for the management of patients with peripheral arterial disease (lower extremity, renal, mesenteric, and abdominal aortic): executive summary a collaborative report [trunc], *J Am Coll Cardiol* 47:1239-1312, 2006.

Jackson JL, O'Malley PG, Kroenke K: Evaluation of knee pain in primary care, *Ann Intern Med* 139:575-588, 2003.

Jacobson JA, Daffner RH, Weissman BN, et al: *Expert Panel on Musculoskeletal Imaging, ACR Appropriateness Criteria®: chronic ankle pain*, Reston, VA, American College of Radiology, 2009. Available at http://www.acr.org/SecondaryMainMenuCategories/quality_safety/app_criteria/pdf/ExpertPanelonMusculoskeletalImaging/ChronicAnklePainDoc5.aspx.

Lichota DK: Anterior knee pain: symptom or syndrome? *Curr Women's Health Rep* 3:81-86, 2003.

Ramzi DW, Leeper KV: DVT and pulmonary embolism, part I: diagnosis, *Am Fam Physician* 69:2829-2836, 2004.

Resnik CS, Daffner RH, Weissman BN, et al: *Expert Panel on Musculoskeletal Imaging, ACR Appropriateness Criteria®: acute trauma to the knee*, American College of Radiology (ACR), 2008. Available at http://www.acr.org/SecondaryMainMenuCategories/quality_safety/app_criteria/pdf/ExpertPanelonMusculoskeletalImaging/AcuteTraumatotheKneeDoc2.aspx.

Shea KG, Pfeiffer R, Curtin M: Idiopathic anterior knee pain in adolescents, *Orthop Clin North Am* 34:377-383, 2003.

Toulipolous S, Hershman EB: Lower leg pain—diagnosis and treatment of compartment syndromes and other pain syndromes of the leg, *Sports Med* 27:193-203, 1999.

25 Pain in the Lower Extremity and Limping in Children

The physician should approach leg pain or limp in children as in adults—that is, determine whether it originates in joints or soft tissue. The most common causes of childhood leg pain originating in the soft tissue are unusual or strenuous *exercise* and *trauma*. **Fractures constitute the most common cause of acute limp in children.** Other common causes of leg pain are *growing pains, Legg-Calvé-Perthes disease (epiphysitis of the hip), Osgood-Schlatter disease (an abnormality of the epiphyseal ossification of the tibial tubercle), chondromalacia patellae,* and *ossification of the Achilles insertion. Limping can be due to pain, weakness, or structural abnormality.* It is important to determine the duration and progression of the limp, history of trauma, nature of pain, and any weakness and to observe the gait.

NATURE OF PATIENT

If a limp occurs when a young child begins to walk, *congenital dislocation* of one or both hips should be considered. *Toddler's fracture,* an undisplaced fracture of the distal tibia, may occur when weight bearing first occurs (9 months to 3 years). It may manifest as a limp or the inability to bear weight on the affected leg. In 1- to 5-year old patients, other common causes of limp include toxic synovitis, septic arthritis or osteomyelitis, developmental abnormalities, and juvenile rheumatoid arthritis. In 5- to 10-year-old patients, the more common causes are trauma, toxic synovitis, and infectious joint or bone disease. *Legg-Calvé-Perthes disease* (epiphysitis of the hip) usually occurs between ages 5 and 7 years. In patients 10 to 15 years old, *slipped femoral epiphyses* and *patellar problems* are more common. In children between ages 10 and 12, pain in the heel is most often caused by painful *bursitis* or *irregular ossification* of a *calcaneal apophysis.*

NATURE OF SYMPTOMS

Growing pains is a general diagnosis that is being made less frequently as physicians become more expert in making specific diagnoses. However, growing pains do exist, and they are now thought to be a form of *myalgia*. The aching pain is intermittent and usually located in the leg muscles, particularly in the front of the thigh, the calf, and the back of the knee. The pain is deep and localized to areas outside the joints. It is usually bilateral and typically occurs late in the day, although it may awaken the child from a sound sleep. Growing pains may be exacerbated by excessive running during the day, but exercise is not usually a factor. **The findings that the pain is nonarticular, bilateral, and usually unrelated to activity are essential to the accurate diagnosis of growing pains.** Children with growing pains show no abnormal physical findings.

Most serious diseases that cause leg pain in children (except slipped capital femoral epiphyses) are usually unilateral. Pain in the hip may result from *Legg-Calvé-Perthes disease*, a disturbance of the epiphyseal ossification of the femoral head in children ages 4 to 12 (peak age, 5 to 7 years). It is often associated with a limp. The pain is occasionally referred to the medial aspect of the knee. Transient synovitis of the hip can result from an upper respiratory illness but must be differentiated from septic arthritis and osteomyelitis (both of which require early diagnosis and treatment with intravenous antibiotics). Juvenile *rheumatoid arthritis* (now called *juvenile idiopathic arthritis*) is diagnosed in a child with joint pain for longer than 6 weeks, and a joint effusion, stress pain, limited range of motion, or increased warmth.

The most common causes of knee pain in children are *acute trauma, Osgood-Schlatter disease*, and *chondromalacia patellae*. Osgood-Schlatter disease is an abnormality of the epiphyseal ossification of the tibial tubercle. It is most common in children 10 to 15 years old. This condition involves painful swelling of the tibial tubercle at the insertion of the patellar tendon. The pain is worse with contraction of the quadriceps against resistance. It is exacerbated by activity and relieved by rest.

Chondromalacia patellae is just one of several causes of anterior knee pain. (Some believe the term should be discarded, but its use is still commonplace.) It results from chronic *patellofemoral dysfunction* and is an extremely common syndrome in active children and adolescents. It may be a precursor of adult patellofemoral arthritis.With patellofemoral dysfunction, patellar cartilage degenerates, not because of primary cartilaginous disease but from abnormal mechanical forces acting on it.

These abnormal forces may result from direct or indirect trauma. Direct injury may occur when force is applied to the anterior aspect of the patella; this usually results from a fall on the flexed knee. Indirect trauma is more common and is usually the result of strenuous or repetitive quadriceps activity to which the patient is unaccustomed (e.g., hiking, jogging, calisthenics, skiing). **The most characteristic symptom of indirect trauma is pain in the lower pole of the patella** and adjacent patellar tendon that is precipitated by strenuous activity, especially running, jumping, and squatting. After resting with the knee flexed, patients with indirect trauma experience a marked increase in pain when they initially extend the knee and begin to move around, but they usually find some relief after standing still or walking a short distance. Patients often describe a grating sensation that may be detected on physical examination when the knee is flexed and extended. The grating is noted particularly when the knee is extended against resistance. Radiographic findings are usually normal but may include fragmentation of the lower pole of the patella.

Chondromalacia patellae must be differentiated from *patellar osteochondritis, jumper's knee,* and *partial rupture of the patellar tendon.* Children with chondromalacia patellae usually have localized tenderness at the lower pole of the patella and the adjacent patellar tendon (see Fig. 24-2). The physician may occasionally note separation of the patellar tendon from the lower pole and a palpable defect at that point.

Other conditions that give rise to knee pain are *patellar subluxation, patellar dislocation,* and *meniscal injuries.* Although they are uncommon, *rheumatoid arthritis* and *popliteal cysts* can occur in children.

Limping is a common complaint among children. It is never normal, although its causes are many, ranging from poorly fitting shoes to a sprained ankle to the earliest manifestation of a malignant tumor. To determine the exact cause of limping, the physician must approach the problem methodically and thoroughly, obtaining a detailed history and performing a careful examination of the child's gait.

ASSOCIATED SYMPTOMS

Although limping is often caused by trauma and the most common cause of leg pain is traumatic injury to the joints or soft tissue, these facts may be misleading in some cases. In general, when pain or limp is caused by mild trauma, the symptoms should disappear within 2 to 3 weeks. Despite a history of trauma, if the symptoms do **not** disappear in 3 weeks, the physician must obtain a thorough history and perform a complete physical examination to rule out more serious conditions. The physician must determine whether the limp is:
1. Intermittent or constant
2. Present at the end of the day or in the morning
3. Made worse by climbing stairs
4. Present only after vigorous exercise (which may be the first clue to an impending stress fracture)

The location of leg pain often provides clues to its cause, *particularly in cases of referred pain.* In lower back pathology pain is most commonly referred to the buttocks and lateral thigh, whereas in hip pathology, pain is often referred to the groin, medial thigh, or knee. For example, Legg-Calvé-Perthes disease is a common cause of knee pain and limp in children.

A painless limp may be due to a difference in leg length or dysplasia of the hip. Fever suggests an infectious or inflammatory process. Recurrent fever, limp, joint pain, and morning stiffness suggest rheumatoid arthritis.

PHYSICAL FINDINGS

Range of motion of each joint from the hip down should be noted and compared with that of the opposite side, with careful attention given to the patellae. Leg length should be measured; a discrepancy of 1.25 cm (½ inch) or more can cause a *pelvic tilt* and subsequent limp.

When the patient complains of lower leg pain, particularly with a limp, the gait should be examined first. Gait consists of two phases: stance and swing. In the stance phase, the foot is in contact with the floor, and one limb bears all the body weight. In the swing phase, the foot is not touching the floor. This phase begins when the toe comes off the floor and ends with a heel strike. A child with a stiff hip would have a short swing phase because of limited hip joint movement. During each phase, the physician should observe one or two of the involved anatomic components: first the feet and then the knees, pelvis, and trunk. The sound of the walk may suggest a steppage gait, with slapping of the foot from footdrop. The shoes should be inspected for abnormal wear. Excessive wear of the toes of the shoes suggests *toe walking*, and excessive wear of the medial aspects of the shoes indicates severe *flatfoot*.

Pain in one extremity that causes the patient to shorten the stance phases on that side, resulting in an increased swing, produces an *antalgic gait*. It is usually caused by infection or trauma. A *Trendelenburg gait* occurs when the pelvis tilts downward and away from the affected hip during the swing phase. It is usually caused by weakness of the contralateral gluteus medius. The Trendelenburg gait is most commonly seen in children with Legg-Calvé-Perthes disease and slipped capital femoral epiphysis. A *steppage (equinus) gait* is seen in children with neuromuscular disease (i.e., cerebral palsy). There is exaggerated hip and knee flexion during the swing phase to compensate for an inability to dorsiflex the ankle.

With joint effusion the physician must suspect an infectious process, especially if there are systemic signs. Infections may be caused by gonococci, staphylococci, *Haemophilus* spp., and, in endemic areas, Lyme disease.

DIAGNOSTIC STUDIES

A complete blood count and erythrocyte sedimentation rate (ESR) measurement should be ordered. An erythrocyte sedimentation rate greater than 50 mm/hr in a child with a limp suggests a serious disease. In selected cases a Lyme titer, a test for rheumatoid factor or human leukocyte antigen (HLA) B27, or a culture of joint effusion may be diagnostic. Plain radiographs (ordered first), a bone scan, ultrasonography, computed tomography, or magnetic resonance imaging may also be diagnostic. Magnetic resonance imaging is as sensitive as, and more specific for diagnosing osteomyelitis than, bone scan.

Differential Diagnosis of Lower Extremity Pain and Limp in Children

CAUSE	NATURE OF PATIENT	NATURE OF SYMPTOMS	ASSOCIATED SYMPTOMS	PRECIPITATING AND AGGRAVATING FACTORS	AMELIORATING FACTORS	PHYSICAL FINDINGS	DIAGNOSTIC STUDIES
Epiphysitis of hip (Legg-Calvé-Perthes disease)	Ages 4-12 yr (peak incidence 5-7yr) Usually male Rare in African Americans	Unilateral hip pain often referred to medial aspect of knee	Limp			Antalgic or Trendelenburg gait Limitation of hip motion	Radiography of hip Bone scintigraphy
Epiphysitis of knee (Osgood-Schlatter disease)	Ages 10-15 yr	Painful swelling of tibial tubercle		Quadriceps contraction against resistance	Rest		Radiography of knee
Chondromalacia patellae	Children and adolescents	Pain in lower pole of patella and adjacent patellar tendon		Running Jumping Squatting	Quiet standing or walking	Grating of knee with flexion and extension	Radiography of knee
Trauma	History of sports participation	Joint or soft tissue			2-3 wk of rest	Local tenderness Antalgic gait	Ultrasonography for synovitis of hip
Growing pains		Intermittent myalgia, especially in front of thigh, calf, and back of knee Nonarticular and bilateral Not related to activity				No abnormal findings	
Slipped capital femoral epiphysis	Usually males ages 12-15 More common in African Americans	Hip pain Only knee pain in 25%	Limp			Bilateral in 25% Trendelenburg gait	Radiography of hip Bone scintigraphy

LESS COMMON DIAGNOSTIC CONSIDERATIONS

Rheumatoid arthritis, popliteal cysts, quadriceps malalignment, supracondylar cortical avulsion, and traumatic epiphyseal injury may cause leg pain, limp, or both. Although it is uncommon in children, *herpes zoster* frequently involves the lower extremity and may cause pain, burning, or itching before the typical herpetic lesion appears. Usually, children with herpes zoster of the leg have only a rash and experience no pain. On rare occasions, spinal problems, appendicitis, and hernias may cause a limp. Although it is rare, pernicious anemia in a child may manifest as ataxia, which may be confused with limping.

Selected References

Barkin RM, Barkin SZ, Barkin AZ: The limping child, *J Emerg Med* 18:331-339, 2000.

Calmbach WL, Hutchens HG: Evaluation of patients presenting with knee pain, part 2: differential diagnosis, *Am Fam Physician* 68:917-922, 2003.

DeBocck H, Vorlat P: Limping in childhood, *Acta Orthop Belg* 69:301-310, 2003.

Fordham L, Gunderman R, Blatt ER, et al: *Expert Panel on Pediatric Imaging: Limping child—ages 0-5 years,* American College of Radiology (ACR), 2007. Available at http://www.acr.org/SecondaryMainMenuCategories/quality_safety/app_criteria/pdf/ExpertPanelonPediatricImaging/LimpingChildUpdateinProgressDoc6.aspx.

Leet AI, Skaggs DL: Evaluation of the acutely limping child, *Am Fam Physician* 61:1011-1021, 2000.

Leung AKC, Lemay JF: The limping child, *J Pediatr Health Care* 18:219-223, 2004.

Sawyer J, Kapoor M: The limping child: a systematic approach to diagnosis, *Am Fam Physician* 79:215-224, 2009.

Tse S, Laxer R: Approach to acute limb pain in childhood, *Pediatri Rev* 27:170-179, 2006.

Pain in the Upper Extremity

26

SHOULDER

After backache, upper extremity pain is the next most common type of musculoskeletal pain. It usually occurs in the joints (shoulder, elbow, and wrist), with the shoulder being the most common site. Subacromial impingement syndrome and rotator cuff tears are the most common disorders. Arm pain is frequently caused by occupational *repetitive strain injury*. Shoulder pain can be referred from the neck, chest, or diaphragmatic region; it is usually caused by a local process. On rare occasions, systemic disease affecting the viscera may cause pain referred to the shoulder (Fig. 26-1). The "shoulder joint" consists of three large bones (clavicle, scapula, humerus) and four joints (sternoclavicular, acromioclavicular, glenohumeral, thoracoscapular) (Figs. 26-2 to 26-4).

Terms used to describe painful disorders of the shoulder refer to variations of the same basic process and include *supraspinatus tendinitis, rotator cuff tendinitis, subacromial bursitis, bicipital tendinitis, painful arc syndrome, impingement syndrome, calcific tendinitis, calcific bursitis,* and *calcific bicipital tendinitis.*

Pain may originate in the bursa as well as in the shoulder joint. Many writers suggest that the only significant bursa in the shoulder is the subacromial bursa and that the subdeltoid, subcoracoid, and supraspinatus bursae are extensions of the subacromial bursa.

The initial process with shoulder pain is usually *supraspinatus tendinitis* with extension to other muscles of the rotator cuff. With severe or continuing damage, the inflammatory process spreads first to the subacromial bursa and then to the joint capsule and intra-articular and extra-articular structures. **The greater the area of pain in the arm and shoulder and the greater the spontaneity of pain (i.e., onset without aggravating events), the greater the likelihood of an extensive lesion.**

Pain in the shoulder (as well as in the elbow and wrist) can be caused by *tendinitis, bursitis, trauma, arthritis,* or *referred pain.* Cartilage and bone are not very sensitive to pain. The following are listed in order of decreasing pain sensitivity: tendons, bursae, ligaments, synovial tissue, capsular reinforcements, and muscles.

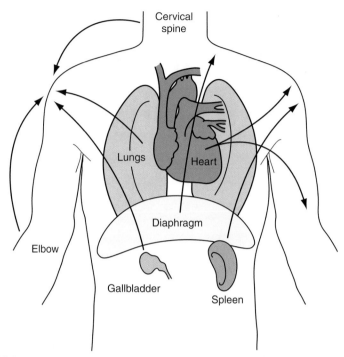

Figure 26-1. Potential site for the referral of pain from the viscera. (Reprinted from McGee DJ: Orthopedic Physical Assessment, 2nd ed. New York , Churchill Livingstone, 1992, p 125 [with permission].)

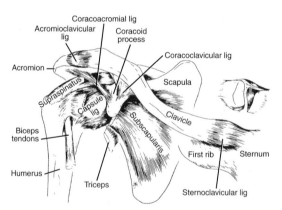

Figure 26-2. Glenohumeral, acromioclavicular, and sternoclavicular joints. The thoracoscapular joint is between the anterior scapular surface and the chest wall. (From Bland JH, Merrit JA, Boushey DR: The painful shoulder. Semin Arthritis Rheum 7:21-47, 1977.)

Nature of Patient

It is important to note the patient's age, dominant hand, occupation, and sports activity.

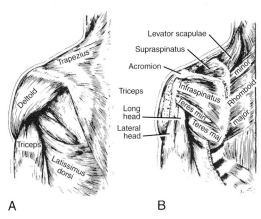

Figure 26-3. Posterior view of the shoulder. **A,** Surface muscles (all groups). **B,** Rotator cuff; subscapularis not shown (medial rotator). Note that the rhomboids and levator scapulae displace the scapula medially toward the midline, whereas the scapulohumeral group rotates the humerus laterally. (From Bland JH, Merrit JA, Boushey DR: The painful shoulder. Semin Arthritis Rheum 7:21-47, 1977.)

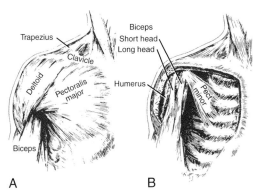

Figure 26-4. Anterior view of the shoulder. **A,** Surface muscles. **B,** Deep layer of muscles. (From Bland JH, Merrit JA, Boushey DR: The painful shoulder. Semin Arthritis Rheum 7:21-47, 1977.)

Acute subacromial bursitis, which is painful enough to cause marked limitation of movement, is more common in younger patients. *Calcific tendinitis* is also more common in younger people and is seldom associated with tears; it is more often seen as a sequela to acute bursitis. A *supraspinatus tear,* which permits some movement, is more common in people 40 years and older. *Dislocation of the shoulder* is also more common in people older than 50 years. First-time dislocations after ages 40 to 50 have a much higher incidence of a rotator cuff tear, which is rare before age 40 years.

Nature of Symptoms

In general, most shoulder problems cause pain in the fifth cervical (C5) dermatome, particularly around the deltoid insertion. The exception is the acromioclavicular joint, which causes pain in the C4 dermatome, especially on the superior aspect of the shoulder or the joint itself. *Intracapsular lesions* of the glenohumeral joint, such as those resulting from arthritis or capsulitis, typically restrict active and passive ranges of motion. The more common *extracapsular lesions*, such as rotator cuff injuries and tendinitis, cause pain on active or resisted motion, whereas passive motion is usually maintained. When *impingement* causes inflammation of the superior part of the cuff, pain develops with resisted abduction and external rotation.

Shoulder pain, referred from the cervical spine, is not affected by shoulder movement but may be influenced by neck movement. The pain may also be felt in the neck and radiate down the arm to an area below the elbow.

Involvement of Supraspinatus Tendon. Shoulder pain is most often located in the lower part of the deltoid region; this is the referral area for pain originating in the supraspinatus tendon. When a dull ache in the region of the deltoid insertion is exacerbated with abduction to 60 degrees or more (painful arc), internal rotation, reaching overhead, or putting on a coat, the physician should suspect *supraspinatus tendinitis*. Characteristically, patients report that the pain is worse at night or when they lie on the affected shoulder.

Involvement of Teres Minor, Infraspinatus, and Subscapularis Muscles. If the shoulder is diffusely tender and moving the humerus posteriorly causes pain, teres minor or infraspinatus muscle involvement should be suspected. If there is pain with resisted medial rotation, the subscapularis muscle may be involved. In patients with teres minor, infraspinatus, and subscapularis involvement with diffuse shoulder tenderness, pain does not usually radiate into the arm or neck and is usually absent or minimal when the arm is dependent.

Tears and Ruptures of Rotator Cuff. If the patient has a sudden onset of shoulder pain in the deltoid area that intensifies within 6 to 12 hours after the initial trauma, a rotator cuff tear should be suspected. The patient may have extreme tenderness over the greater tuberosity as well as pain and restricted motion in one plane of movement at the glenohumeral joint. Patients with these findings and recurrent, severe pain that awakens them at night may have a rotator cuff tear, even if the arthrographic findings are normal. In cases of complete rotator cuff rupture, the patient has severe pain and is totally unable to abduct the arm.

Calcific Tendinitis. After a rotator cuff tear, calcification and calcific tendinitis of the rotator cuff may develop. Calcification has been reported in the rotator cuff in 8% of the asymptomatic population older than 30 years. Nevertheless, studies have shown that 35% of all patients with calcific tendinitis have had symptoms at some time. If 8% of the population has calcific tendinitis and 35% of these people experience symptoms, about 3% of patients older than 30 years eventually present with pain referable to calcific tendinitis. Some studies have related the extent of the symptoms to the size of the calcific area. In the patient in whom the diameter of the calcific mass reaches 1 to 1.5 cm (about ½ inch), symptoms invariably develop. Such a patient has an abrupt onset of severe, aching pain and finds all shoulder movement painful.

Bicipital and Tricipital Tendinitis. When the patient has generalized tenderness anteriorly in the region of the long head of the biceps (the region of the anterior subacromial bursa), particularly if the pain seems to be worse at night, bicipital tendinitis should be suspected. This pain resembles that of adhesive capsulitis, except that the patient with bicipital tendinitis has relative freedom of abduction and forward flexion. Resisted forearm supination causing anterior shoulder pain is a hallmark of bicipital tendinitis. If there is pain in the triceps region with resisted extension of the elbow, tricipital tendinitis is probable.

Bursitis. When the patient has point tenderness over the subacromial bursa (often associated with swelling and warmth), subacromial bursitis is probable. Pain in the acromioclavicular joint suggests that this joint is the source of pain. Patients with subacromial bursitis experience particular pain while performing activities such as lifting objects and combing hair. Virtually all cases of subacromial bursitis are preceded by tendinitis or tenosynovitis in the rotator cuff, biceps, or biceps tendon sheath. When acute onset of excruciating pain occurs in the subdeltoid region of such severity that shoulder movement is totally limited, *calcific bursitis* is probable. Friction of an inflamed bursal surface may be detected with passive motion if the patient is unable to abduct or rotate the upper arm. This acute inflammatory process is probably secondary to calcific deposits in the coracoacromial arch, which ultimately ruptures into the bursal sac, leading to acute bursitis.

Frozen Shoulder. A frozen shoulder should be suspected when the patient has gradual onset of pain with limitation of motion at both the glenohumeral and scapulothoracic joints and has limitation of abduction, external rotation, and forward flexion. Although a frozen shoulder is most often caused by inflammation of the capsule or rotator cuff, it has many other possible causes. The hallmark of frozen shoulder is a spontaneous onset of pain that worsens gradually and insidiously. The pain may radiate into the neck and arm, but pain below the elbow is unusual.

Subluxation or Dislocation. When pain in the shoulder follows severe trauma (as opposed to the minor trauma of everyday activity and routine athletic endeavors), it may be caused by subluxation or dislocation of the shoulder joint. The patient may state that the shoulder "doesn't feel right," that "something popped," or that "something feels out of place." If this problem occurs in a child, particularly with other evidence of external trauma, child abuse should be considered.

Impingement Syndrome. An impingement syndrome secondary to sports trauma usually occurs in the vulnerable avascular region of the supraspinatus and biceps tendon. It usually starts as an irritation in the avascular region of the supraspinatus tendon and progresses to an inflammatory response (tendinitis) that involves the biceps tendon and subacromial bursa and then the acromioclavicular joint. This inflammation may finally result in rotator cuff tears and calcification. The most reliable sign of an impingement syndrome is that the pain is reproduced when the arm is flexed forward forcibly against resistance with the elbow extended (Fig. 26-5). Magnetic resonance imaging (MRI) suggests that subacromial bursitis, supraspinatus tendinitis, and impingement syndrome are variants of a single entity.

Site of Pain. The location of pain is also useful in differential diagnosis (Fig. 26-6). Pain in the acromioclavicular joint suggests that the source of pain is that joint. Pain that occurs in any other part of the arm, shoulder, or neck or in the C5 dermatome may be caused by many other shoulder lesions. With supraspinatus tendinitis, the initial symptom frequently is pain in the deltoid insertion area that is precipitated by abduction. As the inflammation spreads to the subacromial bursa, the pain may extend to the distal arm and occasionally into the forearm. Pain that involves the forearm as far as the wrist suggests that the inflammatory process has spread to the capsule and has been present for 3 to 6 months. If the entire arm is painful and motion is extremely limited, the inflammation has spread to involve the capsule and synovium (frozen shoulder). Diffuse trigger points around the shoulder may indicate fibromyalgia. Burning and tingling in the neck and radiating down the arm past the elbow may indicate cervical disc pathology.

Pain from Vigorous Physical Activity. Although they recognize the traumatic aspects of severe falls and motor vehicle accidents and the recurrent trauma

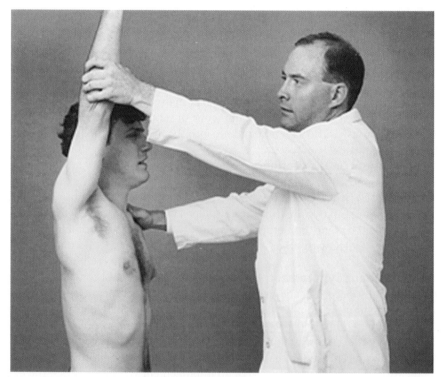

Figure 26-5. Presence of impingement sign. The examiner forcibly flexes the humerus forward, jamming the greater tuberosity against the anterior inferior acromial surface. The patient's facial expression on reproduction of the pain confirms the presence of impingement. This may be relieved by the injection of lidocaine directly into the subacromial bursa. (From Reider B: Orthopaedic Physical Exam, 2nd ed. Philadelphia, WB Saunders, 2005, p 47.)

of competitive sports (e.g., swimming, tennis), examiners may overlook the possibility that shoulder trauma results from ordinary vigorous physical activity (e.g., polishing a car for a few hours). Such physical exertion may cause rotator cuff injuries or subacromial bursitis and severe pain. At rest the pain may be poorly localized; the physician can better determine the source of pain by having the patient repeat the type of activity that apparently induced the pain.

Arthritis.   Arthritis of the shoulder is uncommon but is usually superimposed on a previous injury. With arthritis of the acromioclavicular joint, the pain worsens with adduction of the arm across the chest or with circumduction.

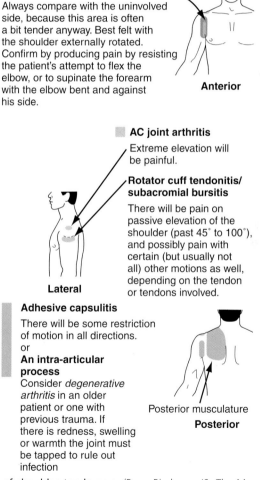

Biceps tendonitis
Always compare with the uninvolved side, because this area is often a bit tender anyway. Best felt with the shoulder externally rotated. Confirm by producing pain by resisting the patient's attempt to flex the elbow, or to supinate the forearm with the elbow bent and against his side.

Anterior

AC joint arthritis
Extreme elevation will be painful.

Rotator cuff tendonitis/ subacromial bursitis
There will be pain on passive elevation of the shoulder (past 45° to 100°), and possibly pain with certain (but usually not all) other motions as well, depending on the tendon or tendons involved.

Lateral

Adhesive capsulitis
There will be some restriction of motion in all directions.
or
An intra-articular process
Consider *degenerative arthritis* in an older patient or one with previous trauma. If there is redness, swelling or warmth the joint must be tapped to rule out infection

Posterior musculature

Posterior

Figure 26-6. Sites of shoulder tenderness. (From Birnbaum JS: The Musculoskeletal Manual, 2nd ed. Philadelphia, WB Saunders, 1986.)

As with other forms of degenerative arthritis, this pain is often worse in the morning and improves as the day progresses.

Nonarticular Pain.   Nonarticular arm pain is most often caused by *overuse syndromes (repetitive strain injury)*. Other common causes are *thoracic outlet, cervical disc*, and *carpal tunnel syndromes* (Table 26-1).

Associated Symptoms

Weakness and atrophy of muscles are uncommon with *supraspinatus tendinitis*. With *rotator cuff tears*, supraspinatus and infraspinatus atrophy may occur in about 3 weeks. With prolonged *frozen shoulder*, several shoulder muscles may atrophy. Patients with *acute bursitis* resist any passive or active shoulder motion.

TABLE 26-1.   Differential Diagnosis of Thoracic Outlet, Cervical Disc, and Carpal Tunnel Syndromes

SYMPTOMS	THORACIC OUTLET	CERVICAL DISC	CARPAL TUNNEL
Symptoms			
Pain	Neck, shoulder, and arm (intermittent)	Neck, shoulder, and arm (constant)	Wrist; volar forearm; fingers 1, 2, and 3 (intermittent)
Numbness	Ulnar nerve or whole hand or arm	Radial nerve (dorsal web between fingers 1 and 2)	Median nerve; fingers 2, 3, and 4
Awkwardness	All fingers or 4 and 5	Thumb	Fingers 1, 2, and 3
Aggravation	Arm elevation	Neck turn or arm stretch	Sustained grasp, pinch
Color	Normal, pallid, cyanotic, or splotchy	Normal or splotchy	Normal, red, or splotchy
Edema	May be present	Absent	May be present
Signs			
Pain on percussion	Brachial plexus	Neck at disc level	Tinel's sign (volar wrist)
Pain on compression	Brachial plexus	Neck and brachial plexus	Phalen's sign (wrist flexion)
Symptoms reproduced by	Arm elevation and brachial plexus compression	Head turn and tilt, cranial compression	Wrist and finger flexion
Nerve conduction test result	Positive or negative (unreliable if negative)		Positive or negative (unreliable if negative)
Radiographic finding	Normal, ling C7 process, anomalies (venoarteriogram)	Degenerative arthritis; disc space narrowed to 85% of normal on myelogram	Normal, arthritis, or old trauma

Modified from Stabile MJ, Warfield CA: Differential diagnosis of arm pain. Hosp Pract 25:5-58, 61, 64, 1990.

Arthritis should be suspected if other joints are involved. If paresthesia or hyperesthesia in the region of C8 or T1 (first thoracic) is noted, especially with atrophy of the hypothenar eminence, *thoracic outlet syndrome* should be suspected. Patients with this condition may also demonstrate Raynaud's phenomenon.

Precipitating and Aggravating Factors
Prolonged and sustained immobilization with the arm at the side may lead to a *frozen shoulder*. This immobilization may have been recommended by the physician, or the patient may have avoided movement for some other reason for a prolonged period. *Impingement syndrome* is often precipitated by repetitive use of the arm above the horizontal position (as in throwing a baseball or in football, swimming, or tennis). Isolated arthritis of the sternoclavicular joint may be caused by trauma or weightlifting. *Septic arthritis of the sternoclavicular joint* has been reported in heroin users and patients with gonococcal arthritis.

Ameliorating Factors
Full trunk and hip flexion that allows the arm to hang limp or supports the forearm in flexion may help alleviate the pain of *rotator cuff tears*. This finding may also help the physician establish the diagnosis.

Physical Findings
A careful physical examination, including resisted adduction, resisted medial rotation, resisted lateral rotation, and resisted abduction, with implementation of specific maneuvers, is essential to the effective diagnosis and management of pain in the upper extremity. Both active and passive ranges of motion of the neck and shoulder joint are indicated. In most cases the diagnosis can be made without radiography or arthrography. No pain on resisted adduction rules out problems in four muscles: pectoralis major, latissimus dorsi, teres major, and teres minor. Pain on resisted medial rotation suggests a problem with the subscapularis tendon, an uncommon cause of shoulder pain. Exacerbation of pain with resisted lateral rotation suggests a problem in the infraspinatus tendon. Patients with *supraspinatus tendinitis* have pain on resisted abduction, limitation of joint motion (with or without disruption of the scapulohumeral rhythm), and a normal passive range of motion. Pain is absent or minimal when the arm is dependent. Pain is usually located in the deltoid region, where the supraspinatus tendon inserts.

Patients with *rotator cuff tears* usually have a full range of passive movement and experience pain at extremes of motion. They have pain and restricted movement at the glenohumeral joint and experience pain and weakness with resisted movement. These patients may also demonstrate the *drop arm* sign: weak ability to maintain abduction after passive abduction support is removed. Radiographs may show that the humeral head is high in the glenoid when the arm is in full adduction. Patients with *calcific rotator cuff tendinitis* experience pain with all movements of the shoulder. They usually have associated muscle spasm throughout the shoulder.

Patients with *bicipital tendinitis* experience exacerbation of pain on resisted forearm supination, which causes anterior shoulder pain. Likewise, pain occurs with resisted flexion of the shoulder at about 80 degrees.

ELBOW

Overuse syndromes may involve the elbow. These muscle strains may be vocational or recreational due to weightlifting, throwing, or racquet sports. *Tennis elbow* is *lateral (forehand) epicondylitis* of the humerus that may appear in tennis players of any age or level of expertise, especially those older than 40 years. *Medial (backhand) epicondylitis* also occurs in tennis players and golfers. Epicondylitis may occur in people who do not play tennis. Lateral epicondylitis is caused by overexertion of the finger and wrist extensors, which originate in the region of the lateral epicondyle. Pain and acute tenderness arise at the origin of the forearm extensor muscles, which attach just distal to the lateral epicondyle of the humerus. The pain may radiate down the back of the forearm. Patients with epicondylitis also experience pain while performing an activity such as opening a door or lifting a cup or glass.

Lateral epicondylitis has been referred to as *backhand tennis elbow,* and medial epicondylitis as *forehand tennis elbow*. Medial epicondylitis also occurs in golfers and baseball pitchers (Fig. 26-7).

If pain and swelling are noted in the posterior aspect of the elbow, *olecranon bursitis* should be suspected. This may occur after a forced, vigorous extension of the elbow joint or from repeated microtrauma. Acute olecranon bursitis can be differentiated from acute arthritis of the elbow in that passive extension is unimpaired in bursitis. Patients with septic olecranon bursitis are usually febrile and have a skin lesion overlying the bursa, with bursal tenderness. If a child experiences pain in the elbow after being swung around by the hand or after having the elbow pulled suddenly while the arm is pronated and extended, *radial head dislocation* is probable. *Rheumatoid arthritis* occasionally involves the elbow (Fig. 26-8).

HAND AND WRIST

Pain at the base of the thumb aggravated by movement of the wrist or thumb and reproducible by flexion of the thumb is called *de Quervain's disease* (Fig. 26-9), which is *tenosynovitis* of the thumb abductors and extensors. This is different from osteoarthritis at the base of the thumb, which is most common in postmenopausal women. Pain in the palm at the base of the third and fourth digits, often associated with a "catching" sensation or with fixation of the fingers in flexion, is known as *Dupuytren's contracture*. Examination reveals painless thickening of the palmar fascia or tendon sheath. If the pain is in the anatomic snuff box, it can be assumed to be due to *navicular bone fracture* unless another cause is determined. Pain or numbness of the fingers is seen in *Raynaud's disease* and associated conditions, including *Buerger's disease, systemic lupus erythematosus* (SLE), and *scleroderma*.

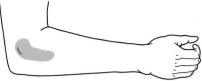

Lateral epicondylitis
There will be pain here as you resist the
patient's effort to extend (dorsiflex) his
wrist and/or supinate his forearm.

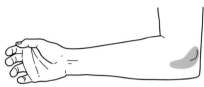

Medial epicondylitis
There will be pain here as you resist the
patient's effort to flex his wrist and/or
pronate his forearm.

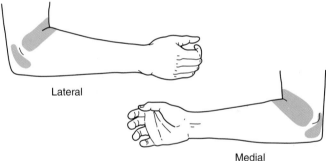

Lateral

Medial

An intra-articular process
Consider **degenerative arthritis** in an older
patient or one with previous trauma; if there
is redness swelling, or warmth, the joint must
be tapped to rule out infection.

Figure 26-7. Sites of elbow tenderness. (From Birnbaum JS: The Musculoskeletal Manual,
2nd ed. Philadelphia, WB Saunders, 1986.)

Peripheral nerve entrapment syndromes such as carpal tunnel syndrome
(median nerve) may cause pain, numbness, or both in the wrist, hand, or forearm. *Carpal tunnel syndrome* is the most common cause of nocturnal hand
pain and often occurs in the later stages of pregnancy and rheumatoid arthritis.
Result of the Phalen test (flexion of the wrist) is usually positive.

Thoracic outlet syndrome (previously referred to as scalenus anticus syndrome, neurovascular compression syndrome, and hyperabduction syndrome)

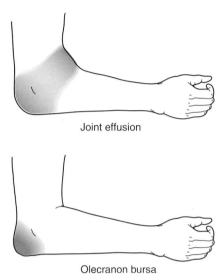

Joint effusion

Olecranon bursa

Figure 26-8. **Elbow swelling.** (From Birnbaum JS: The Musculoskeletal Manual, 2nd ed. Philadelphia, WB Saunders, 1986.)

is most common in middle-aged women and usually occurs on the left side. This syndrome manifests as intermittent pain, numbness, or weakness in the hand (occasionally the forearm) after the arm or arms have been in a hyperabducted state for a prolonged period. Patients often experience this discomfort after working for an extended period with the arms over the head or after sleeping with the arms folded behind the neck. Physical findings are normal except when specific maneuvers are employed. For example, forcing the shoulders back and down while the patient is in forced inspiration may obliterate the radial pulse on the affected side. Likewise, the radial pulse may be obliterated by the Adson maneuver.

Degenerative arthritis usually involves the distal interphalangeal joints, whereas *rheumatoid arthritis* most often involves the proximal interphalangeal and metacarpophalangeal joints. Rheumatoid arthritis can also involve the elbow and wrist; it seldom involves the shoulder. Patients with active rheumatoid arthritis usually have joint stiffness as well as warmth, swelling, and tenderness. The pain is usually polyarticular and migratory rather than monoarticular.

Pain in the wrist is most often caused by *trauma*. Wrist sprains and, less commonly, fractures are occurring more frequently with the increased popularity of in-line skating and home trampolines. A fall on the outstretched arm with the wrist extended often results in a *scaphoid bone fracture*. Classically, there is pain in the anatomic snuff box, but early radiographic findings may be negative, and special scaphoid views, a bone scan, or MRI may be required. **Because the symptoms may be mild and radiographic findings negative, this diagnosis must be kept in mind, because an overlooked scaphoid fracture is a common cause of litigation.**

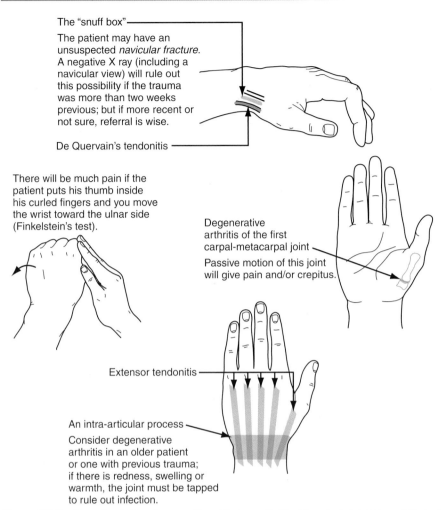

The "snuff box"—
The patient may have an unsuspected *navicular fracture*. A negative X ray (including a navicular view) will rule out this possibility if the trauma was more than two weeks previous; but if more recent or not sure, referral is wise.

De Quervain's tendonitis —

There will be much pain if the patient puts his thumb inside his curled fingers and you move the wrist toward the ulnar side (Finkelstein's test).

Degenerative arthritis of the first carpal-metacarpal joint —
Passive motion of this joint will give pain and/or crepitus.

Extensor tendonitis —

An intra-articular process —
Consider degenerative arthritis in an older patient or one with previous trauma; if there is redness, swelling or warmth, the joint must be tapped to rule out infection.

Figure 26-9. **Sites of wrist tenderness.** (From Birnbaum JS: The Musculoskeletal Manual, 2nd ed. Philadelphia, WB Saunders, 1986.)

DIAGNOSTIC STUDIES

Precise clinical examination is more useful than radiography in the evaluation of soft tissue injuries. Arthroscopy, ultrasonography, MRI, and magnetic resonance arthrography are all useful in the diagnosis of shoulder disorders. Ultrasonography is most readily available and often the most cost-effective. Radiographs and occasionally bone scans should be obtained if fracture is suspected. Electromyography and nerve conduction studies are helpful tools in the diagnosis of neural entrapment syndromes such as carpal tunnel syndrome.

LESS COMMON DIAGNOSTIC CONSIDERATIONS

Less common sources of pain in the upper extremity include some types of local discomfort and referred pain. Apical lung tumors (Pancoast's tumor), cervical disk disease, and cervical spondylosis can all produce shoulder pain. *Cervical spondylosis* can result from intervertebral disk protrusion or primary spondylosis. If radiculitis is present, the pain is sharp and well localized. The patient may have paresthesias and numbness in the sensory distribution of the compromised nerve root. Fasciculations may also be present, and the pain may be exacerbated by movement of the cervical spine. Despite shoulder pain, a full range of motion may be possible. Cervical spondylosis can often be identified by tenderness over the motor point (where the motor nerve enters the muscle).

Sternoclavicular joint arthritis is rare but occurs in a small number of patients with rheumatic diseases as well as in weightlifters. This pain is usually an anterior chest discomfort that may radiate to the shoulder or arm. In the patient with significant soft tissue swelling and warmth in a wide area around the joint, the possibility of septic arthritis, particularly gonococcal, must be considered. Osteoarthritis of the acromioclavicular joint, though rare, may be confused with an impingement syndrome.

Shoulder pain can be referred from *neck* and *visceral lesions*, including mediastinal disease, subphrenic abscess, and gallbladder disease. *Neural entrapment syndromes* (e.g., median and ulnar nerve compression) cause pain in the distribution of the involved nerves. Median nerve compression syndrome is caused by compression of the median nerve as it passes beneath the flexor retinaculum, and its symptoms are those of carpal tunnel syndrome. This condition is most common in middle-aged and elderly women. Patients usually complain of pain and paresthesias in the thumb and in the index and middle fingers. They may also report that they feel clumsy when performing fine movements such as sewing and picking up small objects. Patients may have a sensory loss of median nerve distribution and weakness of the thenar muscles. Both the pain and the paresthesia may be worse at night and on awakening. Suprascapular neuropathy, often misdiagnosed as subacromial impingement syndrome, can be correctly diagnosed with electrophysiologic testing.

Cervical spine and *cervical cord lesions* (rarely thoracic discs) often produce referred pain in the upper extremity. Herniation of the disk at C5-C6 or C6-C7 causes pain from the back of the neck, across the back of the shoulder, and down the arm and forearm to the wrist. The patients may have a history of a recurrent stiff neck. The pain is often aggravated by movement, particularly flexion, of the neck. There may also be paresthesias of the thumb and index finger.

Cervical spine spondylosis can cause pain and stiffness in the neck and a radicular distribution of pain in one or both arms. Compression of the cervical cord can cause weakness, wasting, and fibrillations in the upper limbs; paresthesias in the arms or legs; and occasional evidence of pyramidal involvement (e.g., weakness, spasticity, increased deep tendon reflexes, and presence of Babinski's sign).

Differential Diagnosis of Upper Extremity Pain

CAUSE	NATURE OF PATIENT	NATURE OF SYMPTOMS	ASSOCIATED SYMPTOMS	PRECIPITATING AND AGGRAVATING FACTORS	AMELIORATING FACTORS	PHYSICAL FINDINGS
Shoulder						
Supraspinatus tendinitis	Age >40 yr	Pain in lower part of deltoid region, which is referral area for pain from supraspinatus tendon		Reaching overhead and lying on affected shoulder		Pain worse with resisted abduction and abduction to 60 degrees and internal rotation
Subacromial bursitis	Age <40 yr	Severe pain with marked limitation of motion Pain may radiate to distal arm and even forearm		Lifting objects or combing hair		Point tenderness over subacromial bursa, which may be warm and swollen
Bicipital tendinitis		Generalized tenderness anteriorly in region of long head of biceps (anterior subacromial bursa)				Resisted forearm supination causes anterior shoulder pain Free abduction and forward flexion
Calcific tendinitis	Younger adults	Usually a sequela to acute bursitis	Recurrent pain			
Rotator cuff tear	Adults	Sudden onset Pain in deltoid area that intensifies 6 to 12 hr after initial trauma			Arm hanging limp	Restricted motion in one plane at glenohumeral joint Weakness and atrophy of supraspinatus and infraspinatus Pain over greater tuberosity

Continued

Differential Diagnosis of Upper Extremity Pain—cont'd

CAUSE	NATURE OF PATIENT	NATURE OF SYMPTOMS	ASSOCIATED SYMPTOMS	PRECIPITATING AND AGGRAVATING FACTORS	AMELIORATING FACTORS	PHYSICAL FINDINGS
Teres minor or infraspinatus tendinitis		Diffuse shoulder pain	No pain radiation into arm or neck		Arm dependent	Pain worse with resisted lateral rotation Pain on moving humerus posteriorly
Subscapularis tendinitis		Diffuse shoulder pain	No pain radiation into arm or neck		Arm dependent	Pain with resisted medial rotation
Frozen shoulder		Gradual onset of pain with limitation of motion at glenohumeral and scapulothoracic joints Limitation of abduction, extension, rotation, and forward flexion Pain may radiate into neck and down arm to elbow	Some atrophy of shoulder muscles	Prolonged immobilization		Marked restriction of motion of shoulder in all directions

Secondary impingement syndrome	Athletes (e.g., baseball, swimming, tennis)	Tendinitis of biceps and/or supraspinatus tendon progressing to subacromial bursitis and inflammation of acromioclavicular joint		Pain on forward flexion of arm with elbow extended
Lesion of cervical spine and cord	Referred pain to upper extremity: back of neck, back of shoulder, down arm, forearm			Pain and hypesthesia along dermatome distribution
Elbow				
Lateral epicondylitis: "forehand"	Often in tennis players, especially those older than 40 yr	Pain over lateral epicondyle that may radiate down back of forearm	Resisted extension of wrist and supination of forearm	Tender on palpation over lateral epicondyle
Lateral epicondylitis: "backhand"	Golfers, tennis players	Medial epicondylitis Pain in back of elbow		Tender over medial epicondyle

Continued

Differential Diagnosis of Upper Extremity Pain—cont'd

CAUSE	NATURE OF PATIENT	NATURE OF SYMPTOMS	ASSOCIATED SYMPTOMS	PRECIPITATING AND AGGRAVATING FACTORS	AMELIORATING FACTORS	PHYSICAL FINDINGS
Bursitis						Swelling, warmth, and tenderness over back of elbow
Radial head dislocation	Child			Being swung around by arms		Radial head palpable in displaced position
Hand and Wrist						
Tenosynovitis of abductors and extensors of wrist (de Quervain's disease)		Pain at base of thumb		Flexing thumb		
Tenosynovitis of flexors of fingers (Dupuytren's contracture)		Pain in palm at base of third and fourth digits				Catching or fixation of third or fourth digits in flexion Painless thickening of palmar fascia or tendon sheath
Thoracic outlet syndrome	More common in middle-aged women	Hand pain, weakness, or numbness (usually left) after arms are hyperabducted or on awakening	Numbness of ulnar distribution or whole hand	Prolonged hyperabduction		Decreased radial pulse with Adson and other maneuvers

Gout and pseudogout	Adults	Wrist often involved in pseudogout		
Carpal tunnel syndrome	More common in women	Pain in wrist radiating to hand and forearm		Results of Tinel and Phalen tests may be positive Thenar wasting
Osteoarthritis at base of thumb	Most common in postmenopausal women	Pain at base of thumb and thenar eminence	Pinching and grasping large objects, opening jar tops, turning doorknobs	Pain and crepitus at the trapeziometacarpal joint Poor correlation of symptoms with radiographic findings

The combination of atrophic weakness in the arms and spastic weakness in the legs may suggest *amyotrophic lateral sclerosis.* Spondylosis can be distinguished from amyotrophic lateral sclerosis by a history of paresthesias and the presence of sensory impairment in the former condition.

Meningeal tumors, Pott's disease, and primary or secondary *vertebral body tumors* may produce upper extremity pain as a result of root compression. On rare occasions, benign and malignant tumors cause pain in the elbow, forearm, and wrist. When this pain occurs in a young athlete, sports injury is often diagnosed erroneously. In elderly patients, *herpes zoster* may cause pain in the arm. Many of patients with this condition have a history of an eruption and residual pigmented scars.

Angina pectoris is a common cause of pain in the arm and shoulder. This pain is most frequently located in the upper left arm and usually associated with precordial pain. A history of pain in the arm with exertion is the major diagnostic clue for angina pectoris.

Arteritis of the great vessels (Norwegian pulseless disease) is a rare condition that can produce intermittent claudication of one or both arms. It is most common in young women and should be considered in those patients who have diminished blood pressure in one or both arms, especially if they also experience transient episodes of blindness or other cerebral incidents. The rare quadrilateral space syndrome (neurovascular compression of the axillary nerve and posterior circumflex humeral artery) may cause shoulder pain radiating to the arm.

Painful swelling of the wrist not due to trauma may be caused by acute *gout* or acute *pseudogout.* Both are more common in adult or elderly individuals.

Selected References

American Academy of Orthopaedic Surgeons: *Clinical guideline on diagnosis of carpal tunnel syndrome,* Rosemont, IL, 2007, American Academy of Orthopaedic Surgeons (AAOS).

Burbank KM, Stevenson JH, Czarnecki GR, et al: Chronic shoulder pain, part I: evaluation and diagnosis, *Am Fam Physician* 77:453-460, 2008.

Chumbley EM, O'Conner FG, Nirschl RP: Evaluation of overuse elbow injuries, *Am Fam Physician* 61:691-700, 2000.

Churgay C: Diagnosis and treatment of biceps tendinitis and tendinosis, *Am Fam Physician* 80: 470-476, 2009.

Ciccotti MC, Schwartz MA, Ciccotti MG: Diagnosis and treatment of medial epicondylitis of the elbow, *Clin Sports Med* 23:693-705, 2004.

Doherty M, Jones A: Fibromyalgia syndrome, *Br Med J* 310:386-389, 1995.

Forman T, Forman S, Rose N: A clinical approach to diagnosing wrist pain, *Am Fam Physician* 72:1753-1758, 2005.

Glickel SZ: Clinical assessment of the thumb trapeziometacarpal joint, *Hand Clin* 17:185-195, 2001.

Neal S, Fields K: Peripheral nerve entrapment and injury in the upper extremity, *Am Fam Physician* 81:147-155, 2010.

Spindler KP, Dovan TT, McCarty EC: Assessment and management of the painful shoulder, *Clin Cornerstone* 3:26-37, 2001.

Stevenson JH, Trojian T: Evaluation of shoulder pain, *J Fam Pract* 51:605-611, 2002.

Tytherleigh-Strong G, Hirahara A, Miniaci A: Rotator cuff disease, *Curr Opin Rheumatol* 13: 135-145, 2001.

Palpitations

27

Palpitations are defined here as sensations of a skipped heartbeat, an irregular heartbeat, a rapid or slow heartbeat, or increased awareness of the heartbeat. A patient's awareness of the heartbeat occurs most frequently at rest (e.g., while watching television or lying in bed). In bed the mattress serves as a resonator; this facilitates an awareness of the heartbeat, which may be fast, slow, irregular, or normal.

The most common causes of palpitations are *anxiety, stimulants* (e.g., caffeine, alcohol), *drugs* (e.g., amphetamines, cocaine, digitalis glycosides, psychotropic agents, thyroid hormone), and *cardiac disease* (e.g., valvular disease, ischemia, myocardiopathy, mitral valve prolapse, and heart failure). Other common causes are *conduction abnormalities* (e.g., Wolff-Parkinson-White syndrome, sick sinus syndrome), *panic disorder, hypoglycemia, reactive hypoglycemia, hyperthyroidism, hypoxia,* and *hyperventilation.*

If the palpitations occur infrequently, are not associated with other symptoms (e.g., chest pain, syncope, dizzy spells), and develop in an otherwise healthy patient, concern or extensive workup is probably unnecessary. **If palpitations are frequent, are disturbing to the patient, are or associated with near-syncope or syncope, dizzy spells, chest pain, activity, or evidence of heart disease, they should be considered more serious and further investigation is required. The studies should include electrocardiography performed with the patient at rest, exercise electrocardiography, and frequent 24-hour Holter monitoring or closed-loop event monitoring.**

NATURE OF PATIENT

In children and adolescents, the complaint of palpitations is most often a sign of *anxiety,* although the congenital form of long QT syndrome must be considered. Caffeine and stimulants in over-the-counter cold remedies may also cause tachyarrhythmias. If a rapid arrhythmia is suspected or the problem is recurrent, the physician should perform electrocardiographic studies and Holter monitoring to determine whether *Wolff-Parkinson-White syndrome* is present.

The most common arrhythmias in children are supraventricular tachycardias. Children, adolescents, and young adults should be specifically questioned about the use of *stimulants,* such as tobacco, snuff, caffeine, alcohol, and street drugs (methamphetamine or cocaine).

In adults who have no clinical evidence of heart disease or other systemic disease, the complaint of palpitations is often only an awareness of their normal heartbeat or an occasional atrial or ventricular contraction. The patient should be questioned carefully about excessive use of tobacco and about stimulants such as caffeine, alcohol, and other agents, including recreational drugs, amphetamines, psychotropic agents, over-the-counter weight-reducing agents, and thyroid replacement therapy. **Increasing age often brings a decreasing tolerance to agents such as caffeine, alcohol, and drugs.** These agents, though previously tolerated without symptoms, may induce palpitations as the patient gets older. Palpitations (often paroxysmal atrial fibrillation) are occasionally noted by a patient during the day after unusual but not necessarily excessive alcohol ingestion, a phenomenon known as *holiday heart syndrome.* The most common causes of palpitations in elderly patients include supraventricular and ventricular premature beats, sick sinus syndrome, and atrial fibrillation.

Patients with known cardiac disease who complain of palpitations are more likely to have serious arrhythmias, such as *atrial fibrillation, ventricular tachycardia,* and *sick sinus syndrome.* If a patient with a wide-complex tachycardia has a history of heart failure, myocardial infarction, or recent-onset angina, the tachycardia is more likely to be ventricular in origin than supraventricular with aberration. Those who have poor left ventricular function are particularly prone to ventricular arrhythmias and sudden death. *Mitral valve prolapse* occurs most frequently in young women. One study revealed that the average age of patients with mitral valve prolapse is 38 years and that 70% of these patients are women.

Palpitations occur more frequently and are of greater clinical significance in patients with the *click-murmur syndrome* than in those with only an echocardiographic diagnosis of mitral value prolapse. Well-conditioned athletes often have a *resting bradycardia* (sometimes marked). This condition may be associated with premature ventricular contractions, first-degree atrioventricular (AV) block, and second-degree atrioventricular block; these arrhythmias disappear with exercise.

NATURE OF SYMPTOMS

All patients should be questioned about the characteristics (fast, slow, irregular, etc.) of the palpitations, mode of onset, mode of termination, precipitating factors, frequency, and results of any prior therapy. Patients may complain of a forceful, fast, slow, or irregular heartbeat. It is often useful to have the patient tap out what the rhythm feels like. If the patient cannot do this, the physician can tap out a selection of rhythms—slow and regular, slow and irregular, fast and regular, and fast and irregular as well as the beat of a premature contraction followed by a compensatory pause—to help the patient describe what s/he means by "palpitations."

The sudden onset of a regular tachycardia with a rate greater than 160 beats per minute suggests a supraventricular tachycardia. A rate of 150 beats per minute suggests atrial flutter with a 2:1 conduction ratio. A rapid, irregularly irregular tachycardia with a pulse deficit suggests atrial fibrillation. The precise nature of the arrhythmia must be documented by electrocardiography or Holter monitoring.

Various types of arrhythmia are typically found at different times in the same patient. Recurrence of arrhythmias in late afternoon and early evening suggests that they are precipitated by *reactive hypoglycemia*. For any patient with unexplained, recurrent arrhythmias that occur several hours after eating, the physician should perform a 5-hour glucose tolerance test to rule out reactive hypoglycemia. These arrhythmias are usually supraventricular in origin. Arrhythmias in insulin-dependent diabetic patients that occur near the time of peak insulin activity are also frequently induced by hypoglycemia. Patients with diabetes often have accelerated coronary artery disease, which is another possible cause of arrhythmias.

ASSOCIATED SYMPTOMS

Fatigue, confusion, and syncope may be noted in patients with *sick sinus syndrome*, which occurs frequently in elderly patients. Sweating, tremors, and other symptoms of *hypoglycemia* suggest that this is contributing to the arrhythmia. Reactive hypoglycemia may also induce arrhythmias. When palpitations are associated with anxiety, dyspnea, dizziness, and tingling in the hands or face, *hyperventilation* may be the cause.

Sticking chest pains that do not usually coincide with the arrhythmia should suggest *mitral valve prolapse*, a condition in which arrhythmias are common. Chest pain, congestive heart failure, syncope, and dizziness all suggest a clinically significant arrhythmia such as *paroxysmal atrial tachycardia, complete heart block*, or *ventricular tachycardia. Generalized anxiety disorder* or *panic attack* should be suspected if the patient with palpitations also complains of symptoms such as shortness of breath, nervousness, gastrointestinal upset, muscle aches, tension, and insomnia.

PRECIPITATING AND AGGRAVATING FACTORS

Although exercise may induce arrhythmias in a normal heart, arrhythmias that increase with exercise are probably caused by *cardiac disease,* especially coronary artery disease, mitral valve prolapse, and cardiomyopathy (both the hypertrophic and dilated forms). When premature ventricular contractions decrease with exercise (and its associated increase in sinus rate), they are probably benign.

Digitalis-induced arrhythmias can be in the form of premature beats, tachyarrhythmias or bradyarrhythmias, supraventricular arrhythmias, supraventricular tachycardia with block, or ventricular tachycardia. Digitalis arrhythmias can be precipitated by increased digitalis dosage, hypokalemia, hypomagnesemia, or decreased renal function. *Antiarrhythmic drugs*, particularly the class I agents (e.g., quinidine, procainamide, lidocaine, disopyramide, phenytoin), can both precipitate and suppress arrhythmias. Their prolongation of the QT interval makes the patient more vulnerable to the torsades de pointes type of ventricular tachycardia, which s/he may perceive as palpitations or dizzy spells. In children, the congenital form of long QT syndrome must be considered. Ventricular arrhythmia can be caused by cocaine, phenothiazines, diphenhydramine, propranolol, propoxyphene, tricyclic antidepressants, amiodarone, and class I agents.

Most of the beta blockers, lithium, many of the antihypertensive agents (e.g., reserpine, methyldopa, clonidine), and the calcium channel blockers cause bradycardia. Hydralazine and minoxidil can cause sinus tachycardia. Sometimes the discontinuation of drugs (e.g., clonidine, phenytoin, beta blockers, antiarrhythmics) is associated with the development of palpitations.

AMELIORATING FACTORS

If the palpitations abate with cessation of stimulants or other drugs, the arrhythmias were most likely caused by the discontinued agent or agents. Some patients find that performing the Valsalva maneuver, pressing on the carotid sinus, or gagging themselves to induce vomiting terminates the arrhythmias. In these patients the arrhythmias are probably supraventricular in origin.

PHYSICAL FINDINGS

Auscultation of a midsystolic click or late systolic murmur is found in patients with *mitral valve prolapse*. Premature atrial or ventricular contractions occur most often in patients with mitral valve prolapse; supraventricular tachycardia or ventricular tachycardia occurs in about 12% of these patients. Signs of dilated cardiomyopathy or congestive heart failure suggest that the palpitations may be ventricular tachycardia or atrial fibrillation. A holosystolic murmur heard at the left sternal border that increases with Valsalva maneuver suggests hypertrophic obstructive cardiomyopathy, which is often associated with ventricular tachycardia and atrial fibrillation.

Many clinical signs and maneuvers (well documented in cardiology texts) may help the physician determine the nature of arrhythmias. **Precise diagnosis requires electrocardiographic documentation.** In anxious patients who complain of palpitations, the arrhythmias may be precipitated by *hyperventilation*. If this is suspected, the physician can instruct the patient to hyperventilate forcibly for 3 or 4 minutes to determine whether this activity induces an arrhythmia that should be recorded. If signs of hyperthyroidism (resting tachycardia, warm sweaty palms, tremor, exophthalmos, or lid lag) are noted, the arrhythmia may be secondary to hyperthyroidism.

Differential Diagnosis of Palpitations

CAUSE	NATURE OF PATIENT	NATURE OF SYMPTOMS	ASSOCIATED SYMPTOMS	PRECIPITATING AND AGGRAVATING FACTORS	PHYSICAL FINDINGS*	DIAGNOSTIC STUDIES†
Anxiety	Most common cause of palpitations in children and adolescents		Sweaty palms	Hyperventilation		
Ingestion of stimulants or drugs (caffeine, alcohol, amphetamines, cocaine)	Patients have decreased tolerance to these agents with increased age		Nervousness Tremor	Caffeine Alcohol Street drugs Drugs (e.g., pseudoephedrine, angiotensin-converting enzyme inhibitors, amphetamines, psychotropic agents, thyroid hormone)	Premature ventricular contractions Tachycardia	Toxicology screening tests
Digitalis glycosides			Nausea Anorexia	Increased digitalis dose Hypokalemia Hypomagnesemia Decreased renal function	Premature ventricular contractions Tachyarrhythmias Bradyarrhythmias Second- or third-degree heart block	Serum digitalis measurement Electrocardio graphy Holter monitoring Serum potassium, magnesium, and creatinine measurements
Beta blockers Antihypertensives Calcium channel blockers	Patients with angina or hypertension				Bradycardia	

Continued

Differential Diagnosis of Palpitations—cont'd

CAUSE	NATURE OF PATIENT	NATURE OF SYMPTOMS	ASSOCIATED SYMPTOMS	PRECIPITATING AND AGGRAVATING FACTORS	PHYSICAL FINDINGS*	DIAGNOSTIC STUDIES†
Hydralazine Minoxidil					Sinus tachycardia	
Hypoglycemia	Insulin-dependent diabetics	Arrhythmias occur near time of peak insulin activity	Sweating Headache Tremor Weakness	Increased insulin Decreased carbohydrates	Premature ventricular contractions Tachycardia	Blood sugar
Hyperthyroidism	More common in older men	Atrial premature contractions May be silent	Nervousness Tremors Weight loss	Heart disease	Atrial fibrillation Premature contractions Tachycardias	Thyroid function tests
Exercise	Normal More frequent in patients with coronary heart disease, hypertension, mitral valve prolapse, and cardiomyopathy			Exercise		
Reactive hypoglycemia		Recurrent arrhythmias in late afternoon and early evening Arrhythmias occur several hours after ingestion of carbohydrates	Sweating Tremors Headache	Anxiety		5-hour glucose tolerance test

Cardiac Diseases

Disease						
Mitral valve prolapse	Most common in young women (average age, 38 years)		Sticking chest pain	Exercise	Midsystolic click Late systolic murmur Premature ventricular contractions or premature atrial contractions Tachycardia	Echocardiography
Wolff-Parkinson-White syndrome	Often detected in children and adolescents	Recurrent palpitations Frequent paroxysmal tachycardia		Exercise Digitalis	Paroxysmal tachycardia	Electrocardiography Holter monitoring
Sick sinus syndrome	Older patients	Bradyarrhythmia Tachyarrhythmia	Chest pain Syncope Congestive heart failure Dizziness	Exercise Digoxin Beta blockers Calcium channel blockers	Bradyarrhythmia Tachyarrhythmia	Electrocardiography Holter monitoring Electrophysiologic studies
Coronary artery disease	Older patients	Palpitations	Angina pectoris Congestive heart failure		Premature ventricular contractions Paroxysmal atrial fibrillation	Exercise electrocardiography Holter monitoring

*Arrhythmias are often absent.
†All arrhythmias should be documented by electrocardiography or Holter monitoring.

DIAGNOSTIC STUDIES

If arrhythmias cannot be documented clinically or electrocardiographically and they occur daily and are associated with dizziness, syncope, or other cardiac symptomatology, 24- to 48-hour Holter monitoring should be performed. When palpitations occur unpredictably, a 2-week course of closed-loop event monitoring must be performed. Trans-telephonic event monitors are more valuable and cost-effective than Holter monitors. Several studies of 24-hour Holter monitoring have shown that a significant number of patients note palpitations when no abnormality is detected on the Holter tape; conversely, many patients demonstrate arrhythmias on the Holter tape but are unaware of palpitations at that time.

Other studies that may help the physician determine the cause of palpitations include thyroid function tests, the 5-hour glucose tolerance test, drug screens, determination of serum digitalis and arterial blood gas levels, echocardiography, invasive cardiac electrophysiologic tests, and (rarely) coronary arteriography. Genetic screening for ion channel disease (short or long QT syndrome) may be life-saving.

LESS COMMON DIAGNOSTIC CONSIDERATIONS

Less common causes of palpitations include *short QT syndrome*, *infiltrative myocardial diseases* such as amyloidosis, sarcoidosis, and tumors. *Hypothyroidism* can cause sinus bradycardia; *hyperthyroidism* can cause sinus tachycardia, paroxysmal atrial tachycardia, and paroxysmal atrial fibrillation.

Selected References

Abbott AV: Diagnostic approach to palpitations, *Am Fam Physician* 71:743-750, 2005:755-756.

Brugada P, Gursoy S, Brugado J, et al: Investigation of palpitations, *Lancet* 341:1254-1258, 1993.

Conway D, Lip GYH: Case book: palpitations, *Practitioner* 245:393-401, 2001.

Giada F, Raviele A: Diagnostic management of patients with palpitations of unknown origin, *Ital Heart J* 5:581-586, 2004.

Kaltman J, Shah M: Evaluation of the child with an arrhythmia, *Pediatr Clin North Am* 51: 1537-1551, 2004.

Kopp DE, Wilber DJ: Palpitations and arrhythmias: separating the benign from the dangerous, *Postgrad Med* 91:241-251, 1992.

Miller MB: Arrhythmias associated with drug toxicity, *Emerg Med Clin North Am* 16:405-417, 1998.

Rajagopalan K, Potts JE, Sanatani S: Minimally invasive approach to the child with palpitations, *Expert Rev Cardiovasc Ther* 4:681-693, 2006.

Rodriguez RD, Schlocken DD: Update on sick sinus syndrome: a cardiac disorder of aging, *Geriatrics* 45:26-30, 1990:33-36.

Schwartz PJ, Crotti L: Ion channel diseases in children: manifestations and management, *Curr Opin Cardiol* 23:184-191, 2008.

Zimetbaum P, Josephson ME: Evaluation of patients with palpitations, *N Engl J Med* 338: 1369-1373, 1998.

Shortness of Breath

28

Dyspnea, or breathlessness, has been defined as patient awareness of respiratory discomfort, unpleasant sensation of labored breathing, or shortness of breath. Dyspnea can be caused by increased rigidity of lung tissue, increased airway resistance, enhanced ventilation during exercise, or any combination of these factors.

Some investigators have suggested that determining the cause of dyspnea is often facilitated by first classifying it into different types, such as wheezing dyspnea, dyspnea on exertion, paroxysmal nocturnal dyspnea, hyperventilation, and dyspnea of cerebral origin. Perhaps a simpler classification is acute, chronic, or recurrent. The common causes of dyspnea include *chronic obstructive pulmonary disease* (COPD), *asthma, congestive heart failure* (CHF), *anxiety, obesity*, and *poor physical condition*.

NATURE OF PATIENT

Acute dyspnea in children is most frequently caused by *asthma, bronchiolitis, croup*, and *epiglottitis*. On rare occasions, it may result from *foreign body aspiration*. An acute onset of dyspnea in a woman who is pregnant or is taking oral contraceptives suggests *pulmonary embolism*. Pulmonary embolism should also be suspected if dyspnea occurs in patients who have recently undergone surgery, in people who have had prolonged recumbency, and in patients who have a history of phlebitis or cardiac arrhythmias (dysrhythmias).

The most common cause of chronic and recurrent shortness of breath in children is asthma. In children, a nocturnal cough or nocturnal wheezing is due to asthma until proven otherwise. In elderly patients, chronic dyspnea is frequently caused by COPD and heart failure, which are rare conditions in patients younger than 30 years. As dyspnea develops in these elderly patients , they decrease their physical activity; the resulting deconditioning confounds the clinical picture.

In the elderly, the most common causes of dyspnea are heart failure, chronic obstructive lung disease, and asthma. Other common causes are pneumonia and parenchymal lung disease. Acute dyspnea in the elderly can be caused by heart failure, asthma, COPD, pulmonary embolism, pneumonia, and pneumothorax.

Chronic dyspnea is more common in people who are heavy smokers, because smoking is one of the most important factors in the development of *emphysema, chronic bronchitis,* and COPD. *Obese* and *physically inactive* patients frequently complain of recurrent dyspnea on minimal exertion because of their poor cardiopulmonary reserve.

NATURE OF SYMPTOMS

The duration of dyspnea, precipitating factors such as exercise and exposure to allergens, nighttime and/or daytime occurrence, the number of pillows used when sleeping, concomitant coughing, chest pain, and palpitations are factors that assist the physician in making an accurate diagnosis.

Acute Dyspnea

In patients with acute dyspnea, the physician should consider the possibility of pulmonary embolus, asthma, upper airway obstruction, foreign body aspiration, panic disorder, hyperventilation, pneumonia, pneumothorax, pulmonary edema, and, occasionally, respiratory failure. Asthma is usually episodic and often precipitated by allergens, exercise, cold exposure, or infections. It is characterized by bilateral wheezing and a decreased respiratory flow rate.

Upper airway obstruction can be caused by *aspiration, vocal cord paralysis, tumors,* and *epiglottic* and *laryngeal edema.* In cases of *foreign body aspiration* (more common in children) the onset of respiratory difficulty is acute. When acute respiratory difficulty occurs during eating, especially in the intoxicated or semiconscious patient, foreign body aspiration is probable. When complete respiratory obstruction occurs, severe respiratory distress, cyanosis, gasping, and loss of consciousness occur quickly. Incomplete respiratory obstruction causes tachypnea, inspiratory stridor, and localized wheezing.

Patients with acute dyspnea due to *hyperventilation* are usually anxious. They often complain of numbness and tingling in the perioral region and the extremities. These patients also often complain of lightheadedness, sighing respiration, and an inability to "get enough air in."

A more gradual onset of shortness of breath occurs in patients with *CHF, anemia, lung tumors,* and *parenchymatous lung disease.*

Chronic Dyspnea

Chronic dyspnea in adults is most often caused by *COPD, chronic CHF,* and *obesity.* It may also be seen with *severe anemia* and *infiltrative pulmonary carcinomatosis.*

When dyspnea occurs in one lateral position but not in the other (trepopnea), unilateral lung disease, pleural effusion, or obstruction of the proximal tracheobronchial tree should be suspected. Dyspnea in the upright position that is relieved by recumbency (platypnea) may be seen in patients with intracardiac shunts, vascular lung shunts, and parenchymal lung shunts.

ASSOCIATED SYMPTOMS

When dyspnea occurs in young children, especially when it is associated with coughing and expectoration, *cystic fibrosis* and *bronchiectasis* should be considered.

Acute Dyspnea

When chest pain accompanies acute dyspnea, *spontaneous pneumothorax, pulmonary embolism, chest trauma,* and *myocardial infarction* should be suspected. Pulmonary embolism is a common cause of acute dyspnea in adults. Patients usually appear severely ill and may also complain of chest pain, faintness, and, occasionally, loss of consciousness. Peripheral cyanosis, low blood pressure, and rales may be present.

When fever, chills, and cough are associated with acute dyspnea, pneumonia is most likely. When dyspnea on exertion, paroxysmal nocturnal dyspnea, and peripheral edema are associated with chronic or acute dyspnea, heart failure is most likely. Pulmonary embolism is most often associated with pleuritic pain, cough, leg swelling, or leg pain and occasionally with wheezing and hemoptysis.

When acute dyspnea is caused by severe *anemia* of acute onset, associated symptoms include dizziness, weakness, and sweating and, possibly, signs of hemorrhage (e.g., hypotension, tachycardia, rapid and shallow respirations). When acute dyspnea is a manifestation of *anxiety* or *panic disorder,* the patient also usually complains of dizziness, lightheadedness, palpitations, and paresthesias. The patients do not appear dyspneic and often complain of "not being able to take in enough air." Patients who complain of dyspnea at rest have either a severe physiologic impairment or anxiety hyperventilation.

The most common causes of chronic dyspnea on exertion are *cardiac* and *pulmonary.* Although paroxysmal nocturnal dyspnea is most frequently caused by cardiac pathology, some asthmatic patients experience symptoms primarily when recumbent, usually at night. Associated findings are often helpful in differentiating pulmonary from cardiac causes of dyspnea. When dyspnea is caused primarily by lung disease, the dyspnea is intensified by effort, there is a daily productive cough, the respirations are shallow and rapid, and postural changes have little or no effect. When dyspnea has a cardiac cause, it is intensified by recumbency and the respirations are shallow but not necessarily rapid.

Other clues also help differentiate pulmonary from cardiac causes of dyspnea on exertion. When the cause is pulmonary, the rate of recovery to normal respiration is fast, and dyspnea abates a few minutes after cessation of exercise. However, patients with dyspnea due to cardiac causes remain dyspneic much longer after cessation of exercise. Likewise, in these patients, the heart rate also takes longer to return to pre-exercise levels. Patients with pulmonary dyspnea do not usually have dyspnea at rest. Patients with severe cardiac dyspnea demonstrate a volume of respiration that is greater than normal at all levels of exercise; they also experience dyspnea sooner after the start of exertion.

PRECIPITATING AND AGGRAVATING FACTORS

Smoking is the most frequent precipitating and aggravating factor of chronic pulmonary dyspnea. When *exercise* precipitates wheezing or dyspnea, *bronchial asthma* or CHF may be the diagnosis. *Exposure to cold* often precipitates wheezing and shortness of breath in asthmatic patients. Bronchial asthma is also probable when *airborne allergens, noxious fumes,* or *respiratory infections* precipitate dyspnea, cough, or wheezing.

Drugs (e.g., beta blockers) may precipitate wheezing or dyspnea in asthmatic patients. Beta blockers and calcium channel blockers may exacerbate dyspnea in cardiac patients. Less common precipitating and aggravating factors include *trauma, shock, hemorrhage,* and *gaseous anesthesia.*

AMELIORATING FACTORS OTHER THAN MEDICAL THERAPY

Some patients with severe COPD obtain relief by leaning forward while seated or by lying supine with the head down. These positions increase the efficiency of diaphragmatic movement and facilitate the use of the accessory muscles of respiration. Performing the Heimlich maneuver (abdominal thrust) may dislodge a foreign body from the upper airway. Trepopnea (dyspnea improves in a lateral decubitus position) with the diseased hemithorax facing up suggests unilateral lung disease or pleural effusion.

PHYSICAL FINDINGS

Patients with *upper airway obstruction* have coarse, sonorous rhonchi and impaired inspiration. Stridor as well as suprasternal retraction may be noted with inspiration. Sibilant, whistling expiratory sounds are usually heard in asthmatic patients. Their expiration appears to be prolonged, whereas inspiration seems to be prolonged in patients with upper airway obstruction. The trachea may be shifted to the opposite side in patients with *pneumothorax* or *large pleural effusion.*

In heart failure the common physical findings include basilar rales, jugular venous distention, tachycardia, gallop rhythm, peripheral edema, and murmurs. In pneumonia the usual physical findings include fever, tachycardia, rhonchi, and decreased breath sounds. In pulmonary embolism, tachycardia, tachypnea, focal rales, and an increased pulmonic second sound are often present.

Wheezing dyspnea at rest associated with rhonchi and a productive cough suggests *asthmatic bronchitis.* In contrast, patients with a history of progressive dyspnea that precedes the development of cough or sputum production often have *emphysema.* The physical findings are a hyperinflated lung, decreased breath sounds, decreased diaphragmatic movement, increased anteroposterior chest diameter, and hyperresonance to percussion. Classically, emphysematous patients have been described as "pink puffers"; patients with chronic bronchitis are called "blue bloaters." Bilateral wheezing is usually heard when acute dyspnea is caused by *asthma*. Bilateral wheezing may also occur with *pulmonary edema*. Wheezing may frequently be heard before the auscultation of rales at the bases and other more classic signs of CHF. Bilateral wheezing may also be heard in patients with *pulmonary emboli*, but more frequently the wheezing is limited to the side of the pulmonary embolus. Unilateral wheezing may also indicate a *bronchial obstruction* by a foreign body, polyp, or mucous plug. Other causes of dyspneic wheezing are *upper airway obstruction*, localized *bronchial obstruction*, and *hypersensitivity pneumonitis*.

DIAGNOSTIC STUDIES

When the cause of dyspnea is not apparent, initial studies should include an electrocardiogram, chest radiograph, hemoglobin, thyroid function tests, creatinine measurement, and spirometry with the use of a bronchodilator. Pulmonary function tests (PFTs) are most helpful and can often be performed in an outpatient setting. **PFTs should be an integral part of the clinical evaluation of all patients with dyspnea.** Patients with *simple acute bronchitis* may have a persistent productive cough but demonstrate no signs of airway narrowing on spirometry. In patients with *chronic bronchitis* and a persistent cough, spirometry may indicate widespread narrowing of the airways, but dyspnea may not be present. *COPD* may be diagnosed with simple spirometry. Occasionally, patients with COPD demonstrate airway narrowing on spirometry without any other symptoms except cough.

Results of PFTs do not provide a specific diagnosis; rather, they demonstrate a pattern of the physiologic abnormality. Typical but not exclusive patterns of physiologic abnormalities are seen in most patients with chronic pulmonary diseases, most people with diseases of the pulmonary circulation, and patients with mild cardiac or valvular disease. PFT findings may help the physician differentiate dyspnea due to hyperventilation or psychological factors from pulmonary dysfunction.

PFTs demonstrate increased obstruction to inspiration with extrathoracic (upper airway) obstructive lesions and increased obstruction to expiration with intrathoracic obstructive lesions. Expiratory airway obstruction is indicated by decreased airflow rates, decreased forced expiratory volume in 1 second (FEV_1), decreased peak flow rate (PFR), decreased maximum midexpiratory flow rate (FEF_{25-75}), decreased maximum voluntary ventilation (MVV), increased tidal volume (TV), and increased residual volume (RV). These findings are often observed in patients with *asthma, bronchitis, emphysema*, and *bronchial adenoma*.

The abnormal findings in bronchospasm can usually be transiently reversed with the inhalation of a bronchodilator drug. Lung volume restriction is indicated by decreased total lung capacity (TLC), increased respiratory minute volume, and decreased compliance, which is found in patients with *fibrosis, sarcoidosis, pneumoconiosis, pulmonary edema, pneumonia, pleural effusion, kyphoscoliosis, obesity,* and *ascites.* Pulmonary vascular disease is evidenced by increased ventilation (V_E) and increased dead space (V_D). An electrocardiogram may show P pulmonale and right ventricular strain. Chest radiographs may show pulmonary parenchymal disease, pleural effusions, tumors, or signs of CHF. Doppler ultrasonography measurement of aortic blood flow during exercise may be helpful in distinguishing CHF from COPD as the cause of dyspnea. Aortic blood flow is significantly lower in patients with CHF than in patients with COPD.

Computed tomography (CT) angiography is currently the standard of care for diagnosing pulmonary embolism, although ventilation and perfusion scanning may be used in patients for whom intravenous contrast agents are contraindicated. The Wells criteria can be used to determine the clinical likelihood of pulmonary embolism. Point values are allotted as follows:

- Clinical symptoms of deep vein thrombosis: 3 points
- Other clinical diagnosis not more likely: 3 points
- Heart rate >100 beats/minute: 1.5 points
- Previous deep vein thrombosis (DVT) or pulmonary embolism (PE): 1.5 points
- Immobilization or surgery within the past 4 weeks: 1.5 points
- Hemoptysis: 1 point
- Malignancy: 1 point

A total score higher than 6 points indicates high risk for pulmonary embolism (78.4%), 2-6 points indicates moderate risk (27.8%), and less than 2 points indicates low risk (3.4%). Serum D-dimer measurement, though not very specific for pulmonary embolism, is sensitive, so a negative D-dimer result in a patient with a low clinical probability of pulmonary embolism has a 95% negative predictive value.

Brain natriuretic peptide values are elevated in heart failure and ventricular dysfunction. A brain natriuretic peptide value lower than 100 pg/mL has a very high negative predictive value for heart failure as a cause of dyspnea.

LESS COMMON DIAGNOSTIC CONSIDERATIONS

Dyspnea is occasionally the presenting symptom in patients with *hyperthyroidism.* *Pregnant* patients may complain of dyspnea. Patients with *idiopathic pulmonary hemosiderosis* may present with dyspnea on exertion, chronic cough, hemoptysis, and recurrent epistaxis. People who work in grain elevators or with hay may also have severe wheezing and dyspnea. Progressive dyspnea and a nonproductive cough may be the presenting symptoms in patients with *interstitial pulmonary fibrosis,* which may result from drugs (e.g., phenytoin), sarcoidosis, and other granulomatous diseases.

Differential Diagnosis of Shortness of Breath

CAUSE	NATURE OF PATIENT	NATURE OF SYMPTOMS	ASSOCIATED SYMPTOMS	PRECIPITATING AND AGGRAVATING FACTORS	AMELIORATING FACTORS	PHYSICAL FINDINGS	DIAGNOSTIC STUDIES
Acute or Recurrent Dyspnea							
Asthma	Most common cause of recurrent dyspnea in children	Acute dyspnea Episodic Patient may rarely be dyspneic only at night	Cough (indicates asthmatic bronchitis)	Allergens Exercise Noxious fumes Respiratory tract infections Recumbency Exposure to cold Beta blockers		Bilateral wheezing Sibilant, whistling sounds Prolonged expiration	PFT results*: Decreased PFR Decreased MVV Increased TV Pre/post-bronchodilator evidence of reversible airway obstruction (>10%)
Pulmonary emboli	Women using birth control pills Patients in postoperative period Patients with long-term recumbency Patients with phlebitis Patients in postpartum period	Acute onset of dyspnea	Pleuritic chest pain Faintness Loss of consciousness Cough Hemoptysis Swollen, painful leg	Oral contraceptives Prolonged recumbency		Tachypnea Peripheral cyanosis Low blood pressure Rales Wheezing (usually only on side of emboli) Pleural friction later with pulmonary infarction	Ventilation and perfusion studies Electrocardiogram showing acute right ventricular strain CT angiography ↓ po₂ Presence of D-dimer

Continued

Differential Diagnosis of Shortness of Breath—cont'd

CAUSE	NATURE OF PATIENT	NATURE OF SYMPTOMS	ASSOCIATED SYMPTOMS	PRECIPITATING AND AGGRAVATING FACTORS	AMELIORATING FACTORS	PHYSICAL FINDINGS	DIAGNOSTIC STUDIES
Hyperventilation and anxiety	Usually anxious	Acute dyspnea "Sighing" respirations	Lightheadedness Palpitations Paresthesias (especially in perioral region and extremities)	Stress Panic		Signs of anxiety but not of dyspnea	PFT results usually normal
Poor physical conditioning	Obese Physically inactive	Dyspnea on minimal exertion				Obesity After exercise, pulse slows very gradually	PFT results: Decreased TLC Increased respiratory minute volume Decreased compliance
Foreign body aspiration	Children most commonly affect Intoxicated or semiconscious people while they are eating	Acute dyspnea			Removal of foreign body Heimlich maneuver	Tachypnea Inspiratory stridor Localized wheezing Suprasternal retraction with respiration Wheezing may be unilateral	Chest radiograph findings: atelectasis or foreign body

Condition	History	Precipitating Factors	Physical Examination	Diagnostic Studies
Heart failure	Acute onset; Episodic; Dyspnea on exertion; Orthopnea; Paroxysmal nocturnal dyspnea		Tachycardia; Gallop rhythm; Rales at bases; Jugular venous distention; Peripheral edema	Decreased ejection fraction; Chest radiograph findings: cardiomegaly with upper lobe redistribution or Kerley B lines; Increased BNP
Pneumothorax	Often has a prior history of similar episode; Pneumothorax may be familial; Acute onset	Cystic fibrosis; COPD	Decrease or absence of breath sounds; Tracheal shift	Chest radiograph findings: pneumothorax
Chronic Dyspnea				
COPD (emphysema and chronic bronchitis)	Older adults; Rarely patients < 30 years old; Most often smokers; Chronic dyspnea; Dyspnea with exertion; Fast recovery to normal respiration after stopping exercise	Smoking; Exertion; Postural changes have little or no effect; Leaning forward while seated	Rapid and shallow respirations	PFTs; Spirometry
Emphysema	Progressive dyspnea precedes onset of cough; Usually no dyspnea at rest	Smoking	"Pink puffers"; Hyperventilated lungs; Decreased breath sounds and diaphragmatic movement; Increased anteroposterior chest diameter; Hyperresonance	PFT results: Decreased PFR; Increased TV; Decreased MVV; Increased RV

Continued

Differential Diagnosis of Shortness of Breath—cont'd

CAUSE	NATURE OF PATIENT	NATURE OF SYMPTOMS	ASSOCIATED SYMPTOMS	PRECIPITATING AND AGGRAVAT- ING FACTORS	AMELIORAT- ING FACTORS	PHYSICAL FINDINGS	DIAGNOSTIC STUDIES
Chronic bronchitis		Dyspnea not necessarily a presenting symptom Cough precedes dyspnea	Persistent, minimally productive cough			"Blue bloaters" Rhonchi	Same as with emphysema Spirometric findings: widespread airway narrowing
CHF	Older patients	Chronic dyspnea with gradual onset Paroxysmal nocturnal dyspnea Dyspnea remains long after stopping exercise	Edema	Exercise Beta blockers Calcium channel blockers Recumbency Trauma Shock Hemorrhage Anesthesia	Nocturnal dyspnea may be relieved by sitting	Shallow respirations (not necessarily rapid) Edema Hepatomegaly Jugular venous distention Third heart sound Basilar rales	Spirometry Respiratory volume greater than normal at all exercise levels Radiograph: pulmonary congestion and cardiomegaly Elevated β-type natriuretic peptide

BNP, Brain natriuretic peptide; *CHF,* Congestive heart failure; *COPD,* chronic obstructive pulmonary disease; *CT,* computed tomography; *MVV,* maximum voluntary ventilation; *PFR,* peak flow rate; *PFTs,* pulmonary function tests; *RV,* residual volume; *TLC,* total lung capacity; *TV,* tidal volume.

Patients with recurrent *pulmonary emboli* may present with recurrent episodes of dyspnea. Patients with *interstitial pulmonary diseases* (e.g., pulmonary fibrosis, pneumoconiosis), as well as those with *constrictive cardiomyopathy* and *constrictive pericarditis,* may present with dyspnea on exertion, chronic cough, and paroxysmal nocturnal dyspnea.

Selected References

Bettmann MA, Lyders EM, Yucel EK, et al: Expert Panel on Cardiac Imaging. Acute chest pain—suspected pulmonary embolism, Reston, VA, American College of Radiology (ACR), 2006. Available at http://www.acr.org/SecondaryMainMenuCategories/quality_safety/app_criteria/pdf/ExpertPanelonCardiovascularImaging/AcuteChestPainSuspectedPulmonaryEmbolismUpdatein ProgressDoc4.aspx.

Dosh SA: Diagnosis of heart failure in adults, *Am Fam Physician* 70:2145-2152, 2004.

Evensen A: Management of COPD exacerbations, *Am Fam Physician* 81:607-613, 2010.

Krafczyk M, Bautista F: When an athlete can't catch his breath, *J Fam Pract* 58:454-459, 2009.

Lim HS, Lip GY: A case of breathlessness, *Practitioner* 247:204-207, 2003.

Mayo D, Colletti J, Kuo D: Brain natriuretic peptide testing in the emergency department, *J Emerg Med* 31:201-210, 2006.

Ponka D, Kirlew M: Top 10 differential diagnoses in family medicine: dyspnea, *Can Fam Physician* 53:1333, 2007.

Ray P, Delerme S, Jourdain P, et al: Differential diagnosis of acute dyspnea: the value of B natriuretic peptides in the emergency department, *QJM* 101:831-843, 2008.

Sarkar S, Amelung P: Evaluation of the dyspneic patient in the office, *Prim Care* 33:643-657, 2006.

Wells PS, Anderson DR, Rodger M, et al: Excluding pulmonary embolism at the bedside without diagnostic imaging: management of patients with suspected pulmonary embolism presenting to the emergency department by using a simple clinical model and D-dimer, *Ann Intern Med* 135: 98-107, 2001.

Yernault JC: Dyspnea in the elderly: a clinical approach to diagnosis, *Drugs Aging* 18:177-187, 2001.

Zoorob RJ, Campbell JS: Acute dyspnea in the office, *Am Fam Physician* 68:1803-1810, 2003.

Skin Problems

29

Skin problems are one of the most common reasons why patients seek medical attention. The 10 most common skin problems leading patients to consult dermatologists are *acne, fungal infections, seborrheic dermatitis, atopic* or *eczematous dermatitis, warts,* benign and malignant *skin tumors, psoriasis, hair disorders, vitiligo,* and *herpes simplex.*

Occupational dermatoses (Table 29-1) most often appear as eczematous *contact dermatitis,* although they occasionally manifest as skin cancers, vitiligo, or infectious lesions. Irritant contact dermatoses are often caused by frequent hand washing, cleansers, solvents, cutting oils used by machinists, and disinfectants. Allergic contact dermatitis is usually caused by frequent exposure to nickel chromates and epoxy resins. Other common lesions are infestations such as *scabies* and *pediculosis, contact dermatitis* (Table 29-2), *pityriasis rosea, herpes zoster,* and *seborrheic keratoses.*

These are not necessarily the most common skin problems; some of the most prevalent are handled by physicians other than dermatologists. About one third of all patients with a primary dermatologic complaint consult a general physician.

This chapter presents the most common dermatologic problems in the table "Differential Diagnosis of Skin Problems" (on page 378). Dermatologic diagnosis is based on the type of lesion, its configuration, and the distribution of the lesions, so the summary table is organized accordingly. See the color insert for illustrations of selected skin conditions. The color photos also portray some common pediatric viral exanthems.

Systemic disease may manifest as skin problems. General pruritus may be caused by anemia, uremia, or liver disease. Erythema nodosum (tender red nodules on the shins) may be associated with sarcoidosis, inflammatory bowel disease, or leukemia. Cutaneous vasculitis may be present in connective tissue disorders such as systemic lupus erythematous or, in an acutely unwell patient, meningococcal meningitis. Café-au-lait spots in children may indicate neurofibromatosis.

Skin tumors are most common later in life. The most common malignant lesions are *basal cell epithelioma* and *squamous epithelioma. Basal cell*

TABLE 29-1. Potential Allergens in Contact Dermatitis from Occupational Exposure

AGENT	WHERE TYPICALLY FOUND	BODY SITE AFFECTED
Nickel	Tools, utensils, musical instruments, machinery parts, batteries, steel-toed work boots, jewelry, clothing snaps	Face, hands, eyelids, waist, umbilicus, tops of toes
Chromates	Engraving devices, lithography and photography processing materials, ceramics, glue and adhesives, shoe polishes, cement, leather, match heads, automobile primer paints, catgut, electroplating solutions	Hands, wrists, forearms, feet
Epoxy resin	Adhesives and glues for industrial and household use, laminates, electrical encapsulators, eyeglass frames, paints and inks, product finishers, surface coatings, handbags	Hands, face (especially eyelids), forearms
Formaldehyde	Photography processing materials, paints, paper products, pathology fertilizers, plastic, resins, insulation, wood composites, permanent-press fabrics, cosmetics, shampoos, medications, leather-tanning agents, smoke from cigarettes, cigars, charcoal, and wood	Axillae, waist, hands, face, scalp
Mercaptobenzothiazole	Rubber products, especially shoes (soles and arch supports), and—less frequently—gloves, cutting oils, antifreeze, anticorrosive agents, cement and adhesives, detergents, fungicides, photographic film emulsion	Feet, hands
Thiuram	Rubber products, especially gloves, and—less frequently—shoes, fungicides, germicides, insecticides, soaps and shampoos, disulfiram	Hands, face, scalp, feet
Mercaptobenzothiazole	Hair dyes, printer's ink, leather, fur dyes (cross-reacts with para-aminobenzoic acid, procaine, benzocaine, thiazides, sulfonamides)	Scalp, face, hands
Ethylenediamine	Aminophylline, hydroxyzine hydrochloride, hydroxyzine pamoate, tripelennamine, rubber products, antifreeze, dyes, fungicides, triamcinolone acetonide/nystatin and other prescription creams	Hands, face, generalized allergic reaction
Acrylates	Construction adhesives, printing materials, textiles, medical products (dental adhesives, artificial joints, heart valves, contact lenses), utensils (plexi-glass, veneer), glues (superadhesive types), artificial nails, nail polish	Hands, face

Continued

TABLE 29-1.   Potential Allergens in Contact Dermatitis from Occupational Exposure—cont'd

AGENT	WHERE TYPICALLY FOUND	BODY SITE AFFECTED
Propylene glycol	Cosmetics, pharmaceuticals (topical corticosteroids, otic preparations, sterile lubricant jelly, electrocardiogram plates, injectables), antifreeze, food coloring, flavoring agents	Face, ears, hands, genitalia, generalized allergic reaction
Polyethylene glycol	Topical medications, suppositories, shampoos, hair dressings, toothpaste, contraceptive jellies, insect repellents, glues, lubricants for rubber molds, textile fibers, used in metal-forming operations	Scalp, face, genitalia, anus, hands
Neomycin	Topical antibiotics (cross-reacts with kanamycin, gentamicin, spectinomycin, tobramycin, bacitracin)	Face, ears, leg ulcers, generalized allergic reaction
Benzocaine	Topical anesthetics (including creams and lozenges) for burns hemorrhoids, poison ivy, and toothaches (cross-reacts with procaine, tetracaine, procainamide, hydrochlorothiazide, sunscreens containing para-aminobenzoic acid, paraphenylenediamine, sulfonamides, sulfonylurea, para-aminosalicylic acid)	Face, genitalia, anus, generalized allergic reaction

From Prawer SE: Occupational dermatoses in primary care: a guide to recognition. Consultant 38:423-444, 1998.

carcinoma is typically described as a pearl-white, dome-shaped papule with raised edges and overlying telangiectasia. *Squamous cell carcinoma* is described as having a red, poorly defined base and an adherent yellow-white cutaneous horn. Sqamous cell carcinomas progress into nodular lesions with necrotic centers and are often found within a background of sun-damaged skin and actinic keratoses. *Melanomas* vary in appearance; 30% develop within existing nevi, and 70% appear de novo. Clinical signs that increase the likelihood that a pigmented lesion is melanoma follow the *ABCD* mnemonic; Asymmetry, Border irregularity, Color variegation, and Diameter > 6 mm. With proper training, office dermoscopy can be used to differentiate between benign and malignant pigmented skin lesions. **If any uncertainty exists about whether a skin lesion is malignant, it should be biopsied.** A full-thickness biopsy (as opposed to a shave biopsy) should be performed for any lesion suspicious for melanoma because depth of penetration determines prognosis and treatment.

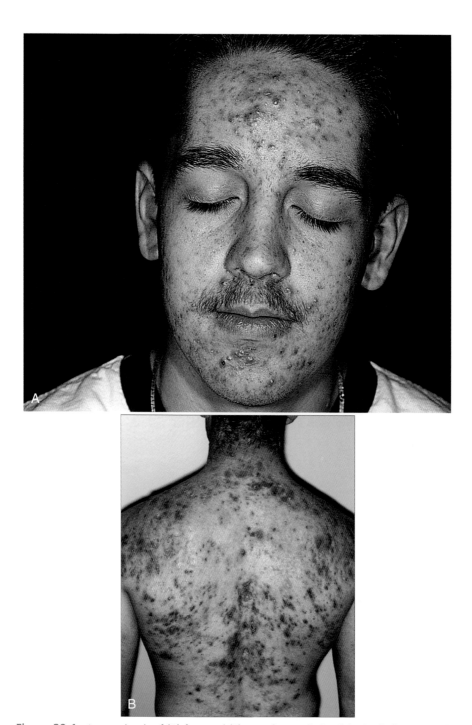

Figure 29-1. Acne vulgaris of (**A**) face and (**B**) pustular psoriasis of the back. (**A** From Callen JP, Greer KE, Paller AS, Swinyer LJ: Color Atlas of Dermatology, 2nd ed. Philadelphia, WB Saunders, 2000, p 10; **B** from James WD, Berger TG, Elston DM: Andrews' Diseases of the Skin: Clinical Dermatology, 10th ed. Philadelphia, Saunders, 2005.)

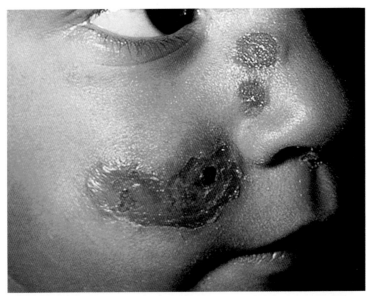

Figure 29-2. Impetigo. Note serous exudation and crusting. Because impetigo is contagious, it can spread to other people and different parts of the body. It is caused usually by *Staphylococcus aureus* and less frequently by *Streptococcus pyogenes (hemolyticus).* (From James WD, Berger TG, Elston DM: Andrews' Diseases of the Skin: Clinical Dermatology, 10th ed. Philadelphia, WB Saunders, 2000, p 256.)

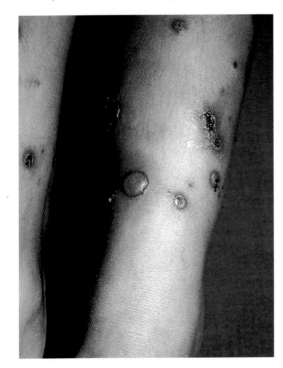

Figure 29-3. Impetigo circinata. Occasionally, the center of an impetiginous lesion heals, leaving a ringed, crusted-edge culture from which the diagnosis can be established. (From James WD, Berger TG, Elston DM: Andrews' Diseases of the Skin: Clinical Dermatology, 10th ed. Philadelphia, WB Saunders, 2000, p 256.)

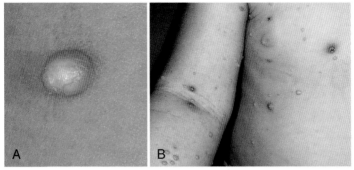

Figure 29-4. Molluscum contagiosum. **A,** Papules with central umbilication. **B,** Typical lesion. (From Paller AS, Mancini AJ: Hurwitz Clinical Pediatric Dermatology, 3rd ed. Philadelphia, WB Saunders, 2006, p 413.)

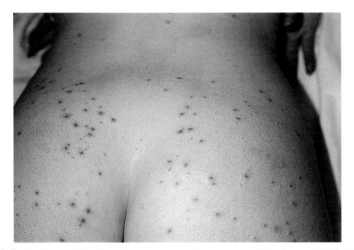

Figure 29-5. Hot tub folliculitis. Papules and pustules due to *Pseudomonas* infection. (From Callen JP, Greer KE, Paller AS, Swinyer LJ: Color Atlas of Dermatology, 2nd ed. Philadelphia, WB Saunders, 2000, p 67.)

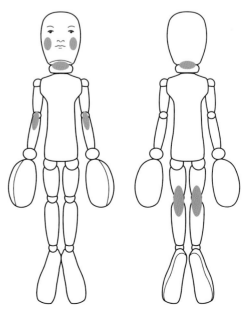

Figure 29-6. Lichenified pruritic areas in flexural regions and on the face are typical locations for adult atopic dermatitis.

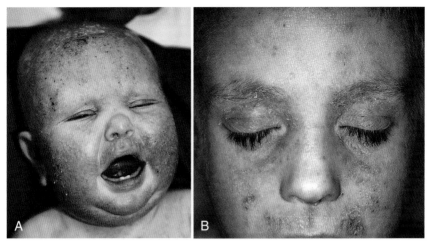

Figure 29-7. Atopic dermatitis. **A,** Characteristic facial appearance. **B,** Chronic excoriated dermatitis, with "sad" and "strained" look. (From Paller AS, Mancini AJ: Hurwitz Clinical Pediatric Dermatology, 3rd ed. Philadelphia, WB Saunders, 2006, pp 51-52.)

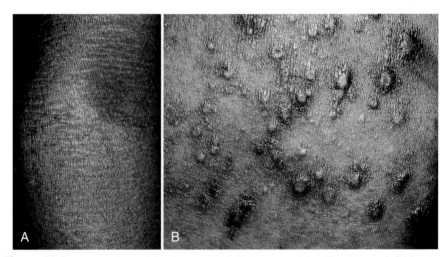

Figure 29-8. Atopic dermatitis: characteristic lesions. **A,** Lichenification and thickening, antecubital fossa. **B,** Prurigo-like papules in adult atopic dermatitis. (From James WD, Berger TG, Elston DM: Andrews' Diseases of the Skin: Clinical Dermatology, 10th ed. Philadelphia, WB Saunders, 2000, p 71.)

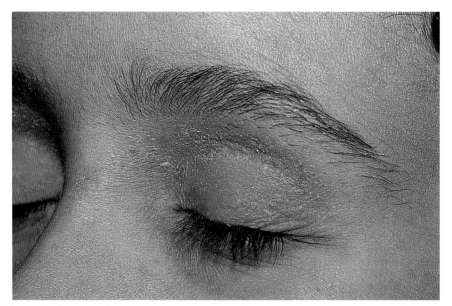

Figure 29-9. Infantile atopic dermatitis of face. (From White GM, Cox NH: Diseases of the Skin: A Color Atlas and Text. London, Mosby, 2002, p 25.)

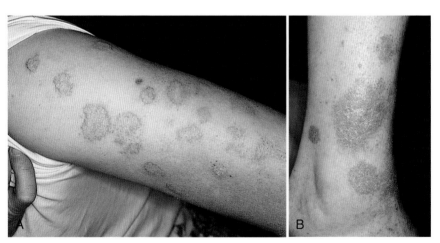

Figure 29-10. Nummular eczema on **(A)** arm and **(B)** ankle. (From Callen JP, Greer KE, Paller AS, Swinyer LJ: Color Atlas of Dermatology, 2nd ed. Philadelphia, WB Saunders, 2000, pp 15, 95, 245.)

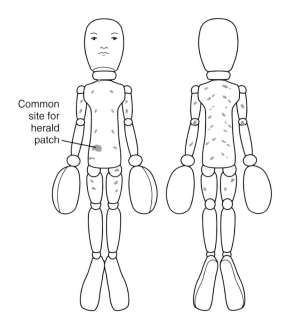

Common
site for
herald
patch

Figure 29-11. Pityriasis rosea typically starts with a "herald patch" and is followed by oval patches in a fernlike or "Christmas tree" pattern.

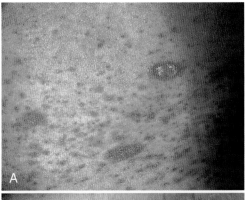

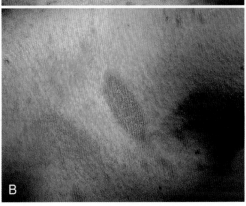

Figure 29-12. Pityriasis rosea. **A,** Discrete papulosquamous lesions. **B,** Larger initial patch in groin (herald lesion). (From James WD, Berger TG, Elston DM: Andrews' Diseases of the Skin: Clinical Dermatology, 10th ed. Philadelphia, WB Saunders, 2000, p 208.)

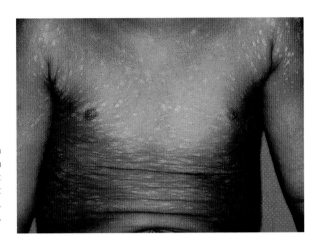

Figure 29-13. Pityriasis rosea on chest and abdomen. (From James WD, Berger TG, Elston DM: Andrews' Diseases of the Skin: Clinical Dermatology, 10th ed. Philadelphia, WB Saunders, 2000, p 208.)

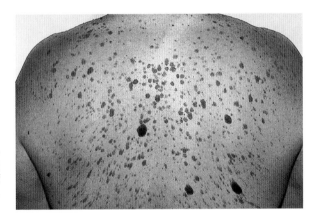

Figure 29-14. Multiple seborrheic dermatoses. (From White GM, Cox NH: Diseases of the Skin: A Color Atlas and Text. London, Mosby, 2002, p 413.)

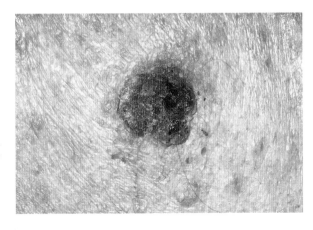

Figure 29-15. Irritated seborrheic dermatoses may become lighter in color. (From Lawrence CM, Cox NH: Physical Signs in Dermatology, 2nd ed. London, Mosby, 2002, p 180.)

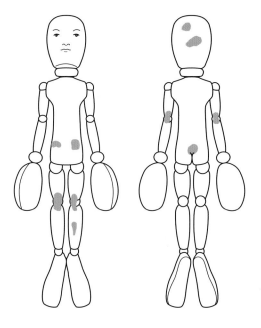

Figure 29-16. Psoriasis tends to be found on extensor surfaces and areas of repeated trauma, such as the waistline.

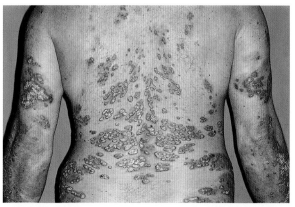

Figure 29-17. Psoriasis vulgaris. (From Callen JP, Greer KE, Paller AS, Swinyer LJ: Color Atlas of Dermatology, 2nd ed. Philadelphia, WB Saunders, 2000, p 280.)

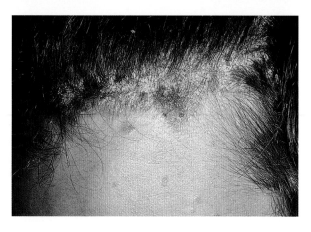

Figure 29-18. Psoriasis of scalp along hair margin and forehead. (From Callen JP, Greer KE, Paller AS, Swinyer LJ: Color Atlas of Dermatology, 2nd ed. Philadelphia, WB Saunders, 2000, p 358.)

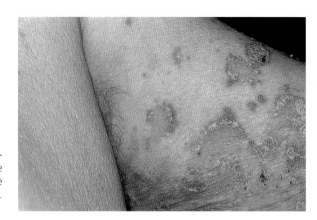

Figure 29-19. Guttate psoriasis of thigh. (From White GM, Cox NH: Diseases of the Skin: A Color Atlas and Text. London, Mosby, 2002, p 51.)

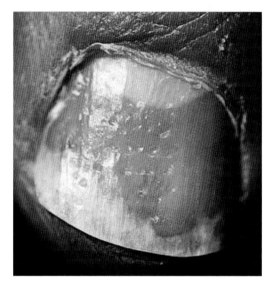

Figure 29-20. Minute pits are typically seen on the surface of nails in patients with psoriasis. (From James WD, Berger TG, Elston DM: Andrews' Diseases of the Skin: Clinical Dermatology, 10th ed. Philadelphia, WB Saunders, 2000, p 193.)

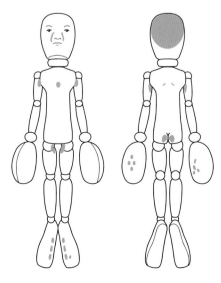

Figure 29-21. Usual location of erythema and scaling in seborrheic dermatitis.

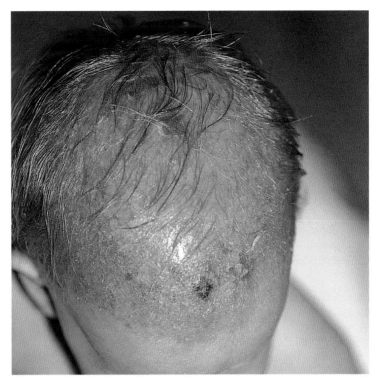

Figure 29-22. "Cradle cap," a form of seborrheic eczema. (From Callen JP, Greer KE, Paller AS, Swinyer LJ: Color Atlas of Dermatology, 2nd ed. Philadelphia, WB Saunders, 2000, p 358.)

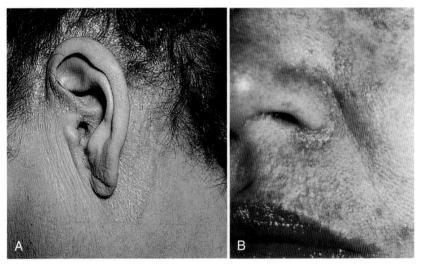

Figure 29-23. Seborrheic dermatitis of the **(A)** postauricular and **(B)** nasolabial regions, both common locations. (**A** from Callen JP, Greer KE, Paller AS, Swinyer LJ: Color Atlas of Dermatology, 2nd ed. Philadelphia, WB Saunders, 2000, p 91; **B** from White GM, Cox NH: Diseases of the Skin: A Color Atlas and Text. London, Mosby, 2002, p 43.)

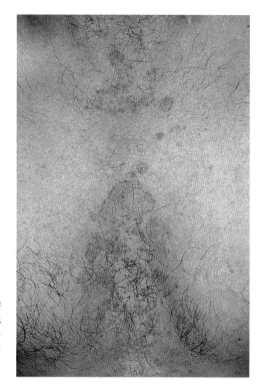

Figure 29-24. Seborrheic dermatitis of the chest and presternal areas. Lesions often appear greasy and scaling. (From Lawrence CM, Cox NH: Physical Signs in Dermatology, 2nd ed. London, Mosby, 2002, p 18.)

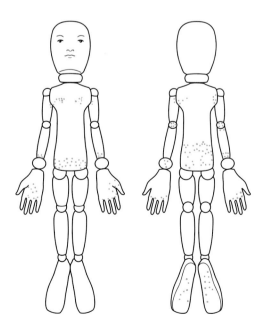

Figure 29-25. Pruritic papules are most prevalent about the waist, pelvis, elbows, hands, and feet in scabies.

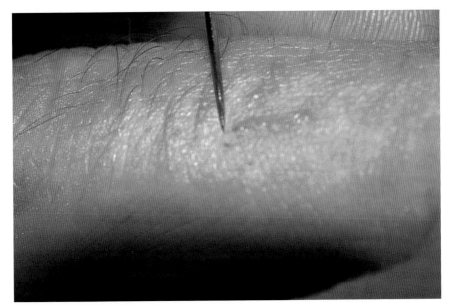

Figure 29-26. Scabies. Itchy papules and burrows occur between the fingers. (From Lawrence CM, Cox NH: Physical Signs in Dermatology, 2nd ed. London, Mosby, 2002, p 276.)

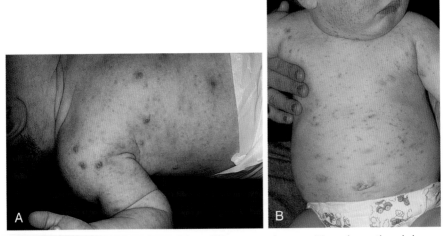

Figure 29-27. Scabies. **A,** Infant with a diffuse, papular, pruritic rash on the abdomen, chest, and axillae. The face is usually spared. **B,** Usual distribution. (**A** from Callen JP, Greer KE, Paller AS, Swinyer LJ: Color Atlas of Dermatology, 2nd ed. Philadelphia, WB Saunders, 2000, p 283; **B** from Lawrence CM, Cox NH: Physical Signs in Dermatology, 2nd ed. London, Mosby, 2002, p 277.)

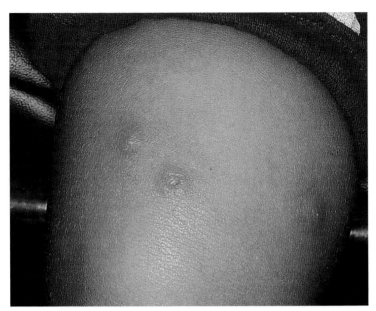

Figure 29-28. Insect bites frequently cause papular urticaria. A pruritic wheal develops at the site of each bite. (From Callen JP, Greer KE, Paller AS, Swinyer LJ: Color Atlas of Dermatology, 2nd ed. Philadelphia, WB Saunders, 2000, p 221.)

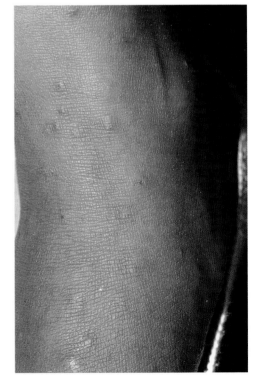

Figure 29-29. Flea bites. They are more common on the ankle and lower leg, because fleas cannot jump higher than 2 feet. (From White GM, Cox NH: Diseases of the Skin: A Color Atlas and Text. London, Mosby, 2002, p 376.)

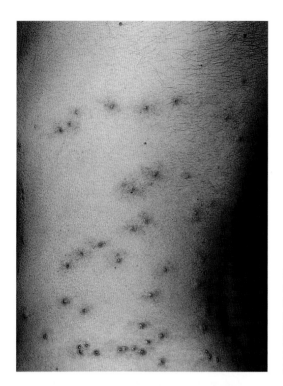

Figure 29-30. Bed bug bites cause erythematous wheals or papules that may itch. They frequently attack exposed areas, especially at night. (From Callen JP, Greer KE, Paller AS, Swinyer LJ: Color Atlas of Dermatology, 2nd ed. Philadelphia, WB Saunders, 2000, p 67.)

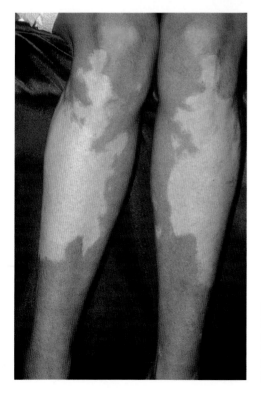

Figure 29-31. Vitiligo. The disease frequently occurs in body folds, such as the axillae and genitalia, and also on the face, legs, and hands. (From White GM, Cox NH: Diseases of the Skin: A Color Atlas and Text. London, Mosby, 2002, p 286.)

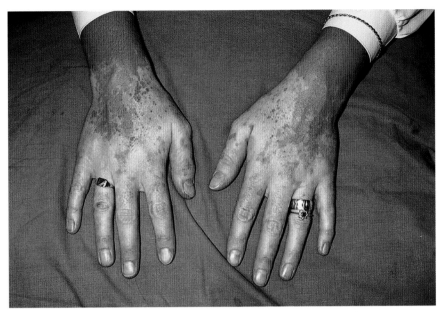

Figure 29-32. Vitiligo frequently involves the dorsal surface of the hand. (From Lawrence CM, Cox NH: Physical Signs in Dermatology, 2nd ed. London, Mosby, 2002, p 52.)

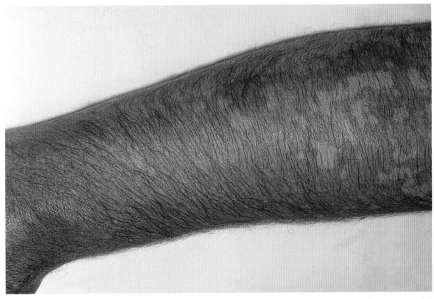

Figure 29-33. Chemicals such as phenols may cause depigmentation. When caused by phenols, the lesions are usually sharply demarcated. (From White GM, Cox NH: Diseases of the Skin: A Color Atlas and Text. London, Mosby, 2002, p 285.)

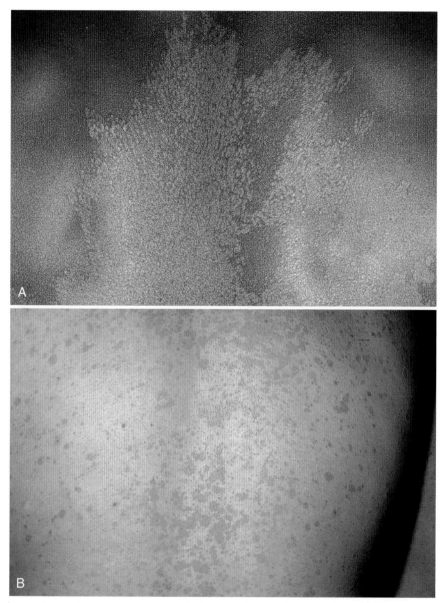

Figure 29-34. Tinea versicolor (pityriasis versicolor). Lesions may be hypopigmented or hyperpigmented, thus the name versicolor. They often manifest as circular scaling areas of **(A)** depigmentation in dark- or tan-skinned patients and **(B)** light brown or fawn colored in light-skinned individuals. (From White GM, Cox NH: Diseases of the Skin: A Color Atlas and Text. London, Mosby, 2002, p 355.)

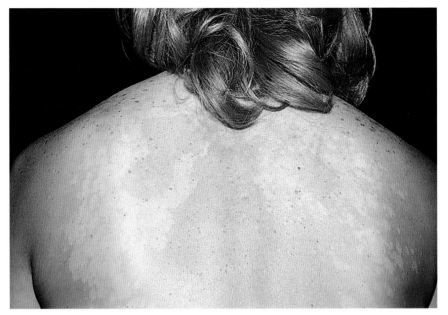

Figure 29-35. Classic presentation of tinea versicolor, with oval or circular areas of depigmentation on tan skin. (From Callen JP, Greer KE, Paller AS, Swinyer LJ: Color Atlas of Dermatology, 2nd ed. Philadelphia, WB Saunders, 2000, p 44.)

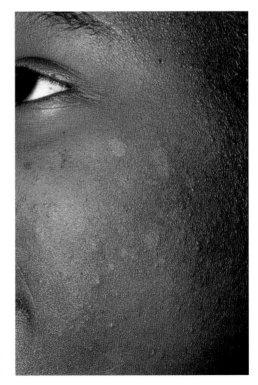

Figure 29-36. Tinea versicolor does not usually occur on the face, but when it does it may cause a significant cosmetic problem in black patients. (From White GM, Cox NH: Diseases of the Skin: A Color Atlas and Text. London, Mosby, 2002, p 356.)

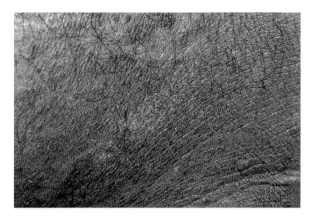

Figure 29-37. Tinea versicolor and many circular scaling lesions that are light brown or fawn colored on an untanned patient with a tan complexion. (From White GM, Cox NH: Diseases of the Skin: A Color Atlas and Text. London, Mosby, 2002, p 356.)

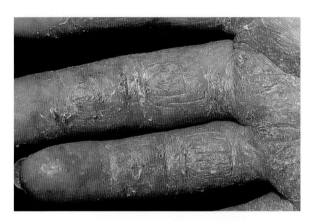

Figure 29-38. Irritant contact dermatitis, particularly of the hands, may occur from frequent exposure to water (e.g., dish washing), hand washing, chemicals (e.g., soaps, cleansers), or cold weather. (From White GM, Cox NH: Diseases of the Skin: A Color Atlas and Text. London, Mosby, 2002, p 35.)

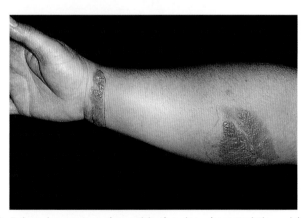

Figure 29-39. Poison ivy contact dermatitis showing characteristic vesicles and blisters, often occurring in a linear pattern and caused by dragging a plant over the skin or scratching a finger. Rhus dermatitis often occurs on the fingers, in the finger webs, or on areas touched by the contaminated fingers, such as the neck or face, but the rash (itching vesicles) may be diffuse. (From Callen JP, Greer KE, Paller AS, Swinyer LJ: Color Atlas of Dermatology, 2nd ed. Philadelphia, WB Saunders, 2000, p 132.)

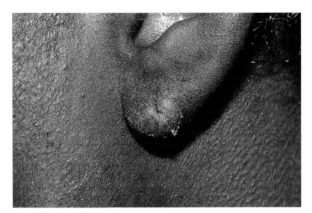

Figure 29-40. Contact dermatitis from nickel in jewelry. The earlobe is a frequently affected site, as is the navel. (From White GM, Cox NH: Diseases of the Skin: A Color Atlas and Text. London, Mosby, 2002, p 41.)

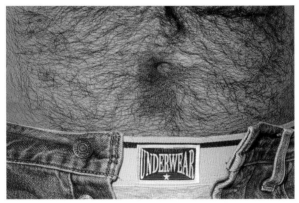

Figure 29-41. Contact dermatitis from nickel in a belt buckle. (From White GM, Cox NH: Diseases of the Skin: A Color Atlas and Text. London, Mosby, 2002, p 42.)

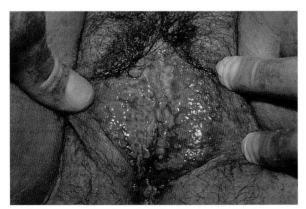

Figure 29-42. Genital herpes caused by herpes simplex type II. (From White GM, Cox NH: Diseases of the Skin: A Color Atlas and Text. London, Mosby, 2002, p 282.)

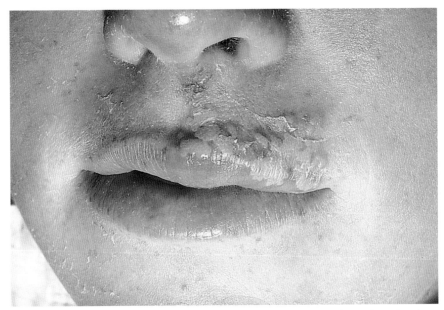

Figure 29-43. Recurrent cold sore (herpes simplex type I) on the lips. There is often a prodrome of itching and/or burning before the development of vesicles on an erythematous base. (From Callen JP, Greer KE, Paller AS, Swinyer LJ: Color Atlas of Dermatology, 2nd ed. Philadelphia, WB Saunders, 2000, p 366.)

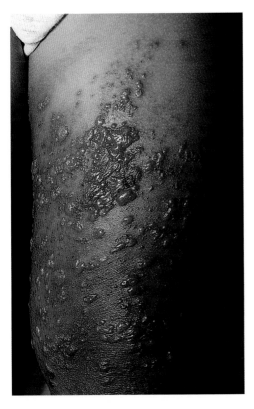

Figure 29-44. Herpes zoster commonly manifests as a painful vesicular eruption involving a single dermatome. It is bilateral in 10% to 20% of cases. (From Callen JP, Greer KE, Paller AS, Swinyer LJ: Color Atlas of Dermatology, 2nd ed. Philadelphia, WB Saunders, 2000, p 144.)

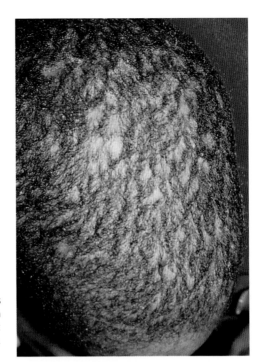

Figure 29-45. Tinea capitis often affects children, causing patches of hair loss with some scaling. (From Zitelli BJ, Davis HW: Atlas of Pediatric Physical Diagnosis, 4th ed. Philadelphia, Mosby, 2002, p 311.)

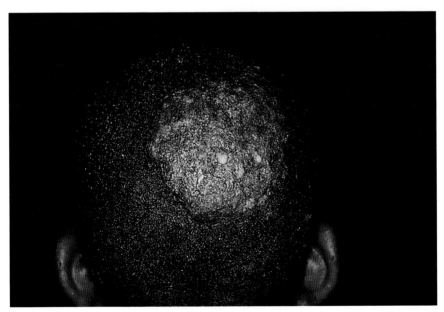

Figure 29-46. Inflammatory tinea capitis involving scalp and neck. Lesions can be pustular and boggy (kerion). (From Callen JP, Greer KE, Paller AS, Swinyer LJ: Color Atlas of Dermatology, 2nd ed. Philadelphia, WB Saunders, 2000, p 156.)

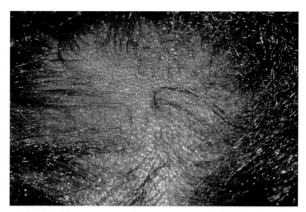

Figure 29-47. Tinea capitis caused by an endothrix infection that invades the hair shaft, causing the hairs to break off and leave a "black dot." If the patient's hair is light colored, the dots are light colored. (From White GM, Cox NH: Diseases of the Skin: A Color Atlas and Text. London, Mosby, 2002, p 364.)

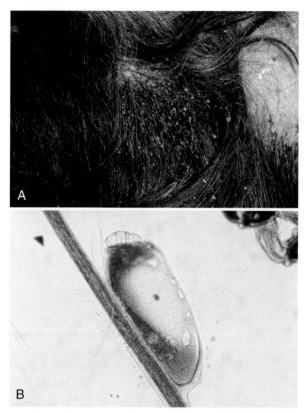

Figure 29-48. A, Pediculosis capitis produces marked irritation and itching of scalp. The nits can be seen attached to the hair shaft. **B,** Nit attached to hair shaft. (From White GM, Cox NH: Diseases of the Skin: A Color Atlas and Text. London, Mosby, 2002, p 373.)

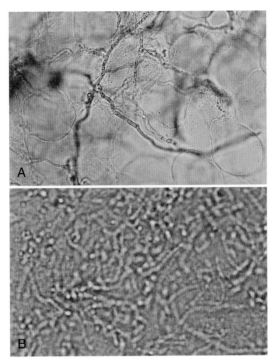

Figure 29-49. **A,** Potassium hydroxide preparation of tinea showing branching filamentous hyphae that are uniform in width. **B,** KOH preparation of *Candida albicans* showing pseudohyphae and oval yeast cells. (**A** from James WD, Berger TG, Elston DM: Andrews' Diseases of the Skin: Clinical Dermatology, 10th ed. Philadelphia, WB Saunders, 2000, p 304; **B** from Zitelli BJ, Davis HW: Atlas of Pediatric Physical Diagnosis, 4th ed. Philadelphia, Mosby, 2002, p 276.)

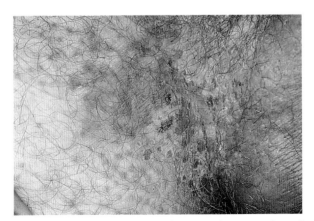

Figure 29-50. Candidiasis of groin. *Candida* infections often occur in moist intertriginous areas. The lesions are red and scaling, often with satellite pustules near the edge of the rash. (From Callen JP, Greer KE, Paller AS, Swinyer LJ: Color Atlas of Dermatology, 2nd ed. Philadelphia, WB Saunders, 2000, p 156.)

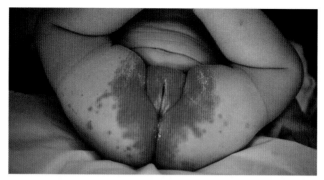

Figure 29-51. Diaper candidiasis showing erythematous folds with satellite pustule. (From Lawrence CM, Cox NH: Physical Signs in Dermatology, 2nd ed. London, Mosby, 2002, p 92.)

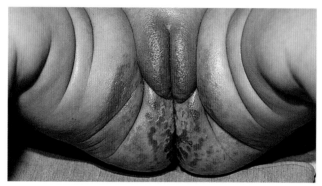

Figure 29-52. Diaper rash, a form of irritant contact dermatitis from prolonged contact with urine and feces in a soiled diaper. (From Callen JP, Greer KE, Paller AS, Swinyer LJ: Color Atlas of Dermatology, 2nd ed. Philadelphia, WB Saunders, 2000, p 303.)

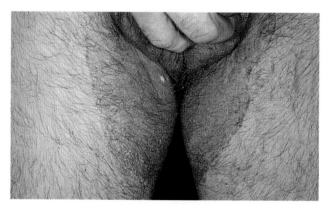

Figure 29-53. Tinea cruris (jock itch) shows an erythematous lesion with a sharp, scaling border. The redness and scaling spread away from the groin and down the inner thigh. (From Callen JP, Greer KE, Paller AS, Swinyer LJ: Color Atlas of Dermatology, 2nd ed. Philadelphia, WB Saunders, 2000, p 303.)

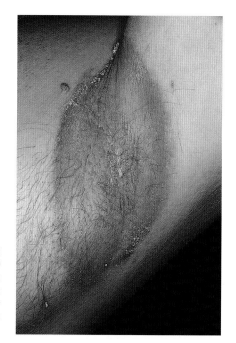

Figure 29-54. Erythrasma is a bacterial infection *(Corynebacterium minutissimum)* that causes a diffuse, scaling, brownish plaque that can be confused with tinea. (From Callen JP, Greer KE, Paller AS, Swinyer LJ: Color Atlas of Dermatology, 2nd ed. Philadelphia, WB Saunders, 2000, p 303.)

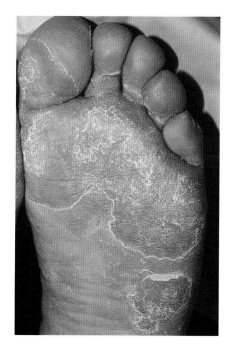

Figure 29-55. Tinea pedis. The infection has spread out of the toe web. (From White GM, Cox NH: Diseases of the Skin: A Color Atlas and Text. London, Mosby, 2002, p 359.)

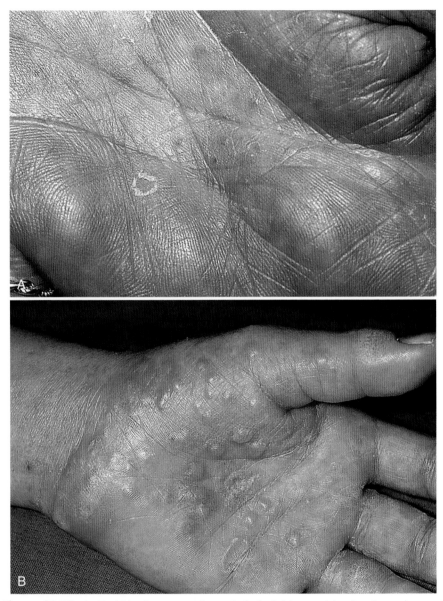

Figure 29-56. **A,** Dyshidrotic eczema (pompholyx). Itching vesicles involve palms and fingers. **B,** Dyshidrotic eczema (pompholyx). Vesicles may become confluent and cause large blotches. This lesion is more common in the summer and is often associated with severe stress. (From White GM, Cox NH: Diseases of the Skin: A Color Atlas and Text. London, Mosby, 2002, p 32.)

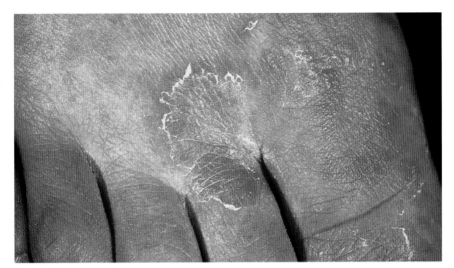

Figure 29-57. Tinea pedis. The skin is oily, scaly (often crescentic in shape), and asymmetrical. The toenails, webs, and dorsum of the foot may be involved. (From Lawrence CM, Cox NH: Physical Signs in Dermatology, 2nd ed. London, Mosby, 2002, p 123.)

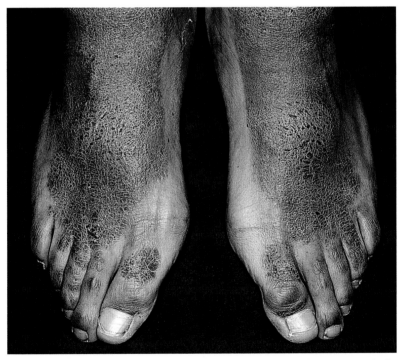

Figure 29-58. Contact dermatitis of the foot due to sensitivity to chromates in the leather. The tops of toes and dorsum of foot are usually involved. The web spaces are spared. (From Callen JP, Greer KE, Paller AS, Swinyer LJ: Color Atlas of Dermatology, 2nd ed. Philadelphia, WB Saunders, 2000, p 19.)

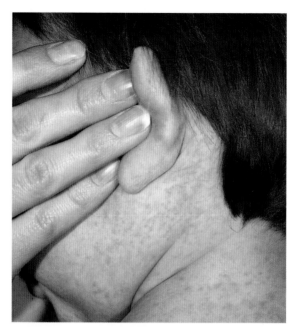

Figure 29-59. Roseola. Pale pink macules may appear first on the neck (From Habif T: Clinical Dermatology, 5th ed., Philadelphia, Mosby, 2010, p. 557.)

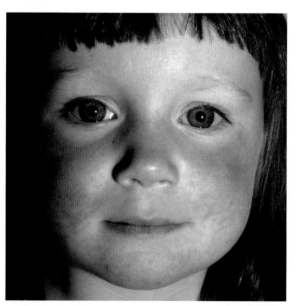

Figure 29-60. Erythema infectiosum. Facial erythema slapped cheek. The red plaque covers the cheek and spares the nasolabial fold and the circumoral region (From Habif T: Clinical Dermatology, 5th ed., Philadelphia, Mosby, 2010, p. 553.)

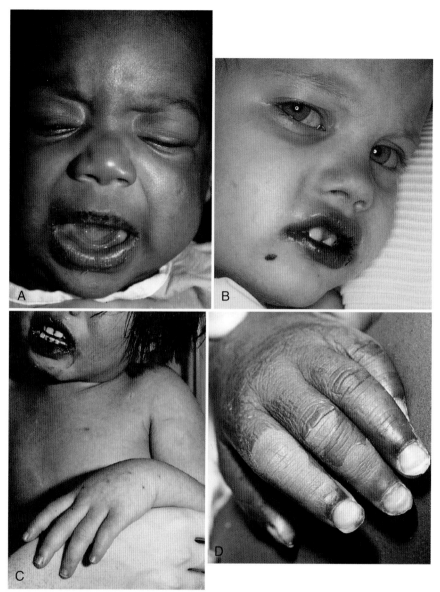

Figure 29-61. Kawasaki disease. A and B, Nonpurulent conjunctival injection and cherry red lips with fissuring and crusting are early signs of the disease. (Courtesy Anne W. Lucky, MD). C and D, The hands become red and swollen; they peel approximately 2 weeks after the onset of fever. (Courtesy Nancy B. Esterly, MD) (A-D From Habif T: Clinical Dermatology, 5th ed., Philadelphia, Mosby, 2010, p. 563.)

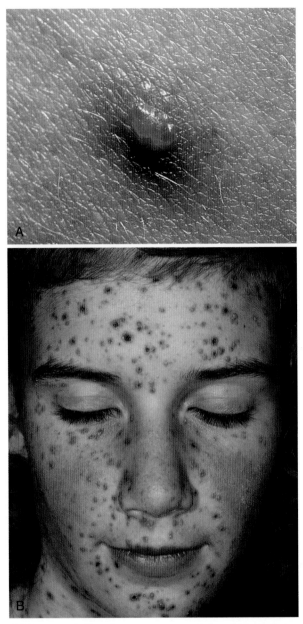

Figure 29-62. Chickenpox. A, Dewdrop on a rose petal; a thick-walled vesicle with clear fluid forms on a red base. B, The disease starts with lesions on the trunk and then spreads to the face and extremities. (From Habif T: Clinical Dermatology, 5th ed., Philadelphia, Mosby, 2010, pp. 474, 475.)

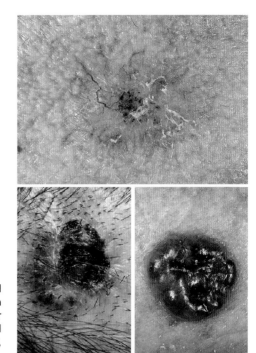

Figure 29-63. Pigmented basal cell carcinoma. Variable amounts of melanin are seen in these special types of nodular basal cell carcinomas (From Habif T: Clinical Dermatology, 5th ed., Philadelphia, Mosby, 2010, p. 806.)

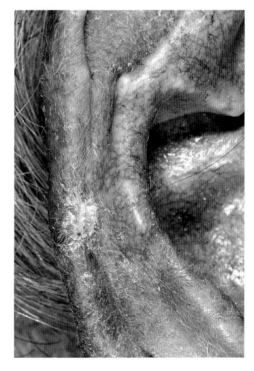

Figure 29-64. Squamous cell carcinoma. A red, keratotic papule with dense surface scale. Lesions may be misinterpreted as actinic keratosis. Cryotherapy may destroy the surface but leave deeper malignant cells untreated. Check draining lymph nodes. (From Habif T: Clinical Dermatology, 5th ed., Philadelphia, Mosby, 2010, p. 826.)

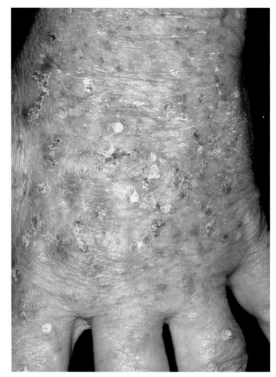

Figure 29-65. Actinic keratosis. Several oval-to-round, red, indurated lesions with adherent scale (From Habif T: Clinical Dermatology, 5th ed., Philadelphia, Mosby, 2010, p. 812.)

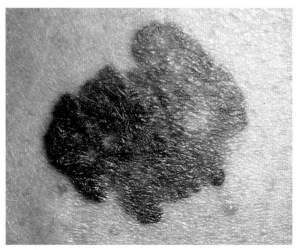

Figure 29-66. Superficial spreading melanomas (From Habif T: Clinical Dermatology, 5th ed., Philadelphia, Mosby, 2010, p. 865.)

TABLE 29-2.   Common Areas of Involvement and Causes of Allergic Contact Dermatitis

AREA	CAUSES
Ear lobes	Earrings (nickel)
Postauricular area	Hair dye (paraphenylenediamine) Shampoos (formalin) Hearing aids or glasses (nickel or plastic)
Ear canal	Medications
Face	Hair dye (paraphenylenediamine) Poison ivy Cosmetics Sprays or any airborne contactants
Eyelids	Sprays or any airborne contactants Cosmetics Eyelash curlers (rubber accelerators or nickel) Any contactant on the hands (topical medications, formalin in nail polish)
Perioral area	Lipstick Toothpaste
Neck	Jewelry (nickel) Perfumes Sprays or any airborne contactants
Axillae	Deodorants Clothing (formalin)
Chest	Brassieres (rubber accelerators) Metal objects carried in pockets (nickel)
Back	Metal fasteners (nickel)
Waist	Belt buckles or snaps (nickel) Waist bands or girdles (rubber accelerators)
Extremities	Poison ivy Airborne contactants
Wrists	Jewelry (nickel)
Hands	Rings (nickel) Gloves (rubber accelerators)
Feet	Components of shoes (rubber accelerators, dichromates in leather)
Scrotum	Any contactant on the hands or agent applied to the groin (topical medication)

From Huff JC, Weston WL: Eczematous dermatitis. Maj Probl Clin Pediatr 19:86-122, 1978.

Differential Diagnosis of Skin Problems

NATURE OF LESION	DISTRIBUTION OF LESION	ASSOCIATED FINDINGS	NATURE OF PATIENT	LESIONS WITH SIMILAR APPEARANCE	DIAGNOSIS
Papules and pustules	Face, back, and chest	Comedones	Start at puberty and last several years		Acne (Fig. 29-1)
Papules, vesicles, and pustules	Face, head, and neck Occasionally diaper area in infants	Oozing, honeycomb-colored crusting	Mostly children	Molluscum contagiosum (Fig. 29-4) Folliculitis (Fig. 29-5)	Impetigo (Figs. 29-2 and 29-3)
Scaling and lichenification	Face, extensor surfaces, and exposed areas in children Flexural folds (antecubital, popliteal), wrists, neck, upper arms, and thighs in adults Symmetrical	Often a family history of hay fever or asthma Itching, erythema, often lichenification In African Americans, rash tends to be more papular 10% of general population has atopic dermatitis Erythematous or with plaques Rash in adults is usually localized, dry, excoriated, or lichenified	Often begin in infancy at age 5 mo Often clear spontaneously at age 5 yr Rare in elderly people	Seborrheic dermatitis (different locations and yellow scales) Psoriasis (typical locations and silvery scales) Contact dermatitis is usually asymmetrical	Atopic dermatitis or eczema (Figs. 29-6 to 29-9)
Scaling plaques	Mostly extensor surface of extremities, back, buttocks, and hands, but can occur anywhere	Coin-shaped lesions Itching Oozing	Children and adults	Ringworm (positive KOH test result) Contact dermatitis (exposed areas) Psoriasis (elbows and knees)	Nummular eczema or nummular dermatitis (Fig. 29-10)
Scaling plaques or patches	Trunk and proximal extremities	Herald patch (2 × 6 cm), usually on trunk, precedes generalized lesion More common in winter Salmon-colored May itch Oval patches (1 × 2 cm) with long axis along skin lines, giving Christmas tree pattern Collarette scaling	Children Young adults	Fungus Psoriasis Secondary syphilis Drug eruptions	Pityriasis rosea (Figs. 29-11 to 29-13)

Morphology	Distribution	Characteristics	Age	Differential	Diagnosis
Plaques	Usually on covered parts of body and face Often multiple	Irregular, greasy surface Superficial, on top of skin ("stuck to skin") Yellow, tan, dark brown, or (rarely) black Sharply defined edges	Adults (mostly elderly)	Actinic keratoses occur in sun-exposed areas and are smaller	Seborrheic keratoses (Figs. 29-14 and 29-15)
Erythematous plaques	Extensor surfaces, especially knees and elbows Scalp Coccygeal region Nails Rare on face	Silvery, loosely adherent scales Occasional itching Arthritis, especially in distal interphalangeal joints Sharp margins Scalp lesions usually stop at hairline	Adults Rare in young children	Seborrheic dermatitis can involve scalp but extends beyond hairline Nummular eczema	Psoriasis (Figs. 29-16 to 29-20)
Scaling patches	Scalp Eyebrows Nasolabial fold Midchest Umbilicus	Yellow, greasy scaling Greasy scaling with poor margin Some erythema	More common in adults "Cradle cap" in infants	Dandruff with little erythema; no other areas involved Psoriasis involves extensor surfaces Psoriasis of scalp usually stops at hairline with well defined plaques	Seborrheic dermatitis (Figs. 29-21 to 29-24)
Papules inflamed, with excoriation and crusting Linear burrows not always seen	Finger webs Wrists Antecubital Elbows Areolar Umbilicus Lower abdomen Genitalia Gluteal cleft	Itching (worse at night) Excoriation Weeping Others in household may have same problem	Adults and children	Pediculosis pubis Nits attached to hair Lice often seen on skin	Scabies (Figs. 29-25 to 29-27)
Papules inflamed	Usually on trunk Grouped	Itching; flea bites often grouped	In adults, sand flies and fleas on lower legs In children, flea bites can be anywhere	Scabies Drug eruptions Lymphoma	Insect bites (Figs. 29-28 to 29-30)

Continued

Differential Diagnosis of Skin Problems—cont'd

NATURE OF LESION	DISTRIBUTION OF LESION	ASSOCIATED FINDINGS	NATURE OF PATIENT	LESIONS WITH SIMILAR APPEARANCE	DIAGNOSIS
Depigmenta-tion	Orifices Eyes Extensor surfaces Areas of trauma	Positive Wood's light reaction (bright white) Increased familial incidence	Familial Thyroid disease Addison's disease	Postinflammatory hypopigmentation Tinea versicolor alba Exposure to phenolic compounds	Vitiligo (Figs. 29-31 to 29-33)
Depigmenta-tion and pink-red-brown macules	Mainly trunk Upper arms	Positive Wood's light reaction (pale yellow) Pink-red-brown macules Scaling Positive KOH test result Mild itching	Young adults	Postinflammatory hypopigmentation (e.g., seborrheic dermatitis, pityriasis rosea, especially in African Americans) Other fungi	Tinea versicolor (pityriasis versicolor) (Figs. 29-34 to 29-37)
Vesicles	Anywhere (often asymmetrical exposed areas) Hands Axillae	Itching, oozing May occur hours to a few days after exposure	Adults and children	Allergy to systemic medications Atopic dermatitis	Contact dermatitis (see Table 29-2) Detergents Chemicals (Fig. 29-38) Deodorant
On erythema-tous areas	Exposed areas (especially extremities)	Lesions often in streaks	Adults and children	Eczema	Plants (ivy, oak, sumac) (Fig. 29-39)
	Near hands, zippers, jewelry (e.g., wrist, earlobe)	Itching	Adults and children	Eczema	Nickel (Figs. 29-40 and 29-41)
	Where medication is applied (e.g., eye, hair, face, neck) Hands, other exposed areas Genital region Buttocks	Itching	Adults and children	Eczema	Medications, hair preparations, cosmetics Industrial agents (see Table 29-1)

Signs/Symptoms	Distribution	Characteristics	Occurs in	Possible diagnoses	Probable diagnosis
With erythematous base	Genital area	Pain, not itch; Positive Tzanck test result	Adults; Neonates	Acute contact dermatitis	Herpes progenitalis (simplex II) (Fig. 29-42)
	Cold sore (rarely in genital area)	Pain; Systemic symptoms; Positive Tzanck test result/PCR	Adults; Neonates	Erythema multiforme	Herpes simplex I (Fig. 29-43)
With dermatomal distribution	Leg most common site in children	Tingling; Occasional itching; Pain (usually not in children); Often sciatic distribution	Adults and children	Contact dermatitis (usually itches); Cellulitis	Herpes zoster (Fig. 29-44)
Patchy alopecia	Scalp	Hairs broken and short; Positive KOH test result; Does not fluoresce; Culture in DTM; Microsporum audouinii and canis give apple-green Wood's light reaction	Preadolescents and adults	Alopecia areata	Fungal infections mostly Trichophyton tonsurans (Figs. 29-45 to 29-47)
Patchy alopecia (possibly scarring)	Scalp	Pustular lesion; Boggy scalp; Culture in DTM	Most common in children	Fungal infection	Bacterial infection
	Scalp	Pinhead-sized nits on hair shaft; Bacterial infection may be superimposed; Itching	More common in children but can occur in adults	Seborrheic dermatitis; Bacterial infection	Pediculosis capitis (Fig. 29-48)
Erythematous; Some scaling; Occasional maceration and oozing	Groin	Border not sharp; pustules at edge; Positive KOH test result; Moist	Children; Diabetics	May all look similar (KOH test required for differentiation) (Fig. 29-49)	Candidiasis (Figs. 29-50 and 29-51); Diaper rash (Fig. 29-52)
	Under breast	Border sharp and accentuated; Itching; No pustular edge; Positive KOH test result; Moist			Tinea cruris (Fig. 29-53)

Continued

Differential Diagnosis of Skin Problems—cont'd

NATURE OF LESION	DISTRIBUTION OF LESION	ASSOCIATED FINDINGS	NATURE OF PATIENT	LESIONS WITH SIMILAR APPEARANCE	DIAGNOSIS
	Groin	Border sharp Positive Wood's light reaction (coral red) Reddish brown macules	Often complicates simple herpes rash More common in males Not seen in children Obese adults Adults		Seborrheic intertrigo Erythrasma (Corynebacterium) (Fig. 29-54)
Scaling, vesicles	Feet (soles)	Scaling Itching (worse in summer) Positive KOH test result	Adults and children	May coexist*	Tinea pedis (dyshidrotic form) (Fig. 29-55)
Vesicles	Feet (soles, sides, dorsum)	Negative KOH test result Often associated with similar process in hands	Adults	May coexist*	Dyshidrotic eczema (Fig. 29-56)
Maceration	Feet (between toes, mainly 4th and 3rd spaces)	Itching (worse in summer) Positive KOH test result	Adults and children	May coexist*	Tinea pedis (intertriginous form) (Fig. 29-57)
Scaling	Face or feet (soles)	Erythema and fissuring Negative KOH test result; spares toe webs	Children		Juvenile plantar dermatitis
Erythema scaling	Feet (dorsum and toes; toe webs and soles not involved)	Negative KOH test result	Adults and children	Tinea pedis	Shoe dermatitis due to chrome used in leather tanning (Fig. 29-58)

Tumor					
	Most common on face and other sun-exposed areas	Smooth surface Atrophic center Pearly edge Round shape Tannish brown Telangiectasia on border	Elderly people Those often exposed to sun	Squamous cell cancer Melanoma Sebaceous nevi	Basal cell carcinoma
	Most common on sun-exposed areas (especially hands, face, and ears)	Smooth or irregular surface Firm Irregular edge May be scaling Tannish brown	Elderly people Those often exposed to sun	Basal cell carcinoma Warts Actinic keratoses	Squamous cell carcinoma
	Men: mostly on trunk (47%) Women: mostly on legs (39%)	Pigmented, often with different colors in same lesion (blue, purple, white, tan) Irregular border Change in size Satellites	Adults	Mole (melanocytic nevus) Pigmented lesions Seborrheic keratosis Dermatofibroma Angiokeratoma Lentigo	Malignant melanoma

DTM, Dermatology test medium; *KOH,* potassium hydroxide.
*Different forms of tinea pedis may exist with one another as well as with dyshidrotic eczema.

Selected References

Adam R: Skin care of the diaper area, *Pediatr Dermatol* 25, 2008:427-33.

Ali I, Dawber R: Hirsutism: diagnosis and management, *Hosp Med* 65:293-297, 2004.

Bart BJ: Annular skin eruptions: not every ring on the skin is ringworm, *Postgrad Med* 96:37-50, 1994.

Beacham BE: Common dermatoses in the elderly, *Am Fam Physician* 47:1445-1450, 1993.

Berger TG, Obuch ML, Goldschmidt RH: Dermatologic manifestations of HIV infection, *Am Fam Physician* 41:1729-1743, 1990.

Browning J: An update on pityriasis rosea and other similar childhood exanthems, *Curr Opin Pediatr* 21:481-485, 2009.

Carter KF, Dufour LT, Ballard CN: Identifying primary skin lesions, *Nursing* 33:68-69, 2003.

Davidson CL: Occupational contact dermatitis of the upper extremity, *Occup Med State Art Rev* 9:59-74, 1994.

du Vivier A: *Atlas of Clinical Dermatology*, ed 3, London, 2002, Churchill Livingstone.

Fawcett RS, Linford S, Stulberg DL: Nail abnormalities: clues to systemic disease, *Am Fam Physician* 69:1417-1424, 2004.

Gropper CA: An approach to clinical dermatologic diagnosis based on morphologic reaction patterns, *Clin Cornerstones* 4:1-14, 2001.

Habif TP: *Clinical dermatology: a color guide to diagnosis and therapy*, ed 4, Philadelphia, 2004, Mosby.

Habif T, Campbell J, Chapman MS, et al: *Skin disease: diagnosis and treatment*, ed 2, Philadelphia, 2005, Elsevier.

Karthikeyan K: Scabies in children, *Arch Dis Chil Educ Pract Ed* 92:65-69, 2007.

Lee A: Skin manifestations of systemic disease, *Aust Fam Physician* 38:498-505, 2009.

Luba M, Bangs S, Mohler A, et al: Common benign skin tumors, *Am Fam Physician* 67:729-738, 2003.

Luggen AS: Wrinkles and beyond: skin problems in older adults, *Adv Nurse Pract* 11(60):55-58, 2003:62.

Malvehy J, Puig S, Argenziano G, et al: Dermoscopy report: proposal for standardization, *J Am Acad Dermatol* 57:84-95, 2007.

O'Connor N, McLaughlin M, Ham P: Newborn skin, part 1: common rashes, *Am Fam Physician* 77:47-52, 2008.

Prawer SE: Occupational dermatoses in primary care: a guide to recognition, *Consultant* 38:423-444, 1998.

Sahl WJ, Mathewson RJ: Common facial skin lesions in children, *Quintessence Int* 24:475-481, 1993.

Shah K: The diagnostic and clinical significance of cafe-au-lait macules, *Pediatr Clin North Am* 57:1131-1153, 2010.

Usatine R: Diagnosis and management of contact dermatitis, *Am Fam Physician* 82:249-255, 2010.

Usatine R, Sandy N: Dermatologic emergencies, *Am Fam Physician* 82:773-780, 2010.

30 Sore Throat

This chapter defines *sore throat* as pain in the throat at rest that often worsens with swallowing. The most common causes (70% to 80%) of sore throat without pharyngeal ulcers include *viral pharyngitis (rhinovirus, adenovirus, influenza, respiratory syncytial virus, coxsackie virus, herpes virus, and Epstein-Barr virus), bacterial pharyngitis* and *tonsillitis, allergic pharyngitis, pharyngitis secondary to sinusitis,* and *infectious mononucleosis.* Common causes of sore throat with pharyngeal ulceration include *herpangina, aphthous stomatitis, herpes simplex, fusospirochetal infection, candidiasis, herpes zoster,* and *chickenpox* (varicella). The less common primary and secondary syphilitic ulcerations are usually not painful.

Pharyngitis is a vexing problem because it is extremely prevalent (1.1% of visits in primary care settings) and because a precise diagnosis is difficult to establish. The annual cost of laboratory tests and medications ordered for patients with sore throats is about $300 million. Even though viral and streptococcal pharyngitis (including infectious mononucleosis) are the most common causes of sore throat, studies have shown that even with careful diagnostic techniques, a precise cause can be determined in only about 50% of patients. *Mycoplasma pneumoniae* is being recognized more frequently as a cause of pharyngitis in children.

Prompt diagnosis and treatment of *streptococcal pharyngitis* (group A beta-hemolytic streptococcus [GABHS]) are essential to reducing its spread to close contacts; treatment also prevents acute rheumatic fever. In addition, prompt antibiotic therapy shortens the clinical course and decreases morbidity. Rapid screening tests (rapid antigen detection testing [RADT]) for streptococcal antigens are useful in patients with signs and symptoms of acute pharyngitis. **Because of improvement in RADT, a throat culture is not necessary unless the RADT result is negative, symptoms do not improve, or the patient shows no response to appropriate antibiotics.** This statement does not mean that throat cultures are of no value, but it does reinforce the need for sound clinical judgment in the diagnosis and treatment of patients with sore throats (Table 30-1).

TABLE 30-1.   Probabilities of Streptococcal Isolation in Four Series
with Different Clinical Predictors*

	Probability (%)			
PREDICTOR	**PRESENT SERIES**	**WALSH ET AL**	**CRAWFORD ET AL**	**CENTOR ET AL**
Number of subjects (n)	693	418	472	234
Tonsillar exudate	25.4	19.9	18.5	18.9
Anterior cervical adenopathy	13.8	12.6	15.3	16.5
Temperature >100° F	22.2	14.3	NR	NR
Temperature >101° F	26.1	23.9	25.0	19.5
History of recent exposure to streptococcus	11.1	18.8	20.0	NR
No cough	15.0	14.8	14.7	19.3
No rhinorrhea	14.8	13.4	NR	11.9
At "high risk" according to Walsh algorithm†	26.4	19.0	22.7	NR

*Probabilities in all series adjusted to an assumed prevalence rate of 10% using Bayes' theorem.
†"High-risk" patients are those with enlarged or tender cervical nodes *and* pharyngeal exudate or history of recent exposure to someone with diagnosed streptococcal infection.
NR, not reported.
Adapted from Komaroff A, Pass TM, Aronson MD, et al: The prediction of streptococcal pharyngitis in adults. J Gen Intern Med 1:1-7, 1986.

NATURE OF PATIENT

Streptococcal pharyngitis is most prevalent in patients younger than 25 years, particularly those between ages 5 and 15 years. Likewise, *herpangina, herpes simplex, fusospirochetal infections,* and *candidiasis* are more common in children. As a cause of pharyngitis, *infectious mononucleosis* is most prevalent in adolescents and young adults. It does occur, though less frequently, in patients older than 60 years. It is particularly notable that 70% of elderly patients with infectious mononucleosis do not experience pharyngitis, adenopathy, or splenomegaly.

Chlamydia trachomatis and *Neisseria gonorrhoeae* manifesting as oropharyngeal symptoms are becoming more common as causes of pharyngitis but are often unrecognized. *Neisseria* has been cultured from the throat in 10% of patients with anogenital gonorrhea. Of those with positive culture results, most do not have pharyngeal symptoms. It is more common in people who engage in orogenital sex. Male homosexuals have a higher incidence of oropharyngeal gonorrheal infections than other groups.

Common ulcerative and vesicular pharyngeal lesions include *recurrent aphthous stomatitis, herpes zoster, herpes simplex, fusospirochetal infections,* and *candidiasis* (particularly if the patient is immunosuppressed or taking antibiotics [Table 30-2]). Oral ulcers may occur with periodic fever and PFAPA

Table 30-2. Common Infections Causing Oropharyngeal Ulceration

DISEASE	LOCATION	VESICULATION	PAIN	SIZE OF LESION (MM)	DIAGNOSTIC CRITERIA
Local herpangina	Tonsils, pillars, uvula	Yes	Yes	1-2	Characteristic clinical presentation, coxsackievirus in culture of lesion exudate, positive serologic test result
Herpes simplex	Lips, gingivae, buccal mucosa, tongue	Yes	Yes	1-2	Multinuclear giant cell with ballooning degeneration in Tzanck smear of ulcer-crater exudate
Fusospirochetal infection	Gingivae, may spread diffusely	No	Yes	2-30	Characteristic lesions, foul breath, anaerobic forms and spirochetes in smear of lesion exudate
Candidiasis	All parts of oropharynx	No	Yes	3-10	Candida albicans in gram-stained smear and culture of scrapings
Primary syphilis	Lips, tonsils, tongue	No	No	5-15	Indurated "heaped-up" lesion, positive serologic test result (periodic evaluation necessary)
Herpes zoster	Unilateral involvement	Yes	Yes	2-4	Unilateral involvement, painful prodromes, giant cells in Tzanck smear of lesion exudate
Systemic hand-foot- and-mouth disease	All parts of oropharynx	Yes	Yes	1-10	Exanthem on hands and feet, coxsackievirus in culture of lesion exudate, positive serologic test result
Varicella	All parts of oropharynx	Yes	No	2-4	Characteristic exanthem
Secondary syphilis	Symmetrical involvement of all parts of mouth and oropharynx	No	No	2-10	Other evidence of secondary syphilis, positive serologic test result, spirochetes visible on dark-field microscopy

From Brown RB, Clinton D: Vesicular and ulcerative infections of the mouth and oropharynx. Postgrad Med 67:107-116, 1980.

(periodic fever, aphthae, pharyngitis, cervical adenopathy), a rare childhood disease. Although they are rare, primary and secondary syphilitic lesions are seen in adults. They should be suspected if a lesion is not painful and the usual accompanying symptoms of upper respiratory infection (URI) are absent.

NATURE OF SYMPTOMS

Marked pain in the throat (frequently associated with dysphagia), tonsillopharyngeal exudate, an oral temperature exceeding 100° F to 101° F (37.7° C to 38.3° C), chills, age 5 to 15 years, and a rapid onset of symptoms suggest the probability of *streptococcal pharyngitis*.

Sore throat and the presence of a low-grade fever, myalgia, conjunctivitis, coryza, malaise, diarrhea, or fatigue suggest **viral pharyngitis**. When children (2-6 years) have three or more episodes of nonstreptococcal pharyngitis in a 6-month period, *M. pneumoniae* pharyngitis should be suspected. A low-grade temperature, gradual onset of pharyngeal symptoms, and systemic symptoms (particularly fatigue) that are more persistent suggest *infectious mononucleosis*. In reality, it is difficult for the physician to determine the cause of pharyngitis on the basis of the nature of the chief complaint; predisposing factors and physical findings are frequently more useful indicators.

ASSOCIATED SYMPTOMS

Headache, nausea, vomiting, and abdominal pain may occur with sore throat, especially in children with streptococcal pharyngitis.

PREDISPOSING FACTORS

Herpangina, herpes simplex, and *candidiasis* are most common in immunosuppressed patients. Candidiasis is also most prevalent in diabetic patients and in patients taking broad-spectrum antibiotics. Inhaled and nasal steroids predispose an individual to *Candida pharyngitis*. Herpangina is most common in children and shows a strong seasonal propensity for summer and autumn, whereas *streptococcal pharyngitis* is most prevalent in the winter and early spring. Aphthous stomatitis is associated with Behçet's disease, Crohn's disease, ulcerative colitis, malabsorption syndrome, gluten-sensitive enteropathy, PFAPA syndrome, and human immunodeficiency virus (HIV) infection.

PHYSICAL FINDINGS

Marked erythema and swelling of the throat (often associated with exudative pharyngitis or tonsillitis), tender anterior cervical adenopathy, temperature higher than 101° F, tachycardia, and occurrence between September and April all strongly suggest *streptococcal pharyngitis*. Likewise, a history of streptococcal exposure within the patient's family during the past week, prior history of acute rheumatic fever, diabetes, tender anterior cervical nodes, or a scarlatiniform rash increases the likelihood that streptococcal pharyngitis is the correct diagnosis. The presence of cough mitigates against a GABHS infection. Streptococcal pharyngitis is rare after age 30 years and is most common between ages 5 and 15 years.

Although many writers stress an association between tonsillopharyngeal exudate and streptococcal pharyngitis, only 50% of the patients with proven streptococcal pharyngitis have an exudate, and only 50% of all patients with a pharyngeal exudate have streptococcal pharyngitis. A nonadherent pharyngeal exudate is a sensitive but nonspecific indicator of streptococcal pharyngitis, because an exudate is found in many other bacterial and viral infections. Despite this fact, many physicians presume a streptococcal cause if a tonsillar exudate is present and one or more of the following signs are demonstrated: temperature higher than 101° F, tender anterior cervical nodes, and duration of sore throat for more than 6 days, particularly with no cough (see Table 30-1).

Studies have shown that when the patient is 15 years of age or older, the presence of all four criteria (tonsillar exudate, tender anterior cervical adenopathy, temperature higher than 101° F, absence of cough) suggests a GABHS infection with a probability of 50% to 60%.

The absence of fever or the presence of conjunctivitis, cough, hoarseness, coryza, anterior stomatitis, ulcerative oral lesions, viral exanthem, and diarrhea mitigates against a diagnosis of a streptococcal infection.

Viral infection **is the most common cause of pharyngitis and, unlike streptococcal pharyngitis, has no particular distribution with regard to age or time of year, although it is slightly more frequent in the winter months.** Patients with viral pharyngitis usually have less severe pharyngeal symptoms and more severe systemic symptoms. These patients are less likely to have an exudate or marked erythema of the pharynx, which is usually slightly injected but may also appear swollen, boggy, or pale. Exudate or follicular tonsillitis is not usually present, but systemic symptoms (malaise, fever, cough, headache, fatigue) are more prominent than they are with streptococcal pharyngitis.

Patients with the pharyngitis of *infectious mononucleosis* may present with an exudate, although most do not. The enanthem of infectious mononucleosis (palatine petechiae) is almost diagnostic. The petechiae resemble small, red, raised grains of sand surrounded by 0.5-mm pale bases. The pharyngitis of infectious mononucleosis is almost invariably (90% of cases) accompanied by posterior cervical adenopathy. Some writers are reluctant to diagnose infectious mononucleosis in the absence of posterior cervical adenopathy.

Epiglottitis, which may occur in children but is rare in adults, is usually caused by a *Haemophilus* infection. When epiglottitis is suspected, appropriate cultures should be performed, and antibiotics should be administered promptly. *Gingivitis* is most often seen in patients with poor oral hygiene. In some cases it can involve the entire oropharynx. The most common presentation of *ulcerative gingivitis (trench mouth)* is an acute onset of painful, bloody gums; foul breath; and a grayish exudate covering the interdental papillae. Ulcerative gingivitis is a *fusospirochetal infection* that responds well to improved oral hygiene and appropriate antibiotics. Pharyngeal involvement with fusospirochetal organisms *(Vincent's angina)* may occur primarily or may be secondary to a spread of fusospirochetal infection from anterior sites. In patients with this infection, sore throat is the most common complaint, and necrotic, gray, ulcerative lesions may develop about the tonsillar pillars. If the "pseudomembrane" is removed, bleeding of the undersurface usually occurs. Although in most cases involvement is initially unilateral, it often spreads and becomes bilateral.

Patients who have frequent sore throats without evidence of pharyngitis or fever may have *allergic pharyngitis*. This condition is often associated with an intermittent postnasal drip that leads to minor irritation and inflammation of the posterior pharynx. Some patients with recurrent or chronic low-grade *sinusitis* may present with a sore throat induced by a postnasal drip from the affected sinuses. **When a patient complains of a sore throat that becomes worse with swallowing and the physical findings of the oropharynx are normal, the physician should suspect thyroiditis and palpate the thyroid for swelling or pain.** This presentation is common for the uncommon illness thyroiditis.

Retropharyngeal abscess is most common in infants and young children, but it does occur infrequently in adults. The patient may have an unexplained fever, upper respiratory infection, loss of appetite, difficulty in swallowing, and stridor. The last sign is particularly common in children. Retropharyngeal abscess is a medical emergency and should be evaluated promptly. The study of choice is computed tomography (CT). Some investigators believe that earlier treatment with antibiotics reduces the incidence of this complication and the need for surgical intervention.

Sore throat may be the presenting complaint in children with a *peritonsillar abscess*. This complication of tonsillitis is more common in older children and adolescents. Dysphagia, odynophagia, and trismus may be associated with it, but the tonsil may be without significant inflammation or exudate. The tonsil is usually displaced medially.

The presence of oropharyngeal ulcerations, with or without vesiculation, is often helpful in differential diagnosis (see Table 30-2). In patients with *herpangina*, usually children, the painful ulcerations measure 1 to 2 mm and appear on the tonsils, pillars, and uvula. The pharyngeal ulcers (2 to 30 mm) due to *fusospirochetal infections* are usually present on the gingivae, but they may spread diffusely throughout the oropharynx. These lesions are usually painful, but there is no associated vesiculation. In adults and children with *herpes simplex*, the painful ulcers measure 1 to 2 mm and can occur on the lips, gingivae, buccal mucosa, or (rarely) the tongue. The painful ulcerations of *herpes zoster* are usually unilateral and involve the tongue, lip, or buccal mucosa. These lesions are usually 2 to 4 mm and associated with vesiculation. In infants and adults with *candidiasis*, the ulcerations measure 3 to 11 mm and can involve any part of the oropharynx. Vesiculation does not occur with candidiasis.

DIAGNOSTIC STUDIES

Tests that are often helpful in the differential diagnosis of sore throat are a complete blood count (CBC) with differential count, throat cultures, rapid "strep" tests, and the monospot test. With the advent of RADT for streptococcal antigens, the latest recommendation is treatment if the result is positive. If the result is negative in a child, a throat culture should be performed and treatment should be given if the culture result is positive. In an adult, the physician should do nothing. One approach recommends culture if any one of the following is present: age less than 25 years, definite streptococcal exposure during the previous week, a history of acute rheumatic fever, diabetes, a known epidemic of streptococcal pharyngitis, oral temperature higher than 99.5° F, exudate, tender anterior cervical nodes, and a scarlatiniform rash.

Difficulty with follow-up, a known epidemic of nephritogenic streptococcal infections, or the presence of a scarlatiniform rash is an indication for both throat culture and treatment with penicillin. In addition, if there is a history of rheumatic fever or diabetes is present, treatment with penicillin is indicated despite the clinical picture. **A patient with a temperature higher than 101° F, tonsillar exudate, tender anterior cervical nodes, and no cough probably has streptococcal pharyngitis, and immediate treatment is justified.** A complete blood count showing a lymphocytosis of greater than 50% or an absolute lymphocytosis of greater than 4500 lymphocytes per mm^3 with more than 10% atypical lymphocytes suggests *infectious mononucleosis*. This diagnosis can be confirmed by the positive result of a monospot test or heterophile antibody test. **Virtually no false-negative monospot test results exist, although some studies have shown 10% false-positive results.** Most of these characteristic hematologic and serologic abnormalities occur within 1 week from the onset of symptoms in 80% of patients.

LESS COMMON DIAGNOSTIC CONSIDERATIONS

Patients with *thyroiditis* may present with sore throat, dysphagia, or both. In a patient complaining of a sore throat whose throat findings are negative, the thyroid gland should be palpated. If it is tender, thyroiditis should be suspected. Patients with *hypothyroidism* may complain of sore throat or hoarseness regardless of whether a goiter is present. Some patients with seasonal *allergy* present with sore throat. Most such patients have minimal pharyngeal swelling. A postnasal drip is occasionally seen, and other allergic symptoms can usually be elicited as well.

Lemierre's syndrome (tonsillitis, thrombosis of the external jugular vein, and septic emboli) is a rare complication of tonsillitis.

Kawasaki's disease usually affects children less than 5 years of age. They typically have a sore throat, fever, conjunctivitis, anterior cervical adenopathy, strawberry tongue, an erythematous rash, cracked lips, and erythema of the

Differential Diagnosis of Sore Throat

TYPE OF PHARYNGITIS	NATURE OF PATIENT	NATURE OF SYMPTOMS	PREDISPOSING FACTORS	PHYSICAL FINDINGS	DIAGNOSTIC STUDIES
Without Pharyngeal Ulcers					
Viral	All ages	Pain in throat Rapid onset Systemic symptoms		Exudate less likely than with streptococcal infections	
Infectious mononucleosis	Adolescents and young adults Uncommon in elderly	Gradual onset		Low-grade temperature Occasional exudate Enanthem Posterior cervical adenopathy Hepatosplenomegaly	Monospot test
Streptococcal pharyngitis	Patients younger than 25 yr, especially ages 6-12 yr	Pain in throat Rapid onset Few systemic symptoms	Fall and winter Streptococcal infection in family Diabetes	Marked erythema and throat swelling Temperature >101° F Tender anterior cervical nodes Scarlatiniform rash Tonsillar exudate more likely than with viral infection	Culture Rapid streptococcal antigen screening Increased ASO titer
Gonococcal pharyngitis	Most common in male homosexuals and people with anogenital gonorrhea	Often no symptoms	Orogenital sex		Culture
Sinusitis with postnasal drip	Adults	Mild throat soreness Symptoms often worse with recumbency		Evidence of sinusitis Postnasal drip	Sinus radiographs

Allergic pharyngitis		Seasonal allergies	No fever; Intermittent postnasal drip; Swollen pharynx with minimal injection	Eosinophils in nasal secretions
With Pharyngeal Ulcers				
Herpangina	More common in children	Painful ulcers on tonsils, pillars, or uvula	Immunosuppression; Summer and autumn	Vesicles; 1- to 2-mm ulcers	Serologic tests
Fusospirochetal infection (Vincent's angina)	Children and people with poor oral hygiene	Painful ulcers; Bleeding gums; Foul breath		No vesicles; Ulcerative gingivitis; Gray, necrotic ulcers; 2- to 30=mm ulcers; Pseudomembrane	Gram stain: spirochetes
Candidiasis	Children; Immunosuppressed patients; Those taking antibiotics		Immunosuppression; Antibiotics; Inhaled steroids	3- to 11-mm ulcers; No vesicles	KOH smear: *Candida*; Culture
Herpes simplex	Most common in children	Not usually a cause of sore throat	Immunosuppression	1- to 2-mm painful ulcers; Vesicles present on lips, gingivae, buccal mucosa, or tongue	Tzanck smear shows multinucleated giant cells, viral culture, PCR, HSV antibody assay

ASO, (serum) Antistreptolysin-O; *KOH,* potassium hydroxide.

hands and feet. The dermatologic findings appear 3 days after the onset of fever. PFAPA syndrome is a rare, benign cause of aphthous stomatitis that is seen in children.

Patients who have swallowed a coarse *foreign body* such as a bone, rough vegetable, or piece of meat may complain of sore throat with or without dysphagia, even if they have successfully swallowed the object. If this complaint persists or is severe, the possibility that a foreign body is lodged in the posterior pharynx or proximal esophagus should be considered.

Patients with *leukemia, agranulocytosis,* or *diphtheria* may also present with sore throat.

Selected References

Bisno AL, Gerber MA, Gwaltney JM Jr, et al: Practice guidelines for the diagnosis and management of group A streptococcal pharyngitis, *Clin Infect Dis* 35:113-125, 2002.

Colletti T, Robinson P: Strep throat: guidelines for diagnosis and treatment, *JAAPA* 18:38-44, 2005.

Esposito S, Cavagna R, Bosis S, et al: Emerging role of *Mycoplasma pneumoniae* in children with acute pharyngitis, *Eur J Clin Microbiol Infect Dis* 21:607-610, 2002.

Femiano F, Lanza A, Buonaiuto C, et al: Oral aphthous-like lesions, PFAPA syndrome: a review, *J Oral Pathol Med* 37:319-323, 2008.

Gieseker KE, Roe MH, MacKenzie T, et al: Evaluating the American Academy of Pediatrics diagnostic standard for *Streptococcus pyogenes* pharyngitis: backup culture *versus* repeat rapid antigen testing, *Pediatrics* 111:666-670, 2003.

McIsaac WJ, Goel V, Slaughter PM, et al: Reconsidering sore throats, part 2: alternative approach and practical office tool, *Can Fam Physician* 43:495-500, 1997.

Middleton DB: Pharyngitis, *Prim Care* 23:719-739, 1996.

Neuner JM, McCarthy EP, Davis RB, et al: Diagnosis and management of adults with pharyngitis: a cost-effective analysis, *Ann Intern Med* 139:113-122, 2003.

Popelars RA, Kizilay P: Pharyngitis in adults, *Adv Nurse Pract* 14:71-72, 2006.

Tewfik TL: Al Garni M: Tonsillopharyngitis: clinical highlights, *J Otolaryngol* 34(Suppl 1):S45-S49, 2005.

Vincent MT, Celestin N, Hussain AN: Pharyngitis, *Am Fam Physician* 69:1465-1470, 2004.

Swelling of the Legs

31

Swelling of one or both legs is a frequent presenting complaint. Common causes are systemic edema states, (heart failure, nephrotic syndrome, and cirrhosis) acute and chronic thrombophlebitis, chronic venous insufficiency, cellulitis, lymphedema, and drugs, as well as mechanical factors, such as dependency and constricting garters or pantyhose. Pulmonary hypertension from intrinsic lung disease (e.g., chronic obstructive pulmonary disease [COPD]) or obstructive sleep apnea may also cause chronic leg swelling. Although the causes are numerous and the pathophysiology complex, diagnosis is simplified by determining whether one or both legs are involved, onset is sudden or gradual, pain is present or absent, and there are other associated symptoms. **Certainly the most common cause of unilateral leg edema is chronic venous insufficiency, and the most common causes of bilateral leg edema are the systemic edema states (heart failure, nephrotic syndrome, and cirrhosis), venous insufficiency, dependency, and primary lymphedema.**

NATURE OF PATIENT

Primary lymphedema is an inherited defect in the lymphatic system caused by hypoplasia, aplasia, or digitation of the lymphatic vessels. In the neonate, unilateral edema of a leg is termed *congenital lymphedema* and is caused by a form of primary lymphedema. If the swelling of the leg becomes apparent around 10 years of age, it is called *lymphedema praecox*. Traumatic thrombophlebitis, cellulitis, arthritis, and *compartment syndromes* also cause unilateral leg edema in children. Also in children, bilateral leg edema is usually caused by a *systemic illness*, such as acute glomerulonephritis, nephrotic syndrome, hypoproteinemia, or primary lymphedema.

Unilateral or bilateral edema in adolescents or older women may be caused by constricting garments such as tight jeans, pantyhose, and (rarely) garters. In a runner, the sudden onset of painful calf swelling suggests a *ruptured gastrocnemius muscle*, whereas intermittent pain and swelling of the upper or lower leg suggest a compartment syndrome. Unilateral or bilateral edema of the lower leg may be caused by elastic bands used for tenodesis.

In obese women, the development of bilateral leg swelling that spares the feet suggests *lipedema,* which occurs almost exclusively in women and is a bilateral and symmetrical deposition of fat in the lower extremities. The foot is not involved in lipedema, whereas in lymphedema the swelling starts in the most distal part of the foot; this pattern differentiates the two conditions.

In a chronic alcoholic, bilateral edema of the leg suggests that it is caused by *cirrhosis* with or without ascites. In a diabetic patient, unilateral and occasional bilateral swelling of the legs suggests *cellulitis,* especially if it is accompanied by warmth and tenderness. Leg swelling due to *venous insufficiency* is more common in women, and there is frequently a history of varicose veins in female relatives of affected women. In patients with *heart failure* or cirrhosis, bilateral leg edema is usually a manifestation of the systemic disease. In patients with *rheumatoid arthritis,* painful unilateral swelling of the calf may result from a ruptured Baker's cyst, sometimes referred to as *pseudophlebitis.* Localized pretibial swelling in a patient with tachycardia, exophthalmos, or other signs or symptoms of hyperthyroidism suggests *pretibial myxedema,* which is a rare finding in hyperthyroidism.

Unilateral swelling of the lower leg may be the presenting complaint in patients with *Kaposi's sarcoma,* which is more common in acquired immunodeficiency syndrome (AIDS).

NATURE OF SYMPTOMS

Unilateral swelling of the lower or upper leg suggests local mechanical or inflammatory processes. These include *lymphedema, venous insufficiency* (the most common cause of unilateral leg edema), *thrombophlebitis, cellulitis,* a *ruptured gastrocnemius muscle, compartment syndrome, ruptured Baker's cyst,* and only rarely an acquired or inherited *arteriovenous fistula.* Bilateral leg swelling is most often caused by systemic conditions, including *heart failure, nephrotic syndrome, cirrhosis, hypoalbuminemia, acute glomerulonephritis, drugs* (Table 31-1), *constricting garments,* and *prolonged dependency* of the legs. Less common causes of bilateral leg swelling include *idiopathic edema, lipedema, primary lymphedema,* and exposure to *extremes of temperature.*

A sudden onset of calf swelling suggests ruptured Baker's cyst, ruptured gastrocnemius muscle, arterial occlusion, thrombophlebitis, cellulitis, or compartment syndrome. Chronic bilateral swelling of the legs occurs in the systemic illnesses mentioned as well as in lymphedema, lipedema, lymphatic obstruction, chronic venous insufficiency, and cellulitis, which may be secondary to bilateral venous stasis dermatitis. The gradual onset of edema that starts in the distal part of the foot and involves the dorsum of the foot and ankle suggests lymphedema. **Painless unilateral leg edema in a woman older than 40 years should prompt suspicion of gynecologic cancer with obstruction of the lymphatics causing secondary lymphedema.**

TABLE **31-1.**   Drugs Associated with Causing Edema

Hormones:
    Estrogens
    Testosterone
    Corticosteroids
    Progesterone
    Androgen

Nonsteroidal anti-inflammatory drugs

Antihypertensives:
    Guanethidine
    Beta blockers
    Calcium channel blockers
    Clonidine
    Hydralazine
    Methyldopa
    Minoxidil
    Reserpine
    Labetalol

Antidepressants:
    Trazodone

Hypoglycemics:
    Pioglitazone
    Rosiglitazone

Cytokines:
    Granulocyte-macrophage colony-stimulating factor
    Granulocyte colony-stimulating factor
    Interleukin-4 (Il-4)
    Il-2
    Interferon-α

Chemotherapeutics:
    Cyclophosphamide
    Cyclosporin
    Mitramycin
    Cytosine arabinoside

Antivirals:
    Acyclovir

Neurotrophic Agents
    Gabapentin
    Pregabalin

Modified from Yale SH, Mazza JJ: Approach to diagnosing lower extremity edema. Comp Ther 27: 242-252, 2001.

ASSOCIATED SYMPTOMS

If warmth, redness, moderate pain, and tenderness on palpation are associated with calf swelling, cellulitis or thrombophlebitis is probable. The absence of pain does not eliminate the diagnosis of thrombophlebitis. If pain is associated with calf swelling, then thrombophlebitis, compartment syndrome, arterial thrombosis, ruptured Baker's cyst, or ruptured gastrocnemius muscle should be suspected.

Dyspnea on exertion, orthopnea, or paroxysmal nocturnal dyspnea suggests heart failure as the cause of leg edema. If spider angioma, palmar erythema, hepatomegaly, or jaundice is present in a patient with swollen legs, cirrhosis should be suspected. Patients with nephrotic syndrome often have generalized edema and swelling of the eyelids, the latter being particularly noticeable after prolonged recumbency. If leg swelling is absent or minimal after recumbency but develops as the day progresses, venous insufficiency is most likely. Snoring or apnea may indicate pulmonary hypertension from obstructive sleep apnea.

PRECIPITATING AND AGGRAVATING FACTORS

Prolonged sitting or standing may cause swelling of the lower extremities, particularly in patients with venous insufficiency. Garments such as jeans or pantyhose that are tight enough to impede venous return may also cause swelling of the legs. Patients may gain weight gradually so that their thighs are fatter yet are not recognized as such by the patient. The garments that have previously fit adequately now impede venous return. Elastic knee bands may be used intermittently by patients with arthritis of the knee for pain relief and tenodesis. They can impede venous return and cause lower leg swelling. The physician should inquire about the use of such bands because the patient may not wear them at the visit.

Trauma to a vein resulting in thrombophlebitis may cause painful unilateral swelling of the leg. Conditions such as pregnancy and large uterine fibroids that increase intra-abdominal pressure may mechanically impede venous return and cause painless unilateral or bilateral swelling of the legs.

Drugs such as estrogens, oral contraceptives, nonsteroidal anti-inflammatory drugs (NSAIDs), psychotropic agents (lithium, tricyclic antidepressants, trazodone), vasodilators (calcium channel blockers, nitrates, prazosin, minoxidil), hypoglycemics (pioglitazone, rosiglitazone), and chemotherapeutics can cause fluid retention, with minimal to moderate painless swelling in both legs. Other drugs that may give rise to gradual bilateral leg swelling are corticosteroids, progesterone, testosterone, methyldopa, hydralazine, and diazoxide. Neurotrophic agents such as Gabapentin and Pregabalin can cause swelling of hands and feet.

AMELIORATING FACTORS

Cessation of salt-retaining and vasodilating drugs alleviates edema if these drugs were the cause. Marked weight loss alleviates some of the swelling of lipedema. Support hose alleviate the edema of venous insufficiency. Muscle activity of the lower legs alleviates the edema of dependency. Edema due to a ruptured gastrocnemius muscle or ruptured Baker's cyst gradually subsides, as does the edema from thrombophlebitis and cellulitis. Diuretics and aldosterone-blocking agents often assist in the mobilization of edema in patients with cirrhosis, nephrosis, and heart failure.

PHYSICAL FINDINGS

Physical examination of the legs should include inspection, measurement, and palpation. The lower leg should be examined in the erect and recumbent positions for dilated superficial veins; perforators; and multiple small, superficial veins on the foot. The patient should be examined to determine the area of the swelling, which may be in the knee, the anserine bursa, or Cooperman's fat pad; swelling in none of these locations causes true edema of the lower extremity. Lipedema excludes the foot and is a deposition of fat in the leg, whereas lymphedema begins at the distal area of the foot and involves the dorsum of the foot with a so-called hump.

The character of the skin in the area of edema is also diagnostically helpful. The patient may typically have pitting edema with acute deep vein thrombosis, chronic venous insufficiency, and conditions of systemic edema, whereas the swelling of lymphedema and lipedema is nonpitting. Thick, taut, fibrotic skin suggests that the causative process is chronic rather than acute. Hemosiderin deposition, particularly along the medial malleolus, is suggestive of venous insufficiency, even in the absence of varicose veins. Redness or lymphangitic streaks suggest cellulitis. Ecchymoses in the dependent part of the ankle, associated with midcalf pain, suggest a tear of the gastrocnemius muscle. Tenderness on palpation over the vein, warmth, low-grade fever, and the presence of Homans' sign suggest thrombophlebitis. Painful swelling in one calf in a patient with the stigmata of rheumatoid arthritis and a popliteal cyst on the opposite side suggest pseudophlebitis (i.e., ruptured Baker's cyst).

Physical findings of systemic illnesses associated with swelling of the legs include pulmonary rales, wheeze or decreased air movement, distended neck veins, tachycardia, gallop rhythm, cardiac enlargement, heart failure, large neck circumference with low palate, hepatomegaly, jaundice, ascites, palmar erythema, gynecomastia, spider angiomas, cirrhosis, hypertension, periorbital edema, nephrotic syndrome, peau d'orange skin, and lymphatic obstruction.

DIAGNOSTIC STUDIES

Although venography is the *gold standard* for the diagnosis of deep vein thrombosis, it is not necessary or advisable in all patients. Duplex ultrasonography or, if that is unavailable, Doppler ultrasonography can be used to confirm the diagnosis of venous thrombosis when invasive or radiographic procedures are contraindicated. Magnetic resonance imaging (MRI) has also been used in pregnant women to evaluate lower leg edema, but its use in the first trimester is not recommended. The Wells clinical prediction rule may also be applied to rule out deep vein thrombosis (DVT). One point is assigned to each of the following clinical features:

- Cancer treatment within 6 months
- Paralysis, paresis, or immobilization of the lower extremity
- Bedridden for more than 3 days because of surgery within the last 4 weeks
- Localized tenderness along the distribution of the deep veins
- Entire leg swollen

- Unilateral calf swelling greater than 3 cm
- Unilateral pitting edema
- Collateral superficial veins
- Alternative diagnosis as likely as or more likely than DVT (2 points for this item)

A score of 3 points or higher indicates high risk for DVT (75%), 1-2 points moderate risk (17%), and zero points AU: low risk (3%). A negative D-dimer test result combined with a low risk assessment effectively rules out DVT.

Computed tomography (CT) and spiral CT venography can be used to determine the distribution of edema in instances of leg swelling: venous obstruction exhibits an increased cross-sectional area of muscle tissue and edema in the muscular and interstitial compartments; obesity and lipedema exhibit increased subcutaneous fat; lymphedema exhibits increased fluid in the interstitial space, with a honeycombed pattern when the condition is chronic; and popliteal cysts exhibit an extension of fluid from the joint space to a location between the muscle planes.

Direct and indirect lymphangiography is used to visualize the lymphatics, which are dilated in instances of congenital and acquired lymphatic obstruction, although lymphangiography has been replaced by CT in most cases. Occasionally, lymphoscintigraphy is helpful in the evaluation of a swollen leg.

Diagnostic studies to investigate systemic causes of edema may include a metabolic profile including creatinine and albumin measurements, liver function tests, urinalysis, brain-natriuretic peptide measurement, chest radiograph, electrocardiography (ECG), and two-dimensional echocardiogram.

LESS COMMON DIAGNOSTIC CONSIDERATIONS

Lipedema is a bilateral, symmetrical deposition of fat (lipodystrophy) in the lower extremities that **spares the foot.** Spontaneous *venous thrombosis* occurs more frequently during pregnancy, parturition, surgical trauma, severe illness, polycythemia, malignant disease, multiple myeloma, and dehydration. *Retroperitoneal fibrosis* (most often induced by the antimigraine drug methysergide) can cause obstruction of lymphatic or venous drainage. The swelling may be unilateral or bilateral.

Calf and/or ankle swelling caused by rupture of the gastrocnemius or soleus muscle and tears or sprains of ankle ligaments usually have a *sudden onset* related to trauma or athletic activities.

Erythema nodosum can cause unilateral or bilateral leg swelling. *Reflex sympathetic dystrophy* can cause leg swelling (usually unilateral), but a precipitating factor usually exists, such as crush injury, trauma, frostbite, myocardial infarction, venous or arterial thrombosis, or infection. Pretibial *myxedema* occurs in patients with hyperthyroidism. Thrombosis of the iliac vein and iliac venous compression by a distended bladder or right common iliac artery (May-Turner syndrome) are other rare causes of *unilateral* edema of the leg.

Cyclic or *idiopathic edema* occurs mostly in obese women and is usually bilateral. Fluid retention of several pounds can develop in these patients in a few days.

Differential Diagnosis of Swelling of the Legs

CAUSE	NATURE OF PATIENT	NATURE OF SYMPTOMS	ASSOCIATED SYMPTOMS	PRECIPITATING AND AGGRAVATING FACTORS	AMELIORATING FACTORS	PHYSICAL FINDINGS	DIAGNOSTIC STUDIES
Systemic							
Heart failure	Hypertension, coronary artery disease	Bilateral	Dyspnea on exertion Orthopnea Paroxysmal nocturnal dyspnea	Myocardial infarction		Pulmonary rales Distended neck veins Tachycardia Cardiac enlargement Gallop	Chest radiograph Echocardio-gram
Cirrhosis	Alcoholic	Bilateral	Ascites Jaundice Abdominal swelling			Hepatomegaly Jaundice Ascites Gynecomastia	Abnormal liver function test results Liver biopsy
Nephrotic syndrome	Often children	Bilateral	Polyuria Eyelid swelling			Edema of eyelids Hypertension	Albuminuria Hypercholes-terolemia Serum protein
Hypopro-teinemia	Malnourished	Bilateral					Electrophoresis
Venous insuffi-ciency	Usually women	Often unilateral	Minimal up on arising		Recumbency Elevation of legs	Varicose veins Pitting edema Weeping skin erosions Soft tissue consistency Often cellulitis Skin ulcers around medial malleolus Involves foot	

Continued

Differential Diagnosis of Swelling of the Legs—cont'd

CAUSE	NATURE OF PATIENT	NATURE OF SYMPTOMS	ASSOCIATED SYMPTOMS	PRECIPITATING AND AGGRAVATING FACTORS	AMELIORATING FACTORS	PHYSICAL FINDINGS	DIAGNOSTIC STUDIES
Thrombo-phlebitis		Usually unilateral Sudden onset of swelling with redness and pain	Pain Warmth Redness	Trauma Immobilization Childbirth Drugs (estrogen, oral contraceptives)		Tender cord Presence of Homans' sign Warmth, low-grade fever	Duplex ultraso-nography Venogram Doppler ultra-sonography CT
Mechanical							
Ruptured gastrocne-mius muscle	Runners	Sudden onset	Pain	Strenuous athletics		Ecchymoses of ankle	CT
Baker's cyst	Rheumatoid arthritis		Arthritis				Arthrogram
Constrictive garments	Usually female		Painless	Weight gain	Weight loss	Fat thigh	
Dependency	After stroke		Impaired mobility	Venous insufficiency	Muscle activity of legs		
Primary lymph-edema	Young adults Adolescents Neonates Usually female	Unilateral				Involves foot	CT
Secondary lymph-edema	Age >40 yr Usually female			Pelvic cancer Radiation therapy		Peau d'orange skin Involves foot Dorsal hump No ulcers	Lymphangiog-raphy CT

Lipedema	Obese, female	Bilateral	Obesity	Weight loss		Spares foot, No ulcers, Rare cellulitis, Nontender, Skin normal	
Drugs		Bilateral		Weight gain	Hormones, Antihypertensives, Hypoglycemics, Chemotherapeutics, Contraceptives, Antivirals, NSAIDs, Lithium, Vasodilators		
Pulmonary hypertension due to sleep apnea	Obese	Bilateral	Snoring, Apnea			Large neck circumference, Low palate	Two-dimensional echocardiogram, Sleep study

CT, Computed tomography; *NSAIDs*, nonsteroidal anti-inflammatory drugs.

Selected References

Brukner P: Calf and ankle swelling, *Austr Fam Physician* 29:35-40, 2000.

Ely J, Osheroff J, Chambliss M, et al: Approach to leg edema of unclear etiology, *J Am Board Fam Med* 19, 2006:148-60.

Merli GJ, Spandorfer J: The outpatient with unilateral leg swelling, *Med Clin North Am* 79: 435-447, 1995.

Monnin-Delhorn ED, Gallix BP, Achard C, et al: High-resolution unenhanced computed tomography in patients with swollen legs, *Lymphology* 35:121-128, 2002.

Ramzi D, Leeper K: DVT and pulmonary embolism, part I: diagnosis, *Am Fam Physician* 69: 2829-2836, 2004.

Tewari A, Chung K-S, Button M, et al: Differential diagnosis, investigation, and current treatment of lower limb lymphedema, *Arch Surg* 138:152-161, 2003.

Wells P, Anderson D, Bormanis J, et al: Value of assessment of pretest probability of deep vein thrombosis in clinical management, *Lancet* 350:1796, 1997.

Yale SH, Mazza JJ: Approach to diagnosing lower extremity edema, *Comp Ther* 27:242-252, 2001.

32 Urethral Discharge and Dysuria

About 2 million cases of urethritis (men and women) occur annually in the United States; more than 60% of these cases are nongonorrheal. *Nongonococcal urethritis* occurs five times more frequently than gonococcal urethritis, largely because of a decline in gonococcal urethritis. *Chlamydia*, which causes nongonorrheal urethritis, is a major cause of sexually transmitted disease (STD) and infertility in the United States. Because of the frequency of complaints of dysuria and urethral discharge, the associated public health problem, and the ease of treatment, it is essential that physicians be expert in recognizing the causes of these symptoms.

Dysuria denotes burning or pain associated with urination and can have several causes. Frequency, hesitancy, urgency, and strangury (slow, painful urination) are other symptoms typically associated with micturition disorders. Urinary urgency occurs as a result of *trigonal* or *posterior urethral irritation* produced by inflammation, stones, or tumor; it most often occurs with *cystitis*. Acute inflammatory processes of the bladder cause pain or urgency when only a small quantity of urine is present in the bladder.

When it is due to bladder problems, frequency of urination occurs either with decreased bladder capacity or with pain on bladder distention. Frequency is caused most often by lesions of the bladder or urethra, although diseases of the nervous system involving the bladder's nerve supply (either centrally as in tabes and multiple sclerosis or peripherally as in diabetic neuropathy) may produce bladder decompensation with voiding abnormalities. Urinary frequency may also be a manifestation of overflow incontinence, which can occur with either *prostatic hypertrophy* or *neurologic bladder disorders*.

Inflammatory lesions of the prostate, bladder, and urethra are the most common cause of dysuria and frequency and include *prostatitis* in men, *urethrotrigonitis* in women, and *bladder* and *urethral infections* in men and women. Both men and women may have *chronic inflammation of the posterior urethra*. In the United States, dysuria accounts for 5% to 15% of visits to family physicians; however, only 50% of women with dysuria have classic cystitis with urine culture bacteria concentrations greater than 10^5 organisms per milliliter. **Several studies indicate that symptomatic women with urinary bacteria counts of fewer** than 10^5 organisms/mL (female urethral syndrome) should be considered to have an infectious cause and should be treated accordingly.

NATURE OF PATIENT

In children, *meatal stenosis* may cause recurrent lower urinary tract infections (UTIs). Up to 20% of children with urinary complaints may have some degree of meatal stenosis. Dysuria and urethral discharge are uncommon in children. When these symptoms occur in young girls, they are frequently caused by *chemical vaginitis* or *mechanical urethritis*. When these findings are seen in young boys, they are often secondary to mechanical urethritis, which can result from continued jarring of the perineum from bicycle riding, horseback riding, a foreign body, or masturbation. *Sexually transmitted diseases* (STDs) must be considered in cases of urethritis or vaginitis that occur in boys or girls. If STDs are discovered in young children, child abuse is usually the cause.

A UTI should be considered in infants and children (2 months to 2 years of age) with an unexplained fever for 2 or more days.

Bacteriuria is rare in school-age boys and occurs in only 0.1% of men. The incidence of bacteriuria increases in men at age 50 years and rises to about 1% at age 60 and to 4% to 15% in later years, coinciding with the onset of prostatic disease. Women younger than 18 years have a 5% incidence of asymptomatic bacteriuria. Having multiple sexual partners increases the likelihood of STDs such as *Chlamydia*, gonorrhea, and herpes.

Women between ages 15 and 34 years account for the majority who present with symptoms of UTIs. A study in Great Britain showed that 20% of women in this age group experienced dysuria and frequency. Dysuria in women is most frequently caused by *cystitis, interstitial cystitis, vaginitis, female urethral syndrome,* and *mechanical irritation of the urethra.* Dysuria in young men is most often caused by *Chlamydia urethritis.* In men older than 35 years, UTI is caused by coliform bacteria; in older men, prostatitis and cystitis resulting in urinary stasis are usually caused by prostatic hypertrophy. Dysuria can also be caused by stones, mechanical urethritis, and medications. Urethral discharge, which is essentially limited to men, is usually caused by *gonorrheal or nongonorrheal urethritis (Chlamydia or Trichomonas).* A male smoker who has culture-negative hematuria and dysuria should be examined for a bladder tumor.

NATURE OF SYMPTOMS

Cystitis

In women who complain of frequency, urgency, and dysuria without clinical evidence of an upper UTI, *bacterial cystitis* is usually suspected. However, several studies have shown that 30% to 50% of women complaining of these symptoms do not have a positive urine culture according to traditional criteria (isolation of a pathogen in concentrations greater than 10^5 bacteria per milliliter of urine in a clean-voided specimen). There are several possible reasons for this.

First, dysuria often represents a vaginal infection rather than a UTI. When carefully questioned, women with dysuria due to cystitis usually describe internal discomfort, whereas women with dysuria due to vaginitis usually describe more external discomfort; their burning sensation appears to be in the vagina or the labia and is caused by urine flow over an inflamed vaginal mucosa. **All women with dysuria should be questioned about an associated vaginal discharge or irritation.**

Second, many women who present with symptoms due to bacterial cystitis (dysuria, frequency) have colony counts of fewer than 10^5 bacteria/mL. **Various studies have shown that if pathogens are found in a concentration of fewer than 10^5/mL in a symptomatic woman, there is probably a significant bacterial infection.**

Third, *Chlamydia trachomatis* is frequently the causative agent. Patients who are infected with this organism have symptoms and pyuria but a negative routine urine culture result. Chlamydial infection of the bladder and urethra in a woman is somewhat analogous to nongonorrheal urethritis in a man; in both, there is pyuria but no growth on routine culture. Although it is rare, *urinary tract tuberculosis* may also manifest as pyuria and a negative routine culture result.

The physician must inquire about the duration and onset of symptoms. Longer duration and gradual onset of symptoms suggest a chlamydial infection, whereas a history of hematuria and sudden onset of symptoms indicate a bacterial infection. Dysuria that is more severe at the end of the stream, particularly if associated with hematuria, suggests *cystitis;* dysuria that is worse at the beginning of the stream is a sign of *urethritis.* Patients with the *female urethral syndrome* often have dysuria, frequency, suprapubic pain, onset of symptoms over 2 to 7 days, and some pyuria. Besides having dysuria, frequency, and suprapubic pain, patients with *cystitis* demonstrate symptoms that develop quickly—pyuria, bacteriuria, and positive urine culture results (Table 32-1). Fever, nausea, back pain, and leukocytosis are uncommon findings in both female urethral syndrome and cystitis. Dysuria at the end of urination, with or without suprapubic pain, suggests cystitis.

Urethritis

Dysuria at the onset of urination suggests urethritis. As stated previously, dysuria at the end of urination, with or without suprapubic pain, suggests cystitis.

Urethral discharge in male patients is accepted as objective evidence of *urethritis*, but patients may have urethritis without a significant urethral discharge. **If the patient has dysuria and more than four polymorphonuclear cells per high-powered microscopic field in a urethral smear, urethritis is probable.** *Nongonorrheal urethritis* is defined to include inflammations in men with negative urethral culture results for *Neisseria gonorrhoeae* and a urethral discharge or more than four cells per field in the urethral smear. *Chlamydia trachomatis* is the most

TABLE 32-1.   Clinical Features of Female Urethral Syndrome and Cystitis

CLINICAL FEATURES	FEMALE URETHRAL SYNDROME	CYSTITIS
Dysuria, frequency, suprapubic pain	+	–
Fever, nausea, back pain, other systemic signs	–	–
Duration of symptoms (days)	2-7	1-2
Leukocytosis	–	–
Urinalysis:		
Pyuria	+ or –	+
Bacteriuria	–	+
Hematuria	–	+ or –
White blood cell casts	–	–
Urine cultures	–	+
Blood cultures	–	–

From Meadows JC: The acute urethral syndrome: diagnosis, management, and prophylaxis. Contin Educ Dec:112-120, 1983.

common isolate from patients with nongonorrheal urethritis (Table 32-2). Other causative organisms are *Mycoplasma*, group D streptococci, *Trichomonas*, and (rarely) *Candida albicans*. In women, urethritis may be caused by *Chlamydia* and gonorrhea as well as vaginitis due to *Candida* or *Trichomonas*.

Although a significant number of patients with nongonorrheal urethritis are asymptomatic, most have mild dysuria, and urethral discharge is minimal or absent. When a discharge does appear, it is usually clear or whitish. In contrast, about 80% of patients with gonorrheal urethritis have a moderate to heavy urethral discharge that is usually purulent. Dysuria with a mucoid or mucopurulent urethral discharge usually develops 1 to 3 weeks after coitus with an infected partner.

Urethral discharges are usually observed on awakening, after a long period without urination, or after penile stripping. Other symptoms include urgency, frequency, and meatal or urethral irritation. The usual presentation of nongonorrheal urethritis is a low-grade inflammation; the symptoms of gonorrheal urethritis tend to be more acute and severe and include a urethral discharge that is purulent, spontaneous, and greater in volume. **It is important to recognize that a patient may have gonorrheal as well as nongonorrheal urethritis at the same time. Both may be contracted simultaneously from the same contact.**

ASSOCIATED SYMPTOMS

Dysuria is often associated with frequency, urgency, and nocturia, but its most common cause is UTI.

TABLE 32-2. Comparison between *Chlamydia trachomatis* and *Neisseria gonorrhoeae* as Sexually Transmitted Disease Agents

FEATURE	*C. TRACHOMATIS*	*N. GONORRHOEAE*
Organism	Obligate intracellular parasite	Gram-negative diplococcus often found within cells (as leukocytes on Gram stain)
Transmission	Sexual	Sexual
Incubation period	8-21 days	2-6 days (can be longer, up to 10-16 days, in rare cases)
Major infection	Urethritis (men); cervicitis (women)	Urethritis (men) Cervicitis (women)
Local complications	Yes: epididymitis, bartholinitis, urethral syndrome, salpingitis, others	Yes: same as for *C. trachomatis* and others, including prostatitis
Systemic complications	Possibly: arthritis, perihepatitis, peritonitis, and endocarditis reported	Well known: gonococcal septicemia, with resulting arthritis, dermatitis, endocarditis, and meningitis; perihepatitis and peritonitis also reported
Pharyngitis	Yes	Yes
Conjunctivitis	Yes	Yes
Proctitis	Cultured from the rectum	Yes: common venereal infection in homosexuals
Maternal infection with effect on neonate or infant	Well known: inclusion conjunctivitis and pneumonia	Less well established
Carrier state	Recognized, especially in women; can last for months	Recognized, especially in women; can last for months
Reservoir	Cervix (male urethra a minor role)	Cervix (male urethra a minor role)
Treatment	Azithromycin, doxycycline	Ceftriaxone, cefixime (treat concurrently for *Chlamydia*)
Treatment of sexual contacts	Yes	Yes

Adapted from Greydanus DE, McAnarney ER: *Chlamydia trachomatis:* an important sexually transmitted disease in adolescents and young adults. J Fam Pract 10:611-615, 1980.

When hematuria accompanies dysuria, *cystitis* is most probable, although the possibility of a *tumor* or *stone* should be considered. A male with a weak stream, split stream, hesitancy, or dribbling probably has benign prostatic hyperplasia. If a middle-aged woman complains of recurrent dysuria associated with bladder pain, urgency, marked frequency, and nocturia, *interstitial cystitis* is most probable. The patient obtains some relief by voiding. Urine culture results are usually sterile, and pyuria is absent. The diagnosis is made by cystoscopy.

If dysuria and frequency are associated with a high fever or chills, an upper UTI such as *pyelonephritis* may be present. When frequency and dysuria are associated with backache or costovertebral angle tenderness, *pyelonephritis* or *prostatitis* should be suspected. Patients who have prostatitis often present with an unexplained backache or rectal pain with or without fever. The physician should perform a gentle rectal examination in any man who complains of frequency, dysuria, and fever, to determine whether the prostate is tender on palpation. Pyelonephritis should be suspected if nausea and vomiting accompany dysuria. Patients who demonstrate prostatic enlargement or experience severe pain on micturition that causes them to resist voiding have outflow obstruction. This condition causes bladder distention, which may also induce nausea, vomiting, or mild ileus, resulting in abdominal distention.

Frequency of urination without discomfort on voiding may be caused by *diminished bladder capacity, overflow incontinence,* or *habit* in patients with a normal bladder. It is also observed in patients who pass a large volume of urine because of diabetes, hypercalcemia, hypokalemia, congestive heart failure, loss of renal concentrating capacity, or use of diuretics. The absence of nocturia in a patient with urinary frequency suggests that the increased frequency of urination may be of psychogenic origin. On rare occasions, it may result from a polyp or irritative lesion in the posterior urethra that is relieved by recumbency.

Testicular pain due to *epididymitis* suggests a chlamydial infection, which is the most common cause of epididymitis in young men.

PRECIPITATING AND AGGRAVATING FACTORS

Patients who have multiple sexual contacts are more likely to experience an STD such as *gonorrheal* or *chlamydial urethritis* or *cervicitis.* An abrupt alteration in the frequency of ejaculation may result in symptoms of *prostatitis.* This condition often occurs on the patient's return from a vacation during which the frequency of intercourse and subsequent ejaculation were increased. The use of vaginal sprays, douches, and bubble baths (particularly in children) may induce *chemical vaginitis* that may manifest as dysuria. It is important for the physician to ask women who complain of dysuria whether a vaginal discharge is present, because *vaginitis* is an unlikely cause of dysuria in the absence of a recognizable discharge.

AMELIORATING FACTORS

Some patients with *cystitis* believe that they can alleviate their pain by avoiding urination; they actually mean that the pain is made worse with micturition, particularly at the end of urination, when the inflamed bladder walls become apposed. Some symptoms of cystitis are ameliorated by warm tub baths. Patients who complain of persistent frequency, nocturia, terminal hematuria, and suprapubic pain relieved by voiding may have *chronic interstitial cystitis,* a condition that is most common in middle-aged women.

If *N. gonorrhoeae* is the offending organism, the symptoms of urethritis occasionally abate without treatment after a few months. In contrast, the symptoms of nongonorrheal urethritis, though of low grade, usually persist if not treated appropriately.

PHYSICAL FINDINGS

Pain on palpation of the prostate suggests prostatitis. A distended bladder detected on abdominal examination suggests outlet obstruction of the bladder.

The physical findings in gonorrheal urethritis in men include a spontaneous urethral discharge or one that can be elicited by penile stripping. The most common physical finding in patients with dysuria due to cystitis is suprapubic tenderness on palpation or percussion. When dysuria is caused by vaginitis, a vaginal discharge is usually apparent on pelvic examination, which should be performed in **all** women with dysuria or vaginal discharge.

DIAGNOSTIC STUDIES

A urine culture should be performed in all infants and children who appear ill and have an unexplained fever for 48 hours.

In men, *urethritis* is present if a urethral smear shows more than four polymorphonuclear cells per high-power microscopic field. The nucleic acid amplification test (NAAT) on a first-void urine sample has replaced cultures and urethral swabs for diagnosing *N. gonorrhea and Chlamydia* in men. Urine cultures should be obtained from all patients with symptoms of cystitis. In uncomplicated cases, some physicians use only reagent test strips, including the leukocyte esterase test strips, before beginning empirical antibiotic therapy. When sterile pyuria is demonstrated on routine culture, the urine should be tested for *Chlamydia* and tuberculosis-causing species of *Mycobacterium. Trichomonas vaginalis* and *C. albicans* are uncommon causes of urethritis and need not be considered at the initial visit. A Gram smear or potassium hydroxide preparation of vaginal or urethral discharge may help identify patients with candidal urethritis, and a saline wet mount should be examined if trichomonal urethritis is suspected.

The following are considered indications for urologic evaluation:
- Initial UTI in a child
- UTI in men
- UTI in pregnant women
- Recurrent UTIs (three per year) in women
- Severe, acute UTI suggesting upper tract involvement
- Painless hematuria

Patients with symptoms of chronic cystitis with no apparent cause should undergo cystoscopic examination to rule out tumor and interstitial cystitis.

Ultrasonography may be used to evaluate the upper tract. Computed tomography (CT) scanning has largely replaced intravenous pyelography (IVP) for evaluation of the upper tract collecting system. Cystoscopy is used to evaluate

Differential Diagnosis of Urethral Discharge and Dysuria

CAUSE	NATURE OF PATIENT	NATURE OF SYMPTOMS	ASSOCIATED SYMPTOMS	PRECIPITATING AND AGGRAVATING FACTORS	AMELIORATING FACTORS	PHYSICAL FINDINGS	DIAGNOSTIC STUDIES
Cystitis	Most common in women ages 15-34 yr	Dysuria (worse at end of flow) Urgency Frequency "Internal" discomfort Acute onset of symptoms with bacterial infection	Hematuria Nocturia Fever	Meatal stenosis may cause recurrent UTI in children Drugs (e.g., NSAIDs, cyclophosphamide)	Avoidance of urinating Warm baths	Suprapubic tenderness on palpation or percussion Fever	Urine culture Cystoscopy Test for *Chlamydia* Pyuria by urinalysis or leukocyte esterase test
Interstitial cystitis	Women ages 20-50 yr	Dysuria Marked frequency of small volume of urine	Nocturia Bladder pain Urgency	Some relief of pain with voiding		Tenderness of bladder base	Urine culture: sterile Cystoscopy: Hunner's ulcers
Female urethral syndrome		Dysuria Urgency Frequency Gradual onset of symptoms over 2-7 days	Suprapubic pain			Suprapubic pain No fever	Minimal pyuria Urine culture result usually negative
Vaginitis (see Chapter 33)	Candidiasis more common in diabetic patients	Dysuria "External burning"	Vaginal itching			Vaginal discharge on pelvic examination	KOH and saline wet mounts for *Candida* and *Trichomonas* Test for gonococci

Condition		Symptoms	Associated Findings	History	Physical Examination	Diagnostic Tests
Chemical vaginitis	Common cause of dysuria and urethral discharge in young girls	Dysuria "External burning" Urethral discharge (minimal)		Bubble baths Vaginal sprays and douches	Vaginitis	
Prostatitis	Men older than 50 yr	Dysuria Frequency	Backache Fever Decreased or intermittent stream	Abrupt change in frequency of ejaculation (e.g., after a vacation)	May be costovertebral tenderness Prostate tender on palpation on rectal examination	Examination and culture of prostatic secretions
Meatal stenosis	Children	Dysuria Recurrent UTI symptoms				
Urethritis:						
Gonorrheal	Most common in men	Sexually transmitted Urethral discharge is moderate to large, purulent, mucoid, or mucopurulent and develops 1-3 wk after coitus with infected partner Dysuria (worse at beginning of urine flow)		Sexual contact	Urethral discharge is spontaneous or elicited by penile stripping	Nucleic acid amplification test

Continued

Differential Diagnosis of Urethral Discharge and Dysuria—cont'd

CAUSE	NATURE OF PATIENT	NATURE OF SYMPTOMS	ASSOCIATED SYMPTOMS	PRECIPITATING AND AGGRAVATING FACTORS	AMELIORATING FACTORS	PHYSICAL FINDINGS	DIAGNOSTIC STUDIES
Nongon-orrheal (chlamydial or tricho-monal)	Most common in men	Sexually transmitted Symptoms usually minimal or absent Discharge (if present) is observed on awakening, thin and clear or whitish Dysuria (ranges in severity) Urgency Frequency	Meatal or urethral irritant	Multiple sexual partners		Thin, scanty, and whitish Urethral discharge appears on penile stripping	Nucleic acid amplification test RNA probe for *Trichomonas*
Mechanical	Most common in young boys and girls	Dysuria Minimal urethral discharge		Horseback or bike riding Masturbation Foreign body			

KOH, Potassium hydroxide; *NSAIDs,* nonsteroidal anti-inflammatory drugs; *UTI,* urinary tract infection.

hematuria. When bladder dysfunction is suspected, urodynamic studies are indicated.

LESS COMMON DIAGNOSTIC CONSIDERATIONS

Less common causes of dysuria and urinary frequency include genital herpes simplex virus, *Trichomonas* infection, and *Candida* urethritis. On rare occasions, frequency is an early symptom of a bladder tumor or carcinoma in situ of the bladder. Drug-induced cystitis is not usually recognized. Nonsteroidal anti-inflammatory drugs (NSAIDs), especially tiaprofenic acid, are the most common offenders, but cyclophosphamide may also cause cystitis.

Relatively uncommon causes of urethritis include infections with *Mycoplasma hominis*. Urethritis secondary to *Mycoplasma* is most common in lower socioeconomic groups and men and women who have multiple sexual partners. *Mycoplasma genitalium* is present in 26% of men with nongonococcal urethritis who are *Chlamydia* negative.

Another uncommon cause of urethritis is *Reiter's syndrome*, which frequently begins with urethritis after sexual contact and is followed in a few days by conjunctivitis, mucocutaneous lesions (including balanitis), and arthritis. This type of urethritis is characterized by mucopurulent discharge and dysuria, but it may be asymptomatic. Sometimes Reiter's syndrome may be initiated by gonorrheal urethritis. In such cases the urethritis responds to a cephalosporin, so the purulent discharge disappears and is replaced by the less purulent, mucoid discharge of nonspecific urethritis.

Selected References

Bremnor JD, Sadovsky R: Evaluation of dysuria in adults, *Am Fam Physician* 65:1589-1596, 2002.

Centers for Disease Control and Prevention: Update to CDC's Sexually transmitted diseases treatment guideline, : fluoroquinolones no longer recommended for treatment of gonococcal infections. Centers for Disease Control, *Morbid Mortal Wkly Rep* 56:332-336, 2006:2007.

Centers for Disease Control and Prevention; Workowski KA, Berman SM: Sexually transmitted diseases treatment guideline, *MMWR Recomm Rep* 55(RR-11):1-94, 2006:2006.

Claudius I: Dysuria in adolescents, *West J Med* 172:201-205, 2000.

Kaur H, Arunkalaivanan A: Urethral pain syndrome and its management, *Obstet Gynecol Surv* 62:348-351, 2007.

Krieger JN: Trichomoniasis in men: old and new issues, *Sex Transm Dis* 22:83-96, 1995.

Lipsky BA: Prostatitis and urinary tract infection in men: what's new; what's true? *Am J Med* 106:327-334, 1999.

Patel J, Chambers C, Gomella L: Hematuria: etiology and evaluation for the primary care physician, *Can J Urol* 15:54-62, 2008.

Roberts RG, Hartlaub PP: Evaluation of dysuria in men, *Am Fam Physician* 60:865-872, 1999.

Yerkes E: Urologic issues in the pediatric and adolescent gynecologic patient, *Obstet Gynecol Clin North Am* 36:69-84, 2008.

Vaginal Discharge and Itching

33

Vaginal discharge, which may be accompanied by vulvar itching or burning, is one of the most common problems seen in the physician's office. These symptoms usually indicate *bacterial vaginosis* (a polymicrobial superficial infection characterized by an increase in aerobic bacteria, especially *Gardnerella*, and a decrease in lactobacilli), *candidiasis (moniliasis) (Candida albicans)*, or *trichomoniasis (Trichomonas* infection). Other common causes of vaginal discharge are *acute cervicitis, gonorrhea,* and *herpes genitalis.* Sexual abuse and sexually transmitted diseases such as gonorrhea *must always* be considered in all prepubescent girls with vaginal discharge.

Vulvar itching (which often accompanies vaginal discharge) is common and can occur by itself. The most common vulvar dermatoses are dermatitis, psoriasis, and lichen sclerosus. Streptococcal vulvovaginitis is seen only in children, whereas chronic vulvovaginal candidiasis occurs only after puberty because it is estrogen dependent.

Many discussions of vaginitis emphasize a *typical* appearance of the discharge: cheesy, frothy, or mucoid. However, appearances may be misleading. **In addition, 15% to 20% of patients in one series had two coexisting infections.** Other studies of patients with vaginitis have shown that 35% had bacterial vaginosis, 25% had candidiasis, and 20% had trichomoniasis. The remaining 20% had less common types of vaginitis.

In contrast to cervicitis, vaginitis is an inflammatory change of the vaginal mucosa in the absence of a profuse discharge from the cervix. A vaginal discharge can be produced by cervicitis without a significant vaginal infection, as can be the case with *gonorrhea. Chlamydia* also causes mucopurulent cervicitis.

NATURE OF PATIENT

Prepubertal Patients
Prepubertal girls may experience a vaginal discharge in association with *vulvovaginitis* or *exocervicitis.* These young girls are particularly susceptible to vulvovaginitis because of the anterior location of the vagina; the proximity of the

vagina to the anus; the lack of labial fat pads; a neutral to alkaline vaginal pH; a thin, atrophic vaginal wall; and, occasionally, poor hygiene.

Trichomonal vaginitis is rare in children and women older than 60 years but does occur in neonates of infected mothers. Conversely, *candidal (monilial) vaginitis* can occur at any age but is uncommon in prepubertal girls unless they have been receiving antibiotics. It is a common cause of vulvovaginitis in postpubescent girls and women. In prepubertal girls, vulvovaginitis is more common than vaginitis. Vulvovaginitis can be caused by bubble baths, other chemical irritants, tight nylon panties, mixed bacterial infections, and foreign bodies.

Bacterial vaginosis is uncommon in premenarchal girls. **Gonorrheal infections in premenarchal children are rare but do occur. In such cases, sexual abuse must be suspected.** Although a girl may be asymptomatic when a gonococcal infection is present, vulvovaginitis and exocervicitis are usually present.

Adolescents

After puberty, a vaginal discharge may be caused by physiologic factors, cervicitis, or vaginitis. Although *trichomonal vaginitis* and *candidal vaginitis* may occur in adolescents, the most common cause of vaginitis with discharge in adolescent girls is *bacterial vaginosis. Candida* infection is the second most common cause of specific leukorrhea in adolescents. There is a high and increasing incidence of chlamydial and gonococcal infections among postpubertal girls. Among young mothers, the growing prevalence of *Chlamydia trachomatis* may increase the incidence of this infection among neonates and some children. It is important to question the patient about genital or urinary tract infections (UTIs) in other family members (male or female) or sexual partners (male or female).

The physician must remember that *physiologic leukorrhea* may occur in menarchal girls. This is not usually profuse or associated with itching. Although these girls may be concerned about a vaginal discharge, they may not present with it as a chief complaint. Therefore, the physician should provide reassurance concerning this and other normal changes that may occur with menarche. The discharges that occur just before and after menarche are often thick, grayish white, and odorless and have a pH of less than 4.5. No signs of inflammation exist because these discharges represent a physiologic reaction to the initial phase of cyclic estrogen production.

Adults

In adult women of reproductive age, the common causes of vaginitis are bacterial vaginosis, *Candida,* and *Trichomonas,* in decreasing order of frequency. The three most common causes of cervicitis are *C. trachomatis, Neisseria gonorrhoeae,* and herpes simplex virus. In elderly postmenopausal women, *senile atrophic vaginitis* often causes a discharge, as do other specific forms of vaginitis.

NATURE OF SYMPTOMS

Vulvovaginitis in premenarchal girls usually causes only minor discomfort, which may consist of perineal pruritus, burning, and a discharge that may be profuse or scanty.

The duration and type of symptoms do not consistently distinguish the common infectious causes of vaginitis. However, certain symptoms and findings strongly suggest the diagnosis. For instance, although an acute onset of vaginal discharge or vulvar irritation indicates that a yeast infection is the probable cause, these symptoms are often unreliable. Likewise, a curdlike discharge (resembling cottage cheese) strongly suggests yeast vaginitis; however, the gross appearance is less sensitive and specific in establishing the diagnosis than microscopic examination of the vaginal discharge. A curdlike appearance virtually eliminates the possibility of trichomonal vaginitis, which usually produces a profuse, frothy, white or grayish green, malodorous discharge. The discharge from *trichomonal vaginitis* is typically described as frothy, whereas the discharge from bacterial vaginosis is described as homogeneous.

Because itching and burning may occur with virtually all forms of vaginitis, these symptoms are not particularly helpful in differentiating the cause. Women who *diagnose themselves* as having a *yeast infection* have been shown to be only 11% to 34% accurate (bacterial vaginosis being the other most likely diagnosis). It is important to differentiate vulvar pain from vulvar itching. Itching is most prominent in *candidal vaginitis* and least prominent in bacterial vaginosis. Itching and burning are uncommon with *gonococcal infections,* but a significant percentage of patients with a gonococcal infection have a combined infection. They may have gonorrhea with their itching that is caused by *Trichomonas* or *Candida.*

Vulvar itching is commonly caused by eczema, dermatitis, and vulvovaginal candidiasis. In prepubertal girls, atopic and irritant dermatitis are the most common causes of vulvar itching. Irritants to vulvar skin can be chemical (soaps, bath oils, bubble baths, douches, perfume, lubricants, antifungal creams, retained sweat, and vaginal secretions) or physical (sanitary pads, tight clothing, synthetic underwear, excessive cleansing, and shaving). Systemic causes of vulvar itching include diabetes, which predisposes to candidiasis, liver disease, polycythemia, psoriasis, seborrheic dermatitis, and medications, such as penicillin, ampicillin, and sulfa drugs.

If a vaginal discharge is sticky, brown, or yellowish and occurs in an elderly woman, *atrophic vaginitis* should be suspected.

ASSOCIATED SYMPTOMS

Dysuria may be a symptom of both a vaginal infection and a UTI. Therefore, all women who complain of dysuria should be asked about the presence of a vaginal discharge, irritation, or both. About 30% of the patients who have vaginitis but no evidence of UTI complain of dysuria. These patients usually complain of *external* dysuria (pain felt in the inflamed vaginal labia as the urinary stream passes) rather than "internal" dysuria (pain felt inside the body). Internal dysuria seems to correlate with UTIs, whereas external dysuria usually corresponds to vaginal infections.

Dyspareunia usually indicates vulvar disease rather than vaginitis. When dyspareunia is associated with a purulent discharge, *acute cervicitis* should be suspected. *Trichomonal vaginitis* is often associated with gonococcal or *Bacteroides* cervicitis. *Trichomonas* and *Chlamydia* may produce vaginitis as well as coexisting urethritis that causes dysuria and increased frequency. If dysuria, rectal infections, or pain on walking or climbing stairs is present, *gonorrhea* should be suspected.

If the patient has symptoms of diabetes is taking birth control pills or antibiotics, *candidal vaginitis* is probable. Refractory fungal vulvovaginitis may be secondary to undiagnosed diabetes.

PRECIPITATING AND AGGRAVATING FACTORS

Oral contraceptives, antibiotics, and pregnancy predispose the patient to *candidal vaginitis*. Uncontrolled diabetes and long-term use of tetracycline for acne increase the intestinal reservoir of *Candida,* predisposing the patient to recurrent vaginitis. *Bacterial vaginosis* is common and increasing in incidence. It is most frequently spread through venereal contact. *Trichomonal vaginitis* is usually transmitted by sexual intercourse; however, in children it may be spread by direct nonsexual contact. The growing incidence of venereal diseases such as gonorrhea, bacterial vaginosis, and trichomoniasis results from sexual activity in younger adolescents, multiple partners, and failure to use protective-barrier contraceptives (e.g., diaphragms, condoms).

In young children and some adults, inappropriate genital hygiene (e.g., wiping the perineal region from back to front) may increase the incidence of recurrent vaginal infections. *Chemical vaginitis* is precipitated by douches, bubble baths, and vaginal sprays. It may be aggravated by powders and by wearing of panties made of synthetic fibers.

PHYSICAL FINDINGS

Physical examination should include a thorough evaluation of the genital and pelvic areas. The appearance of the labia, vulva, entire vagina, and cervix should be noted, and the vaginal discharge should be inspected. *Nonspecific vaginitis,* which occurs particularly in premenarchal girls, does not usually extend above the lower third of the vagina.

Atrophic vaginitis, as well as infections, can occur in premenarchal girls due to insertion of foreign bodies into the vagina. When atrophic vaginitis occurs in postmenopausal women, there is often a sticky, brownish vaginal discharge, and the vaginal mucosa is usually thick, pale, and smooth, demonstrating the loss of normal rugose folds.

The pelvic examination should include adnexal palpation and cervical manipulation so that the physician can determine whether any masses or points of tenderness exist. Adnexal tenderness and pain on motion of the cervix *(chandelier sign)* suggest *pelvic inflammatory disease,* not merely cervicitis. When these findings occur in conjunction with a vaginal discharge, a *gonococcal infection* is probable. In such cases, if the patients test negative for gonorrhea, *Chlamydia* should be suspected and appropriately treated.

DIAGNOSTIC STUDIES

Ninety percent of cases of vaginitis can be classified into one of four major clinical categories on the basis of symptomatology, vaginal pH, and wet smear findings (Table 33-1).

Rapid tests (nucleic acid amplification tests [NAATs]) for gonorrhea and chlamydia are sensitive and specific in adolescents and women and can be done on a regular (not clean-catch) urine sample. NAATs should *not* be used in prepubertal girls because of a significant incidence of false-positive results. Vaginal cultures should be done in prepubescent girls. NAATs in adolescents and women are recommended whenever there is a purulent discharge from the cervical or urethral os. **Simultaneous chlamydial infections are present in 30% to 50% of patients with cervical gonococcal infections.**

In some populations with a high prevalence of asymptomatic chlamydial or gonococcal infections, rapid tests for these organisms are considered appropriate whenever a patient has a pelvic examination.

In all patients with a vaginal discharge, saline and potassium hydroxide wet mounts of the discharge should be examined when available. The saline mount should be inspected for *clue cells* (epithelial cells with bacilli adherent to their surface), which are virtually pathognomonic of *bacterial vaginosis.* The pH range of secretions in patients with bacterial vaginosis is usually greater than 4.5. A positive *whiff test result* (presence of a fishy or amine odor when 10% KOH is added to a sample of the discharge) also indicates bacterial vaginosis. Fulfilling three out of Amsel's four criteria (>20% clue cells, positive whiff test result, thin homogeneous discharge, and pH >4.5) is very sensitive for diagnosing bacterial vaginosis. Cultures may occasionally reveal infections other than those causing bacterial vaginosis.

TABLE 33-1.   Classification of Vaginitis

TYPE OF VAGINITIS	SYMPTOM	PH	WET MOUNT FINDINGS
Candidiasis (moniliasis)	Pruritus	<4.5	Hyphae or spores
Bacterial vaginosis	Malodorous	>4.5	*Clue cells*
Trichomoniasis	Profuse discharge	5.0-6.0	Protozoa, white blood cells
Atrophic vaginitis	Discharge	7	Parabasal cells

The saline wet mount may be used to identify the motile protozoan *Tricho-monas*; however its sensitivity may be as low as 50%. It should be done as soon as possible after the specimen is obtained. The pH of the vaginal secretions in patients with *Trichomonas* infection ranges from 4.9 to 6.0. The Affirm VPIII Microbial Identification Test (BD [Becton, Dickinson and Co.], Franklin Lakes, NJ) is a nucleic acid probe test that evaluates for *T. vaginalis*, *G. vaginalis*, and *C. albicans*.

Candidal vaginitis may be diagnosed by microscopic examination of the discharge in a KOH preparation; this will show the *Candida* mycelia. The pH of the discharge in patients with candidal (monilial) vaginitis is less than 4.5. Although they are the most sensitive, cultures should be reserved for certain circumstances because 15% to 20% will give positive results in asymptomatic, healthy women. The Affirm VPIII Microbial Identification Test can be used to identify candidal infection.

LESS COMMON DIAGNOSTIC CONSIDERATIONS

Increased physiologic leukorrhea has a pH of less than 4.5, an absence of yeast and *Trichomonas,* and a culture with a preponderance of *Lactobacillus.* Dermatoses (e.g., psoriasis, seborrheic dermatitis) and infestations with parasites (e.g., amebiasis, pinworms, lice) can cause vulvar itching in some cases. An allergy to nylon underwear and feminine deodorants, sprays, and douches may cause vulvovaginitis, leading to vaginal discharge or itching. Vaginal and cervical neoplasms can cause a serosanguineous discharge. Systemic dermatosis, like lichen planus or lichen sclerosis, may cause vaginal itching. Poor anal and vulvar hygiene may also produce vaginal discharge and itching. Tuberculosis is a rare cause of vulvovaginitis. In premenarchal girls, particularly young children, coliform bacterial infections may produce vaginitis. This is usually a low-grade, somewhat chronic infection and may be associated with pinworm infestation or insertion of a foreign body into the vagina. Retained tampons and other foreign objects may occasionally be found in adults.

Herpes genitalis is a relatively uncommon cause of vaginal discharge (though a common cause of cervicitis), but it is increasing in frequency. It is most common in adolescents and appears less frequently in patients older than 35 years. Herpetic lesions, which can be excruciating, affect not only the vulva but also adjacent areas (the thighs, buttocks, vagina, and cervix). The lesions begin as vesicles that progress in 5 to 10 days to shallow, exquisitely painful ulcerations with a clear, watery discharge. The ulcers last for 3 to 10 days and are prone to secondary infections, especially with *Streptococcus* and *Candida.*

Unfortunately, genital herpes is often recurrent; some patients experience repeated flare-ups for many years. The presenting symptoms may include pain, vulvar pruritus, burning, and frequently extreme vulvar tenderness that makes intercourse unbearable. Micturition may also be excruciating. Examination reveals widespread clusters of vesicles that may involve the vulvar and perineal

Differential Diagnosis of Vaginal Discharge and Itching

CAUSE	NATURE OF PATIENT	NATURE OF SYMPTOMS	ASSOCIATED SYMPTOMS	PRECIPITATING AND AGGRAVATING FACTORS	PHYSICAL FINDINGS	DIAGNOSTIC STUDIES
Vulvovaginitis due to: Candida Chemical irritants Douches Vaginal sprays Bubble baths Bacteria Foreign bodies Antifungal creams Perfume Lubricants	Most common cause of vaginal discharge in prepubertal girls	Variable discharge (scanty to profuse) Perineal pruritus Burning	Possible "internal" dysuria		Vulvovaginitis does not usually extend above lower third of vagina Thin, atrophic vaginal wall	
Physiologic discharge	Menarchal girls	Discharge: thick, grayish white, and odorless, but not profuse No pruritus		Beginning estrogen effect occurs just before or after menarche	No signs of inflammation	pH of discharge <4.5
Candidiasis (moniliasis)	After puberty Common cause of vulvovaginitis in children Common during reproductive years	Acute onset of discharge or vulvar irritation Discharge is often curdlike (resembles cottage cheese) Pruritus prominent	Possible "external" dysuria	Diabetes Antibiotics Oral contraceptives Pregnancy	Vaginitis	Saline or KOH wet mount hyphae or spores Vaginal pH <4.5 RNA probe

		Vaginal discharge				
Sexual abuse	Any age, including prepubescent	Vaginal discharge	Signs of psychological trauma	Dysfunctional social history Mother has many partners or a new boyfriend	Vulvovaginitis Cervical discharge	
Trichomoniasis	Common cause of vaginal discharge in women of childbearing age Rare in children Rare in women older than 60 yr May occur in neonates of infected mothers	Discharge usually profuse, frothy, grayish green, malodorous Varying degrees of pruritus	May be associated with gonococcal or *Bacteroides* infection Urethritis may cause dysuria and frequency	Often sexually transmitted Multiple sex partners	Vaginitis Vaginal petechiae Mucosal inflammation	Vaginal pH 5.0-6.0 Saline wet mount: white blood cells and motile protozoa RNA probe
Bacterial vaginosis	Most common cause of vaginitis in adolescents Common during reproductive years Rare in premenarchal girls	Discharge is malodorous but not usually frothy Pruritus not prominent	Urethritis may cause dysuria and frequency	Change in vaginal secretions at menarche Sexually transmitted Multiple sex partners	Vaginal mucosa not inflamed Adherent grayish white discharge	Saline wet mount: "clue cells" Vaginal pH >4.5-4.7 Positive "whiff test" result RNA probe
Gonorrhea	Increased incidence in neonates of infected mothers Rare in premenarchal girls (if present, sexual abuse must be suspected)	Itching and burning uncommon Purulent cervical discharge Pelvic pain Fever	Dysuria Rectal infection (often asymptomatic) Pain on walking or climbing stairs	Symptoms often worse near time of menstrual period Sexually transmitted Multiple partners	Cervicitis and cervical discharge Pain with cervical manipulation Adnexal tenderness	Intracellular gram-negative diplococci Positive NAAT results Chlamydial infections common

Continued

Differential Diagnosis of Vaginal Discharge and Itching—cont'd

CAUSE	NATURE OF PATIENT	NATURE OF SYMPTOMS	ASSOCIATED SYMPTOMS	PRECIPITATING AND AGGRAVATING FACTORS	PHYSICAL FINDINGS	DIAGNOSTIC STUDIES
Chlamydia infection	Usually sexually active adolescents Less frequently patients older than 35 yr	Scant vaginal discharge Often asymptomatic	Dysuria	Sexually transmitted Multiple partners	Cervicitis and cervical discharge Pain with cervical manipulation	Tests for chlamydia (NAAT) Often coexists with gonococcal infections
Herpes genitalis		Pain can be excruciating Vulvar pruritus uncommon Burning Vulvar tenderness	Dyspareunia Dysuria	Secondary *Streptococcus* or *Candida* infection	Cervicitis Widespread clusters of vesicles over vulvar and perineal areas, vagina, and cervix *Herpetic lesions:* Affect vulva and adjacent areas Begin as vesicles Progress in 5-10 days to shallow, painful ulcers Ulcers last 3-10 days Recurrent Do not usually produce vaginitis	Tzanck smear, PCR, viral culture, serologic tests Newer rapid tests
Senile atrophic vaginitis	Elderly women	Discharge is sticky, brown, or yellowish		Loss of estrogen effect	Vaginal mucosa: thin, pale, smooth (from loss of rugose folds)	Vaginal pH 7.0 Parabasal cells

KOH, Potassium hydroxide; *NAAT,* nucleic acid amplification test for gonorrhea and *Chlamydia.*

areas as well as the vagina and cervix. The physician must remember that herpes does not usually produce vaginitis, although it may infect the vagina and cervix. A Tzanck smear of a specimen from the base of the vesicle is a simple, definitive diagnostic test for this condition.

On rare occasions, what appears to be a clear, gelatinous vaginal discharge in infants may be due to the leakage of bluish absorbent jelly material from the new generation of diapers that contain this chemical substance to increase absorptive capacity.

Selected References

ACOG Committee on Practice Bulletins—Gynecology: ACOG Practice Bulletin. Clinical management guidelines for obstetrician-gynecologists, *Vaginitis Obstet Gynecol* (5):1195-1206, Monber 72 May 2006:2006.

Centers for Disease Control and Prevention: Update to CDC's Sexually transmitted diseases treatment guideline: fluoroquinolones no longer recommended for treatment of gonococcal infections. Centers for Disease Control, *Morbid Mortal Wkly Rep* 56:332-336, 2006:2007.

Centers for Disease Control and Prevention, Berman SM: Sexually transmitted diseases treatment guideline, *MMWR Recomm Rep* 55(RR-11):1-94, 2006:2006.

Cleveland A: Vaginitis: finding the cause prevents treatment failure, *Cleveland Clin J Med* 67:634-646, 2000.

Evans H: Vaginal discharge in the prepubertal child, *Pediatr Case Rev* 3:194-202, 2003.

Farage M, Miller K, Ledger W: Determining the cause of vulvovaginal symptoms, *Obstet Gynecol Survey* 63:445-464, 2008.

Majeroni BA: Bacterial vaginosis: an update, *Am Fam Physician* 57:1285-1289, 1998.

Pirotta M, Fethers K, Bradshaw C: Bacterial vaginosis, more questions than answers, *Aust Family Physician* 38, 2009:394-97.

Spence D, Melville C: Vaginal discharge, *BMJ* 335:1147-1151, 2007.

Striegel AM, Myers JB, Sorensen MD, et al: Vaginal discharge and bleeding in girls younger than 6 years, *J Urol* 176:2632-2635, 2006.

Welsh B, Howard A, Cook K: Vaginal itch, *Austr Fam Physician* 33:505-510, 2004.

Wilson J: In the clinic: vaginitis and cervicitis, *Ann Intern Med* 151: TC3-1-ITC-3-15, 2009.

Vision Problems and Other Common Eye Problems

34

Patients may think that discomfort in the eyes or noticeable redness is serious. **However, visual symptoms are always more serious than nonvisual ones.** Blurred vision caused by refractive error is the most common visual complaint, but it is often the most difficult visual symptom to evaluate. Other common vision problems are diplopia, unilateral photopsia (floaters, stars, light flashes) usually due to posterior vitreous detachment (PVD), and visual blurring associated with pain or eye soreness. A correct diagnosis requires knowing the patient's age and deciding whether the symptoms are unilateral or bilateral, onset is sudden or gradual, and symptoms are constant or intermittent. The prevalence of severe visual impairment is increased in elderly patients. **In all instances, visual acuity must be determined with the use of a Snellen chart.**

The most common causes of visual symptoms include refractive errors, posterior vitreous detachment (usually due to contraction of the vitreous), migraine, acute angle-closure glaucoma, cataracts, dry eyes, drug side effects, and transient ischemic attacks (TIAs).

Other common problems are ocular allergy, *red eye*, and glaucoma.

NATURE OF PATIENT

In young patients the most common cause of visual blurring is *refractive error*. The two most frequent refractive errors are *myopia* (nearsightedness) in teenagers and *presbyopia* (loss of accommodation) in patients at about age 40 years, when glasses become necessary for reading. Scintillating scotoma, another common visual problem in adolescents and adults, is experienced by patients with *migraine* as a prodrome to their headaches. Some patients note only the scintillating scotoma but do not experience a headache, a condition known as *ophthalmic migraine* or *migraine sans migraine* but currently called migraine aura without headache.

The remainder of the common visual symptoms and causes of vision loss listed in the introduction generally occur in older adults. *Cataracts, glaucoma,* floaters, light flashes, *senile macular degeneration, diabetic retinopathy, TIA, drug side effects,* and *dry eyes* occur almost exclusively in elderly patients. Older women often have dry eyes, which may result in visual blurring sometimes associated with a sense of grittiness and warmth in the eyes. In elderly patients a sudden onset of painless unilateral blurred vision often associated with a relative central scotoma and visual distortion suggests *senile macular degeneration,* the most common cause of blindness after age 55 years.

Two neuro-ophthalmologic vascular emergencies occur in elderly patients: temporal arteritis and third-nerve palsy. *Temporal arteritis* presents as a transient (in some cases progressive) unilateral visual loss often associated with visual field defects. Temporal arteritis is twice as common in elderly women as in elderly men. Patients with *third-nerve palsy* present with a sudden onset of diplopia with pain around the eye or diffusely in the head. Because in approximately 20% of these elderly patients an aneurysm is causing third-nerve palsy, their cases must be investigated promptly.

NATURE OF SYMPTOMS

The physician must inquire whether the blurred vision:
1. Is equal or unequal in the two eyes.
2. Is unilateral or bilateral.
3. Is constant or intermittent.
4. Is present for near or distant vision or both.
5. Had a sudden or gradual onset.
6. Has improved or worsened since it was first noted.

Monocular blurring, particularly of sudden onset, is more likely to be serious and of ocular origin. If the blurring is binocular and has occurred gradually over months in an otherwise healthy individual, a *refractive error* is most likely.

In an elderly patient, when primarily distant vision is blurred, the cause is most often *cataracts,* but if near vision is mainly affected, a *retinal circulatory disturbance* or *macular degeneration* should be suspected. Monocular blurring of sudden origin (days or weeks) is generally not a refractive error. In some patients, monocular blurring due to a refractive error may be long-standing but only recently noted.

Episodic blurring is virtually never caused by a refractive error. In older adults it can result from *glaucoma, multiple sclerosis* (MS), or *TIAs.* Brief episodes of blurred vision or loss of vision, usually monocular but occasionally binocular, are typically caused by transient impairment of retinal circulation resulting from *atherosclerotic emboli* from the carotid circulation or heart, *carotid insufficiency,* or *vertebrobasilar insufficiency.* Patients with the latter condition may have transient diplopia, blurring accompanied by dizziness, or both. Episodic blurring due to carotid insufficiency is often referred to as *amaurosis fugax.* Because visual loss becomes permanent in 11 % of these patients, they should be investigated promptly.

Several types of visual auras are experienced by patients with *migraine.* Scotomas are areas of indistinct or totally obscured vision. A *negative* scotoma is a circumscribed, obscured region in the visual field that appears translucent or as a dark or shimmering area. Negative scotomas most often begin in the central region of the visual field and then expand across the visual field, sometimes encompassing part of the right or left field. Homonymous hemianopsia may be present, or the vision may be totally obscured. Vision may also be obscured by *positive* scotomas, which are often described as bright, shimmering, shooting, or scintillating lights. These also occur initially in the center of the visual field and then expand to fill the entire visual field.

When transient blurring (with associated pain and redness) occurs unilaterally in older patients, *acute angle-closure glaucoma* should be suspected. The sudden loss of central vision in one eye and ocular pain without redness suggest *optic neuritis*. Fifty percent of patients with optic neuritis eventually have MS. Optic neuritis preceding MS is virtually always unilateral, and the blurring may last several days. Ischemic neuropathy, often due to *giant-cell arteritis*, usually manifests as variable blurring and superior or inferior field defects. Visual loss is usually permanent.

Patients often confuse *diplopia* (double vision) with *blurred vision*. Patients with diplopia see two separate objects either side by side or one above the other. Most diplopia in adults is caused by paralysis or weakness in one or more of the extraocular muscles. This paralysis may be caused by *trauma, cerebrovascular lesions, MS, thyroid disease, myasthenia gravis,* or *brain tumors*. Diplopia due to *strabismus* is most common in children and leads to eyes that fail to coordinate. Patients may have intermittent exotropia or esotropia. Young children with these symptoms usually suppress one image and therefore do not complain of double vision. Diplopia due to strabismus is more common in adults when the angle of their squint changes.

Diplopia may be monocular or binocular as well as constant or intermittent. Patients with *monocular* diplopia experience double vision with one eye occluded. It is most often the result of *lens opacities*. A slightly *dislocated lens* associated with *trauma* or *Marfan's syndrome* is a rare cause of monocular diplopia. In an otherwise healthy individual, **monocular diplopia** suggests that the *hysteria* is causing diplopia.

Constant *binocular* diplopia may be caused by *head trauma* or pathology involving the extraocular muscles or their cranial nerves. If the patient has total third-nerve palsy and the pupil is involved, an *aneurysm* is probable.

After blurring, the next most common visual complaints are spots floating in the visual field and light flashes. Floaters and flashes are caused by *contraction of the vitreous* and occur in middle-aged and older patients. *Light flashes* are usually noted in the temporal field, particularly when the patient is in the dark or in poorly illuminated areas. Flashes are caused by the vitreous shrinking away from the retina and thus stimulating it. *Vitreous floaters* are produced when the vitreous pulls away from the retina, thus detaching particles suspended in the vitreous. Patients describe these as black or grey spots in the visual field when they look at a bright background such as the sky or a light-colored wall. Neither light flashes nor vitreous floaters are serious, but they should be investigated by an ophthalmologist because they may signal *retinal detachment*. Likewise, if a peripheral field defect occurs after the patient experiences light flashes and a shower of floaters, *retinal detachment* should be suspected, and the patient should be examined by an ophthalmologist.

Halos around lights are a common symptom in patients with *acute angle-closure glaucoma*. The rapid development of a relative central scotoma associated with visual distortion is often caused by *senile macular degeneration.*

Red eye may be produced by subconjunctival hemorrhage, episcleritis, scleritis, pterygium acute angle-closure glaucoma, superficial keratitis, acute anterior uveitis, and, most frequently, conjunctivitis.

Viral conjunctivitis **which usually begins bilaterally** is the most common cause of red eye. There is conjunctival hyperemia, tearing, and a watery discharge. It may start in one eye but quickly spread to the other, may be highly contagious, and may be associated with an upper respiratory infection. *Bacterial conjunctivitis* has a sudden onset in one eye but usually spreads to the other within 2 days. There is much tearing and usually a mucopurulent discharge, causing matting of the lids that is most prominent on awakening. Patient report of eyes being "glued shut" upon awakening has been associated with an odds ratio of 15:1 for a positive bacterial culture result.

Allergic conjunctivitis, **which usually begins bilaterally** may be the only manifestation of an allergic disorder, but there are usually other manifestations of allergy, such as sneezing, blepharitis, and itching of the eyes and/or roof of the mouth. *Seasonal allergic conjunctivitis* is the most common form of allergic conjunctivitis and is related to the occurrence of airborne pollens from sources such as trees, grasses, and weeds, including ragweed. There is usually tearing; burning; itchy eyes; sneezing and rhinorrhea; and a thin, watery discharge. *Perennial allergic conjunctivitis* causes similar symptoms that often occur year round. It is usually caused by household allergens such as animal dander, dust, and dust mites. If the onset of symptoms corresponds to turning on of forced-air heating, dust mites are often the culprit. *Vernal keratoconjunctivitis* is seasonal, occurs in males between 3 and 20 years of age, and lasts up to 10 years. *Contact ophthalmic conjunctivitis* involves the ocular surface and the eyelids. It is a form of *conjunctivitis medicamentosa* due to the use of ophthalmic medications frequently started to relieve seasonal or perennial allergic eye symptoms. Subconjunctival hemorrhage may be caused by a Valsalva maneuver, induced by lifting a heavy object or a coughing spell and rarely by *trichinosis.*

Loss of vision is more common in the elderly. It is usually caused by age-related *macular degeneration, glaucoma, cataracts,* or *diabetic retinopathy.* Although these conditions may be asymptomatic, their usual presenting symptoms are as follows: macular degeneration: blurred vision, central scotomata, trouble reading; glaucoma: visual field loss' cataracts: glare, halo, blurred vision, monocular diplopia; and diabetic retinopathy: visual field loss, blurred vision, impaired night vision. All patients with loss of vision should be referred to an ophthalmologist for evaluation.

ASSOCIATED SYMPTOMS

If blurred vision or diplopia occurs intermittently and is associated with dizziness, *TIAs* involving the vertebrobasilar system must be suspected. When an older patient complains of difficulty with driving at night because of the glare from headlights or difficulty with daytime driving in bright sunlight, *cataracts* may be present. If blurred vision is associated with halos around lights, pain in the eye, and headache, *glaucoma* is most probable, particularly in elderly patients. In *acute narrow-angle glaucoma* the eye is often red, and nausea and vomiting occur. When intermittent or progressive monocular blurring occurs in an elderly patient and is associated with a nocturnal headache, *temporal arteritis* should be suspected, particularly if there is tenderness on palpation over the temporal artery. Elderly patients who are visually impaired often have an associated restriction of mobility.

When visual disturbances are associated with pain in the eye, iritis and acute glaucoma must also be considered. Pain in the eye without visual symptoms or redness suggests a neurologic etiology such as *trigeminal neuralgia*. Because most serious causes of red eye do not affect both eyes at once, monocular redness is more portentous of serious disease than binocular redness. When a red eye is associated with pain in the eye, *iritis, glaucoma, periorbital cellulitis*, and *corneal abrasion* must be considered. Photophobia and a red eye suggest iritis, *keratopathy*, or glaucoma. A sudden onset of blurred vision in both eyes can be precipitated by sudden changes in blood glucose level such as occur in diabetic patients. Although a sudden onset of blurred vision in both eyes can occur with established diabetes, it can also be the initial symptom.

PRECIPITATING AND AGGRAVATING FACTORS

Many drugs, including anticholinergic, antihypertensive, and psychotropic agents, can cause blurred vision by interfering with *accommodation*. The long-term administration of corticosteroids or phenothiazines predisposes the patient to *cataract* formation, which causes visual blurring. Antihistamines that decrease tear formation as well as hot, dry environments may aggravate the condition of patients with dry eyes. Visual hallucinations and *metamorphopsia* can be caused by *hallucinogenic agents*. Patients with *digitalis toxicity* may report yellow vision or complain that everything seems to be covered with snow. Drugs like sildenafil, used for erectile dysfunction, can cause visual problems that include blue vision. Some drugs, particularly those that dilate the pupil, may precipitate *acute angle-closure glaucoma* and its associated symptoms, pain, redness, and blurred vision.

Amaurosis fugax can be caused by a decrease in blood pressure from drugs, arrhythmias, or decreased cardiac output or by emboli from diseased carotid arteries. Chocolate, red wine, or vasodilator medications may precipitate the visual auras of migraine with or without a headache. Decreased illumination may aggravate the impaired vision associated with *cataracts*.

Some studies have shown that hormone replacement therapy (HRT) increases the incidence of dry eyes, and other studies have shown that it may relieve the symptoms of dry eyes.

AMELIORATING FACTORS

Improvement of visual acuity when the patient looks through a pinhole indicates that retinal function is good and the visual problem is caused by a *refractive error*. If diplopia is improved by the occlusion of one eye, the cause may be paralysis or weakness of the extraocular muscles. This weakness may in turn be caused by *neuropathy,* MS, thyroid disease, myasthenia gravis, diabetes, trauma, or an intracerebral process such as a *tumor* or *aneurysm*. If increasing illumination improves vision, a cataract is probable. If the patient notes that dimming the lights or looking beside rather than directly at an object improves vision, *macular degeneration* should be suspected.

PHYSICAL FINDINGS

It is essential to evaluate visual acuity by using a Snellen chart. If visual acuity is decreased, the test should be repeated with the patient looking through a pinhole made in a paper card. If this maneuver improves visual acuity, a *refractive error* is present. The conjunctivae should be examined for redness, which would suggest an inflammatory or allergic process as well as glaucoma. *Acute glaucoma* may cause corneal edema or corneal haziness.

The patient should be tested for a *relative afferent pupillary defect* (RAPD). This test is performed by having the patient look into the distance and then shining a light into one eye, thus eliciting pupillary constriction in that eye and consensual constriction in the other eye. The light is then quickly moved in front of the other pupil, which normally should constrict further. If this additional constriction does not occur and the pupil dilates instead, RAPD is present. This test must be repeated several times. The presence of RAPD requires further investigation by an ophthalmologist. If RAPD is absent, as it should be, unilateral *optic nerve disease* or widespread *retinal damage* is unlikely. For example, RAPD is absent in *macular degeneration* and *cataracts* but is present in *chronic glaucoma, retinal detachment,* and *optic neuritis*. The size and shape of the pupil should also be evaluated. In *acute glaucoma* the pupil is vertically oval.

When the eye is not inflamed and no RAPD exists, *cataracts, vitreous opacities,* and *macular degeneration* are possible. If a white eye (absence of red eye) and RAPD are present, *chronic glaucoma* should be suspected. In addition, chronic glaucoma should be considered with excessive deepening of the optic disc and narrowing of the peripheral field. If chronic glaucoma is suspected, peripheral fields should be checked because the patient may have advanced narrowing of the visual fields without being aware of it. Tonometry may be diagnostic.

When *senile macular degeneration* is present, funduscopic examination may reveal *drusen* (discrete, round yellow spots of retinal pigment in the region of the macula). Neovascularization and other signs of *diabetic retinopathy* may also be seen. The Schirmer test may reveal decreased tear production in patients with *dry eyes*.

A watery discharge is present in viral and allergic conjunctivitis, whereas a purulent discharge is present in bacterial conjunctivitis. Some disorders of the eyelid that are often accompanied by conjunctivitis include:

- *Blepharitis* (scaling and crusting along the anterior lid)
- *Hordeolum* or *stye* (an acute infection of the Zeis gland near the eyelash)
- *Chalazion* or *internal hordeolum* (a focal inflammation of the lid resulting from a blocked meibomian [oil] gland)

DIAGNOSTIC STUDIES

Tests to rule out systemic disease include complete blood count (CBC); thyroid studies to rule out *hyperthyroidism*, which may give rise to certain oculomotor palsies; and the determination of blood glucose and glycosylated hemoglobin to diagnose *diabetes*, which may give rise to *refractive errors, diabetic retinopathy*, and (rarely) *oculomotor palsies*.

Erythrocyte sedimentation rate (ESR) and temporal artery biopsy should be performed if *temporal arteritis* is suspected.

Tonometry is used to measure intraocular pressure when glaucoma is suspected. CT scanning is used to evaluate ocular trauma and tumors. Fluorescein staining of the eye, followed by an ophthalmoscopic examination with a cobalt blue light, can help identify corneal abrasions and foreign bodies. A slit-lamp examination can be used to examine the anterior chamber of the eye as well as the cornea. Subconjunctival hemorrhage is commonly due to trauma but may be caused by fragile conjunctival vessels, hypertension, anticoagulation, bleeding disorders, and (rarely) trichinosis. The deep redness of a *subconjunctival hemorrhage* stops at the edge of the iris. Visibility of blood in the anterior chamber (hyphema) constitutes an emergency, and the patient should be evaluated by an ophthalmologist.

LESS COMMON DIAGNOSTIC CONSIDERATIONS

Brain tumors and *aneurysms* may cause central vision defects as well as oculomotor palsies. Certain drugs have toxic effects on various parts of the eye, thus impairing vision, whereas other drugs, such as anticholinergics and psychotropic drugs, may impair accommodation. *Central* and *branch retinal artery occlusions* are persistent equivalents of *amaurosis fugax*. Acute and painless loss of vision most often results from *carotid atherosclerosis*, in which pieces of the atheromatous plaques migrate to the retinal arteries. These conditions are much more common in elderly hypertensive patients with hyperlipidemia and prior myocardial infarction.

Differential Diagnosis of Vision Problems and Other Common Eye Problems

CONDITION	NATURE OF PATIENT	NATURE OF SYMPTOMS	ASSOCIATED SYMPTOMS	PRECIPITATING AND AGGRAVATING FACTORS	AMELIORATING FACTORS	PHYSICAL FINDINGS	DIAGNOSTIC STUDIES
Refractive errors:		Blurred vision: bilateral, gradual onset			Looking through pinhole improves visual acuity		Determination of visual acuity by using Snellen's chart in all patients
Myopia	Teenagers						
Presbyopia	Older than 40 yr		Glasses needed for reading				
Cataracts	Older adults	Blurred vision, especially distant vision	Glare, halos	Poor illumination	Increased illumination	Lenticular opacification RAPD absent	
Senile macular degeneration	Older adults	Blurred vision, especially near vision Unilateral at first Painless	Central scotomata Visual distortion Often blindness		Dark environment Looking next to object	RAPD absent Drusen near macula	
Glaucoma:							
Acute angle-closure	Older adults	Usually monocular blurring, which is often episodic	Ocular pain and redness Halos around lights Nausea and vomiting	Dark environment Drugs that dilate pupils		Red eye, corneal edema, or haziness RAPD present Pupil vertically oval	Tonometry

Continued

Differential Diagnosis of Vision Problems and Other Common Eye Problems—cont'd

CONDITION	NATURE OF PATIENT	NATURE OF SYMPTOMS	ASSOCIATED SYMPTOMS	PRECIPITATING AND AGGRAVATING FACTORS	AMELIORATING FACTORS	PHYSICAL FINDINGS	DIAGNOSTIC STUDIES
Chronic						White eye RAPD present Deep optic disk Narrowing of peripheral visual fields	Tonometry
Conjunctivitis:							
Viral	All ages	Starts bilaterally	Tearing URI			Red eye Watery discharge	
Bacterial		Sudden onset Starts unilaterally	Matting of lids			Mucopurulent discharge	
Seasonal allergic		Seasonal May begin at onset of heating season	Eye itching, sneezing, rhinorrhea	Airborne particles (dust), dust mites, pollen		Thin, watery discharge	
Contact ophthalmic	All ages	Often sudden onset after restarting ophthalmic preparations	Tearing	Prior use of ophthalmic preparations	Cessation of ophthalmic preparations	Erythema of ocular surface and eyelids	
Dry eyes	Usually older women	Bilateral visual blurring	Pain, soreness, gritty feeling in eyes	Antihistamines Hot and dry environment		Decreased tear formation	Schirmer test

Subconjunctival hemorrhage			Painless	Valsalva maneuver, coughing	Deep redness that stops at the border of the iris	
Hyphema		Visual blurring, pain		Trauma, tumor, hemoglobinopathy	Blood visible in the anterior chamber	Tonometry Ultrasonography CT
TIAs	Older adults	Episodic monocular visual blurring and/or diplopia	Dizziness	Time	Decreased carotid pulsation or bruit	Carotid Doppler ultrasonographic studies
Drug side effects	All ages, but more common in older adults as they take more medications	Bilateral visual blurring Dry eyes	Dry mouth	Anticholinergics Antihypertensives Psychotropic drugs	Impaired accommodation Pupils may be dilated	
Posterior vitreous detachment	Middle-aged and older adults	Floaters and/or light flashes Usually unilateral and of sudden onset		Floaters usually seen when looking at bright background Light flashes usually noted when in dark environment	RAPD absent Vitreous opacities	
Migraine	All ages Often a family history of bad headaches	Scotomas, often scintillating and as prodrome to headache	Headache (sometimes absent) Nausea, vomiting	Stress Vasodilator drugs Certain foods Menstruation		

RAPD, Relative afferent pupillary defect; *TIAs*, transient ischemic attacks; *URI*, upper respiratory infection.

Giant-cell arteritis, which usually affects the temporal artery, can also affect the vertebrobasilar system, giving rise to diplopia and dizziness. On rare occasions, *cavernous sinus syndromes* and *third-nerve palsies* are caused by aneurysms. Both aneurysms and ischemic conditions can cause *oculomotor nerve palsy*.

Short-lasting *u*nilateral *n*euralgiform headache attacks with *c*onjunctival infection and *t*earing (SUNCT) syndrome usually occurs in men older than 50. years The pain is usually unilateral, sharp, or burning in quality and lasts 10 to 120 seconds. Ipsilateral nasal stuffiness, lacrimation, and increased intraocular pressure may also be associated.

Ophthalmic infection from *Chlamydia trachomatis* (causes trachoma, a major cause of blindness worldwide) is uncommon in adults in the United States, where it causes inclusion conjunctivitis, invariably a sexually transmitted disease.

Selected References

Amos JF: Differential diagnosis of common etiologies of photopsia, *J Am Optom Assoc* 70:485-504, 1999.

Bryant WM: Common toxic effects of systemic drugs on the eye, *Occup Health Nurs* 29:15-17, 1981.

Coote MA: Sticky eye, tricky diagnosis, *Austr Fam Physician* 31:225-231, 2002.

Dinowitz M, Rescigno R, Bielory L: Ocular allergic diseases: differential diagnosis, examination techniques, and testing, *Clin Allergy Immunol* 15:127-150, 2000.

Hodge C, Ng D: Dry eyes, menopause, and hormone therapy, *Austr Fam Physician* 35:931-932, 2004.

Koch J, Sikes K: Getting the red out: primary angle-closure glaucoma, *Nurse Pract* 34:6-9, 2009.

Leibowitz HM: The red eye, *N Engl J Med* 343:345-351, 2005.

Magauran B: Conditions requiring emergency ophthalmologic consultation, *Emerg Med Clinics North Am* 26:233-238, 2008.

Margo CE, Harman LE: Posterior vitreous detachment: how to approach sudden-onset floaters and flashing lights, *Postgrad Med* 117:37-42, 2005.

Rosenberg E, Sperazza L: The visually impaired patient, *Am Fam Physician* 77:1431-1436, 2008.

Sallam A, Taylor S: Ocular emergencies 2: non traumatic, *Br J Hosp Med* 70:M54-M58, 2009.

Sethuraman U, Kamat D: The red eye: evaluation and management, *Clin Pediatr* 48:588-600, 2009.

Tarabishy A, Jeng B: Bacterial conjunctivitis: a review for internists, *Cleve Clin J Med* 75:507-512, 2008.

Vafidis G: When is red eye not just conjunctivitis? *Practitioner* 246:469-480, 2002.

Voiding Disorders and Incontinence

35

Voiding disorders and incontinence are common disorders of micturition that are presented to the physician. They occur more frequently in elderly persons; currently, about 15% of Americans are older than 65 years. Although voiding disorders and incontinence are common problems, patients are often reluctant to bring them to their healthcare providers' attention.

Lower urinary tract (LUT) dysfunction causes lower urinary tract symptoms (LUTS). Newer terminology divides LUTS into several groups: voiding (obstructive), storage (filling/irritative), postmicturition symptoms, overactive bladder syndrome, and bladder outlet obstruction.

Voiding symptoms usually caused by LUT obstruction include intermittent or split stream, slow stream, terminal dribbling, and straining. Storage symptoms include daytime frequency, nocturia, urgency, and incontinence. Postmicturition symptoms include the sensation of incomplete emptying and postmicturition dribbling. The latter suggests benign prostatic obstruction but could be considered a form of urinary incontinence due to a weakness in the pelvic floor muscles.

Voiding dysfunction is the rule rather than the exception in elderly men. Signs and symptoms of *benign prostatic hypertrophy* (BPH) have been found in about 70% of elderly male patients. **Incontinence is so common in women that many patients consider it normal.** Decreased bladder capacity and involuntary bladder contractions have been found in as many as 20% of continent elderly persons. About 10% to 20% of community-dwelling elderly patients have *urinary incontinence* severe enough to be considered a social or health problem. Large-scale studies have reported that one third of people older than 60 years occasionally experience an involuntary loss of urine. An even larger percentage of hospitalized and institutionalized elderly patients are troubled with incontinence.

Childhood enuresis (bed-wetting), whether primary or secondary, should be considered a symptom rather than a specific diagnosis. Most cases represent *primary enuresis,* a maturational delay that is occasionally familial. Secondary enuresis occurs when a child who has been continent demonstrates enuresis. *Secondary enuresis* may result from emotional stress (e.g., birth of a sibling, beginning school) or a urinary tract infection (UTI). In these children, bacteriuria may cause uninhibited bladder contractions. Most children with nocturnal or daytime incontinence (99%) have not an anatomic abnormality but rather a disturbance in urodynamics, such as bladder instability.

NATURE OF PATIENT

Enuresis is common until about 4 to 5 years of age. **In most children with voiding disturbances, no anatomic or neurologic disease is causing their enuresis. UTI should be suspected in children of all ages if they have secondary enuresis or an unexplained fever lasting 48 hours or more.**

Voiding dysfunction is common in elderly men. The amount of prostatic enlargement does not necessarily correlate with the symptoms of *prostatism.* Some young men found not to have prostatic enlargement on rectal examination have symptoms of prostatism, the so-called trapped prostate.

Incontinence is more common in women than men. It occurs more frequently in multiparous and menopausal women, in confused patients, and in those with limited mobility. Age-related changes in bladder function include decreased capacity, increased residual urine, increased involuntary bladder contractions (detrusor muscle instability), and increased nocturnal urine production. **Incontinence has been reported in 26% of women during their reproductive years, but in the postmenopausal years the incidence is 30% to 40%. Patients with neurologic disorders, such as multiple sclerosis and spinal cord injury, may present with symptoms of neurogenic bladder leading to overflow incontinence.**

NATURE OF SYMPTOMS

The symptoms of *prostatism* can be divided into two categories: obstructive symptoms (e.g., weak stream, abdominal straining, hesitancy, intermittency of stream, incomplete emptying, terminal dribbling) and storage symptoms (e.g., daytime frequency, nocturia, urgency). Some patients have symptoms of prostatic enlargement and also have symptoms related to unstable detrusor muscle contractions. The symptoms of *BPH* often wax and wane spontaneously, probably because of changes in dynamic factors, which include bladder tone, bladder neck obstruction, and tone in the prostate and prostatic capsule.

An abrupt onset of symptoms of stress or urge *incontinence* suggests *infection.* The gradual onset of symptoms of stress incontinence, particularly after menopause or oophorectomy, suggests *estrogen deficiency.* When the amount of urine leakage is small to moderate and coincides with increased abdominal pressure, stress incontinence is probable. Large amounts of urine and incontinence associated with the sensation of a full bladder suggest an overactive bladder with detrusor muscle instability. This precipitous loss of large quantities of urine unrelated to increased abdominal pressure suggests involuntary detrusor contractions, as does incontinence associated with an extreme desire to void because of pain, inflammation, or a sense of impending micturition. The symptoms of an overactive bladder (frequency, nocturia, and urgency) can occur with or without incontinence. Moderate dripping suggests a partially incompetent outlet, overflow, or congenital or acquired anomalies. Having the patient keep a bladder diary over a few days, noting leakage frequency, voiding intervals, activity or sensation with leakage, and amount and type of fluid intake, is often helpful in determining the cause of incontinence.

In children the symptoms of functional voiding disorders include increased or decreased frequency of urination, urgency, dysuria, nocturnal enuresis, daytime wetting after toilet training is completed, fever, abdominal pain, perineal pain, constipation, and encopresis. The severity and presence of symptoms vary so much that children with the same voiding disorder frequently have different symptoms. The most common symptoms are increased frequency and urgency. *Dysuria* may be caused by bladder dysfunction without infection, although *UTI* should always be suspected.

Nocturia, the presence of two or more nighttime voidings, increases with age. Studies report a 55% prevalence in men older than 70 years and a 79% prevalence in men older than 80 years. The incidences are similar in men and women, although some studies suggest a slightly higher rate in men. It is one of the most common causes of disturbed sleep.

ASSOCIATED SYMPTOMS

Microscopic or gross hematuria, from the rupture of blood vessels coursing over an enlarged prostate, often occurs in patients with *prostatic hypertrophy*. Cystoscopy and evaluation of the upper urinary tract (with computed tomography [CT] scan or ultrasonography) are indicated to rule out a stone and cancer. *Infection, neurologic disease,* and *bladder carcinoma* may produce hematuria and other symptoms similar to those of BPH. In addition, gradual obstruction from prostatic enlargement or carcinoma may lead to a large, distended bladder with overflow incontinence. Urinary retention is more common when symptoms of prostatism develop in less than 3 months or they are secondary to drugs. Urinary retention is less common when symptoms develop gradually. Recurrent *cystitis* develops more frequently in patients with persistent residual urine due to an atonic bladder, cystocele, prostatic hypertrophy, or diabetes mellitus. Constipation is often the cause of urinary voiding disorders in children owing to pressure on the bladder, stimulation of bladder contraction, and pelvic pain. Both the parents and the child should be questioned carefully about bowel habits when a pediatric patient presents with urinary voiding disorders.

Table 35-1 shows some of the factors that help in differentiating unstable bladder contractions from stress incontinence. Nocturia is rare in stress incontinence but occurs frequently with detrusor instability. Urgency and frequency occasionally occur in patients with stress incontinence but are the rule in patients with detrusor instability. Voluntary inhibition of incontinence is frequently present in patients with stress incontinence but is less probable in patients with detrusor muscle instability.

TABLE 35-1.   Comparison of Presenting Symptoms in Patients with
Genuine Stress Incontinence and Detrusor Instability

SYMPTOMS	GENUINE STRESS INCONTINENCE	DETRUSOR INSTABILITY
Precipitating factor	Cough, lifting, exercise, position change	Preceding urge, position change
Timing of leakage	Immediate	Delayed
Amount of leakage	Small to large	Large
Voluntary inhibition	Frequently	Possibly
Urgency, frequency	Occasionally	Yes
Nocturia	Rarely	Yes
Spontaneous remission	No	Occasionally

From Horbach NS: Problems in the clinical diagnosis of stress incontinence. J Reprod Med 35:751-756, 1990.

PRECIPITATING AND AGGRAVATING FACTORS

Stress incontinence may be precipitated or aggravated by coughing, lifting, exercising, and position change. Incontinence caused by detrusor muscle instability may be precipitated or aggravated by the urge to void, a full bladder, or position change. Detrusor muscle instability is aggravated by bladder wall inflammation and estrogen deficiency.

Drugs that may precipitate or aggravate stress incontinence include methyldopa, prazosin, phenothiazines, diazepam, caffeine, and diuretics. Drugs that may precipitate urinary retention include α-adrenergic agents, calcium channel blockers, anticholinergics, androgens, antihistamines, and sympathomimetic agents such as ephedrine and pseudoephedrine. Psychotropic and sedative agents may diminish alertness and facilitate or precipitate urinary incontinence. Some autonomic agents precipitate incontinence, whereas others precipitate urinary retention.

The time, type, and quantity of fluid ingestion have major effects on nocturia. The presence of primary polydipsia, diabetes, diabetes insipidus, and hypercalcemia aggravate nocturia. Heart failure, venous insufficiency, diuretics, cystitis, decreased bladder capacity, an overactive bladder, sleep apnea, and BPH can also precipitate or aggravate nocturia.

AMELIORATING FACTORS

The obstructive symptoms of benign *prostatic hypertrophy* may spontaneously diminish without appreciable change in the size of the prostate. The symptoms and degree of obstruction vary over time despite the absence of change in prostatic size. Cessation of drugs that aggravate urinary retention or incontinence alleviate symptoms in many adult patients. Discontinuing or reducing the intake of fluids, caffeine, alcohol, and diuretics may also alleviate the symptoms of *incontinence,* nocturia, and polyuria. Systemic and local estrogens often improve the symptoms of stress incontinence, although they may not have been administered for that reason. Antibiotics may improve *cystitis* and thereby reduce detrusor instability. Improvement in mental status or mobility of the patient often ameliorates the symptoms of incontinence. Children with urinary urgency may assume a body position (such as a *curtsy* or pressing the upper legs together) to overcome the urge to urinate.

PHYSICAL FINDINGS

Examination of the patient with voiding disorders or incontinence must include assessment of mental and neurologic status, mobility, and general health. Abdominal examination may reveal a distended bladder. Prostatic enlargement may be detected by rectal examination, although the symptoms of bladder outlet obstruction may occur without the appreciation of prostatic enlargement; in this case, trapped prostate or median bar obstruction may be detected only by cystoscopic examination. It may be helpful to observe voiding.

Neurologic examination may provide clues to sensory or motor dysfunction of the bladder, which is under the control of the second to fourth sacral nerves (S2 to S4). Flexion and extension of the ankle, knee, and hip against resistance, as well as assessment of rectal sphincter tone, should be performed to assess whether S2 to S4 are intact.

Pelvic examination should be performed to assess the patient's estrogen status and to look for a cystocele or rectocele. The strength of the pelvic floor muscles may be assessed on bimanual examination. The urethra, trigone, and vaginal area are all estrogen dependent. A large, distended bladder may be detected on physical examination, although more sophisticated tests are needed to assess the amount of residual urine. The typical patient with urge incontinence has a postvoiding residue of less than 150 mL, whereas a residue greater than 500 mL suggests overflow incontinence.

DIAGNOSTIC STUDIES

A urination diary, in which the time and quantity of each voiding are noted, is helpful in the diagnosis of voiding disorders. Several standardized scales have been validated to assess the *bother* of lower urinary tract symptoms to the patient, but simply asking whether the symptoms are troublesome enough to lead the patient to consider a surgical procedure or daily medication may also help elicit the patient's perspective on the problem. Patients with voiding disturbances or incontinence may have increased residual urine. Postvoiding residual urine can be assessed by abdominal ultrasonography, portable bladder scanners, or by catheterization. The cotton-tipped applicator ("Q-tip") test provides information on the mobility of the urethrovesical junction in the evaluation of stress incontinence. The result is positive if the cotton tip inserted in the urethra

Differential Diagnosis of Voiding Problems and Incontinence

CONDITION	NATURE OF PATIENT	NATURE OF SYMPTOMS	ASSOCIATED SYMPTOMS	PRECIPITATING AND AGGRAVATING FACTORS	AMELIORATING FACTORS	PHYSICAL FINDINGS	DIAGNOSTIC STUDIES
Benign prostatic hypertrophy	Common in older men	Nocturia Dribbling Hesitancy Decreased force of stream Incomplete emptying	Hematuria	Prostatitis Residual urine Alcohol Anticholinergics Decongestants Sympathomimetics Antidepressants Caffeine	Occasional spontaneous remission of symptoms Decreasing type and volume of fluid intake, especially after 4 PM	Enlarged prostate Distended bladder	Urination diary Ultrasonography for prostate size and residual volume Intravenous urography Cystoscopy Urinalysis Serum Creatinine level
Stress incontinence	Multiparous and menopausal women Postprostatectomy men	Small-quantity incontinence with cough, sneezing, laughing, and running	Recurrent cystitis	Cystitis Laughing Coughing Upper respiratory infections		Weakness or laxity of pelvic floor or urethral sphincter Atrophic vagina in elderly women	Urinalysis Residual volume Serum BUN and Creatinine level
Urge incontinence (unstable detrusor contractions)	Elderly men more than women Post-stroke Those with dementia	Uncontrolled urge to void Large-quantity incontinence	Unable to delay voiding long enough to reach toilet	Cystitis Urethritis Bladder calculi Alcohol Diuretics			Cystometry Urodynamics Uroflowmetry Videourody-namics

Overactive bladder syndrome	More common in elderly	Frequency, urgency	50% of patients have associated incontinence Nocturia				Urodynamic studies
Overflow incontinence	Patients with: Multiple sclerosis Severe benign prostatic hypertrophy Atonic bladder Diabetic neuropathy Tabes dorsalis	Small-quantity incontinence, nearly continuous dribbling		Medications, including anticholinergics and sympathomimetics Prostatitis in patients with benign prostatic hypertrophy		Distended bladder Anatomic bladder obstruction from benign prostatic hypertrophy or stricture Spinal cord disease Diabetic neuropathy	
Functional incontinence	Impaired mobility or mental status Dementia	Can void normally with assistance		Deterioration in mental or physical status	Toilet training	Severe mental or physical disability preventing normal toilet habits Normal lower urinary tract function	
Enuresis	Children older than age 5 yr; generally not significant if <4½ yr	Bed-wetting while sleeping	Very sound sleep	Emotional stress Urinary tract infections	Usually spontaneous improvement after age 5 yr	Usually normal	Urinalysis and culture Urodynamics Ultrasonography for hydroure-teronephrosis or residual urine (rarely)

moves 30 degrees or more from the horizontal position with coughing or straining. Patients with voiding disturbances and incontinence should undergo urinalysis to rule out infection or hematuria and a serum BUN and creatinine test to assess renal function. The stress test, in which the patient (with a full bladder) coughs in both the erect and recumbent positions, is also useful.

Cystoscopy allows visualization of the bladder wall and determination of the degree of urethral obstruction. Trabeculation of the bladder wall suggests chronic obstruction. Urodynamic studies assess urine flow and the force of the stream. Urodynamic studies, including cystometry, measure filling pressures and detrusor tone to evaluate bladder function. Videourodynamics combines video of voiding with the simultaneous measurement of intravesicular, perivesicular, and rectal pressures. Transrectal prostatic ultrasonography can be used to determine prostate size and the presence or absence of prostatic nodules. It can be used to guide prostatic biopsies. Serum prostate-specific antigen (PSA) measurement is helpful in screening for prostatic cancer.

LESS COMMON DIAGNOSTIC CONSIDERATIONS

Dysfunctional voiding with *vesicoureteral reflux* may occur in young children.

Multiple sclerosis, spinal cord disease, tumors, trauma, syphilis, and diabetic neuropathy as well as incontinence, usually overflow incontinence, can all cause voiding disorders. Urethral stricture, dyssynergic bladder neck contracture, prostate cancer, chronic prostatitis, and bladder cancer may cause symptoms similar to those of BPH. Urethrovaginal prolapse or prolapse of a large cystocele may cause urethral obstruction.

Nocturnal polyuria syndrome, more common in elderly patients, causes an increased volume of urine and greater frequency of micturition at night.

Selected References

ACOG Committee on Practice Bulletins—Gynecology: ACOG Practice Bulletin No. 51: chronic pelvic pain, *Obstet Gynecol* 103:589-605, 2004.

Brown CT, Das G: Assessment, diagnosis, and management of lower urinary tract symptoms in men, *Int J Clin Pract* 56:591-603, 2002.

Brown JS, Bradley CS, Subak LL, et al: The sensitivity and specificity of a simple test to distinguish between urge and stress urinary incontinence, *Ann Intern Med* 144:715-723, 2006.

Cesario S: Lower urinary tract symptoms in men: differential diagnosis is main challenge, *Adv Nurse Pract* 3:57-60, 90, 2002.

Dwyer PL: Differentiating stress urinary incontinence from urge urinary incontinence, *Int J Gynecol Obstet* 86(Suppl 1):S17-S24, 2004.

Ellsworth P, Caldamone A: Pediatric voiding dysfunction: current evaluation and management, *Urologic Nursing* 28:249-257, 2008.

Gormley E: Evaluation of the patient with incontinence, *Can J Urol* 14:58-62, 2007.

McKertich K: Urinary incontinence, assessment in women: stress, urge or both? *Aust Family Physician* 37:112-117, 2008.

Rosenberg M, Staskin D, Kaplan S, et al: A practical guide to the evaluation at treatment of male lower urinary tract symptoms in the primary care setting, *Int J Clin Pract* 61:1535-1546, 2007.

Takeda M, Araki I, Kamiyama M, et al: Diagnosis and treatment of voiding symptoms, *Urology* 62(Suppl 5B):11-19, 2003.

Wang A, Carr L: Female stress urinary incontinence, *Can J Urol* 15:37-43, 2008.

Wein AJ: Diagnosis and treatment of the overactive bladder, *Urology* 62(Suppl 5B):20-27, 2003.

Wein A, Lose GR, Fonda D: Nocturia in men, women, and the elderly: a practical approach, *Br J Urol Int* 90(Suppl 3):28-31, 2002.

Weiss JP, Blaivas JG: Nocturnal polyuria versus overactive bladder in nocturia, *Urology* 60(Suppl 5A):28-32, 2002.

Yerkes E: Urologic issues in the pediatric and adolescent gynecology patient, *Obstet Gynecol Clin North Am* 36:69-84, 2009.

36

Weight Gain and Weight Loss

WEIGHT GAIN

The most common cause of weight gain is *increased caloric intake,* regardless of what the patient states. Though percentage of body fat as measured with calipers is more accurate than body mass index (body mass index [BMI] = weight in kilograms divided by the square of height in meters [kg/m²]) for defining obesity, BMI is clinically more practical and correlates fairly well with percentage of body fat. In adults, a normal BMI is 18.5 to 24.9 kg/m². A value less than 18.5 kg/m² is considered underweight. A BMI of 25.0 to 29.0 kg/m² is considered overweight, whereas 30 kg/m² and above is considered obese. A BMI of 40 kg/m² or above is extremely obese. Obesity affects around one-third of all adults in the United States; two-thirds of these individuals are considered either overweight or obese. Obesity increases the risk of several chronic conditions, including hypertension, type II diabetes mellitus, hyperlipidemia, heart disease, pulmonary disease, hepatobiliary disease, several cancers, osteoarthritis, gastroesophageal reflux disease, and psychiatric illness.

Weight gain due to *fluid retention* occurs in patients with the nephrotic syndrome, congestive heart failure (CHF), or cirrhosis with ascites; these patients have clear signs of edema. *Hypothyroidism* can lead to decreased metabolic needs and weight gain, but for significant weight gain to occur, hypothyroidism must be pronounced, and it is usually clinically apparent. A *low resting metabolic rate* contributes to obesity in some individuals. *Physiologic weight gain* occurs as a result of pregnancy and premenstrual fluid retention. *Drugs* (e.g., steroids, nonsteroidal anti-inflammatory drugs [NSAIDs], antidepressants, lithium, anabolic steroids, and estrogens) can cause weight gain by promoting salt and water retention or by stimulating appetite.

Nature of Patient

Overweight in children is defined as age and gender-adjusted BMI higher than the 84th percentile but lower than the 95th percentile. *Obesity* is defined as age and gender-adjusted BMI in the 95th percentile or above. Although the most common type of obesity in children is exogenous, this diagnosis requires that the endocrine and genetic causes of obesity be considered. Children with *exogenous obesity* often show accelerated or at least normal linear growth and may reach puberty early. **Most children with endogenous obesity are short for their age and have other associated abnormalities. All obese children with short stature should be evaluated promptly and carefully.** Childhood obesity is an increasingly serious problem in the United States and has been tied to increased fast-food consumption, sweetened beverages, and sedentary lifestyle. It has been estimated that 13.9 % of children 2 to 5 years of age, 18.8% of children 6 to 11 years of age, and 17.4% of adolescents (12-19 years of age) are considered overweight. This increase in childhood obesity has led to an increase in the diagnosis of type II diabetes in children (traditionally thought of as an *adult-onset* disorder). Obesity in adolescents correlates directly with the amount of time spent in front of a computer or television screen. Currently, the American Academy of Pediatrics recommends limiting screen time to 2 hours per day.

Obese patients may experience *depression,* which can be either the result of being overweight or the cause of overeating. Some patients with mild depression due to seasonal affective disorder have a craving for carbohydrates. Their mood improves after carbohydrate ingestion.

Familial obesity probably represents an acquired propensity to overeat; various family members are short and obese. Their obesity tends to be proximal but can have a generalized distribution. Twin studies suggest that heredity plays a significant role in obesity.

Weight increase in patients with *edema syndromes* (e.g., cirrhosis, nephrosis, congestive heart failure) is usually accompanied by symptoms that suggest a deteriorating clinical status.

Nature of Symptoms

Patients may present complaining of weight gain, an uncontrollable appetite, an inability to diet, or garments that fit too tight. Obesity may be caused by binge eating or night-eating syndrome. The weight gain associated with fluid retention in the *premenstrual period* is usually described as bloating and is often accompanied by breast tenderness, breast swelling, or finger swelling. Some patients with *hypothyroidism* comment that their skin seems puffy or that they are unable to lose weight on diets that previously resulted in weight loss.

Associated Symptoms and Ameliorating Factors

Sudden, marked changes in weight that occur over 1 to 2 days are usually related to changes in fluid balance. These changes may range from a few pounds gained because of premenstrual edema or salt-retaining drugs to many pounds added as the result of *cyclic edema.* The weight gain of *premenstrual edema* usually dissipates after menstruation. The fluid retention that occurs with *cyclic edema* is relieved by the patient maintaining a recumbent posture for

48 to 72 hours. The weight gain caused by *salt-retaining drugs* is not continuously progressive; it levels off after a weight increase of several pounds.

When weight gain is progressive and the patient appears to be obese without evidence of edema, it is reasonably certain that the patient's weight gain is caused by *overeating*. Some patients with profound obesity complain of fatigue, which may result from *obstructive sleep apnea*.

Precipitating and Aggravating Factors

Weight gain results from ingestion of more calories than are metabolized. Thus, although weight gain is usually related to increased caloric intake, it can also be produced by reduction of either physical activity or metabolic rate. These weight changes occur gradually.

Although most people eat less when they are tense or upset, 15% to 25% respond to stress with increased caloric intake, or *reactive hyperphagia*. These patients are often overweight. They eat excessively when they are depressed or anxious and likewise celebrate good times with elaborate meals.

Drug ingestion is an important factor in weight gain. *Steroids, nonsteroidal anti-inflammatory drugs, anabolic steroids, estrogens, tricyclic antidepressants, selective serotonin reuptake inhibitors* (SSRIs), and *lithium* may cause fluid retention and/or increased appetite, which can produce a weight gain of several pounds. *Oral contraceptives* increase weight by causing fluid retention, increasing appetite, and creating an anabolic effect. *Psychotropic agents* (e.g., tricyclic antidepressants, some phenothiazines) may produce a craving for carbohydrates in patients taking these drugs. In addition, when antidepressant drugs alleviate the anorexia of depression, a pronounced weight gain may occur. *Beta blockers* may cause weight gain through their induction of hypoglycemia. Smoking cessation may contribute to weight gain equivalent to approximately 200 to 300 kcal per day.

Physical Findings

In obese patients, adipose tissue is usually generally distributed but is occasionally proximally concentrated in the extremities. Proximal obesity associated with a "buffalo hump," hirsutism, hypertension, or diabetes suggests *Cushing's disease*. Marked weight gain due to *edema* is usually associated with pitting edema of the legs, ascites, gallop rhythm, or, in the nephrotic syndrome, swelling of the eyelids and facial edema.

The physical findings of *hypothyroidism* may include somewhat coarse, dry skin; coarse hair; loss of the outer third of the eyebrows; a low, hoarse voice; an enlarged thyroid; and "hung-up" ankle jerks (the delayed contraction and relaxation phases of deep tendon reflexes). The hung-up ankle jerk is often more readily detected when the patient kneels on a bed, chair, or examining table with the feet extended over the edge. Tapping the Achilles tendon with a reflex hammer may show a prompt contraction phase but a more readily perceived slow relaxation phase.

Diagnostic Studies

Although hypothyroidism is an uncommon cause of obesity, it is readily diagnosed by thyroid function tests. Obese patients should be screened for diabetes as well as for fatty liver by performance of a complete metabolic profile. A fasting lipid profile should also be obtained. The United States Preventive Services Task Force recommends calculating BMI in adults annually and screening children for obesity starting at 6 years of age.

Less Common Diagnostic Considerations

The endogenous causes of obesity are rare but can usually be diagnosed by other associated findings. Several causes are associated with short stature. *Pseudohypoparathyroidism* is characterized by short stature, short metacarpals, hypocalcemia, and, occasionally, mental retardation. *Prader-Willi syndrome* is characterized by short stature, mental retardation, and hypogenitalism. *Laurence-Moon syndrome* is characterized by short stature, mental retardation, hypogonadism, and retinal pigmentation.

Other rare causes of obesity that are not particularly associated with short stature include *hypothalamic tumors, Cushing's syndrome,* and *insulinomas.* Patients with insulinomas invariably have symptoms of hypoglycemia. Patients with hypothalamic tumors may present with obesity, but other findings are usually suggestive of an intracranial tumor. Cyclic edema is more common in women than men. Postencephalitic obesity, tumors of the third ventricle, obesity that develops after cerebral trauma, and certain brain tumors (e.g., chromophobe adenomas, craniopharyngiomas) are other rare causes of hyperphagia.

WEIGHT LOSS

Unexplained weight loss of more than 5% of body weight within 6 to 12 months suggests underlying pathology. It is important to differentiate *anorexia* (loss of the desire to eat) from true weight loss, although true weight loss results from anorexia when caloric intake is substantially reduced. *Involuntary weight loss* in the absence of other symptoms is most frequently caused by gastrointestinal (GI) disorders; cancer, especially GI; dysphagia; depression; social factors; alcoholism; and medications.

Likewise, the clinician must differentiate starvation from cachexia. *Starvation* is due to a protein-energy deficiency. Although worldwide starvation is due to insufficient food intake, medical causes (severe dysphagia, malabsorption, and anorexia) predominate in developed countries. *Cachexia* is the cytokine-induced wasting of protein and energy stores seen in inflammatory disease, cancer, chronic pulmonary disease, end-stage renal disease, chronic heart failure, and acquired immunodeficiency syndrome (AIDS). Cachexia develops in 50% to 80%percent of all patients with cancer . It is a poor prognostic indicator and a major cause of death in patients with cancer. Weight loss of more than 10% of body weight in cachectic patients signifies significant depletion. Death is likely when more than 30% of pre-morbid weight is lost. It is important to recognize cachexia in chronically ill patients, yet many clinicians find nutritional assessment outside their area of responsibility.

Significant weight loss may occur in patients with anorexia secondary to psychological, cardiac, pulmonary, hepatic, renal, and metabolic diseases as well as drug ingestion. *Drugs* may decrease the appetite by causing nausea, vomiting, abdominal discomfort, and delayed gastric emptying or through the effects of the central nervous system. Weight loss is often the presenting symptom in patients with cancer (a common cause of unexplained weight loss) and chronic infectious processes. Weight loss with anorexia often occurs in patients with *depression, anxiety, anorexia nervosa,* and *GI disorders,* including malabsorption, regional enteritis, granulomatous colitis, ulcerative colitis, chronic liver disease, and carcinoma of the stomach and pancreas.

Weight loss may occur with a normal appetite and adequate intake in patients with *diabetes mellitus, acquired immunodeficiency syndrome hyperthyroidism,* and *decreased intestinal absorption* (e.g., sprue, short-bowel syndrome, parasitic infestation, inflammatory bowel disease).

In their zest to decrease weight, athletes may have food aversion and experience weight loss. Eating disorders such as anorexia nervosa, bulimia nervosa, and binge-eating disorder are three times more prevalent in women than men, with a median onset of 18 to 21 years. Because patients do not usually present with the chief complaint of an eating disorder, the clinician must be attentive to this possible diagnosis, particularly in young women. Most patients with eating disorders do not have signs on physical examination unless the disorder is advanced; such signs include cardiac arrhythmias, orthostasis, flat affect, sallow skin, gingivitis, loss of tooth enamel, calluses on the dorsum of hands (from induced vomiting), and diminished deep tendon reflexes. Diagnostic criteria for various eating disorders may be found in the American Psychiatric Association's *Diagnostic and Statistical Manual of Mental Disorders* (2000). Premenstrual girls may have a history of poor weight gain and growth retardation. Older girls with an eating disorder may have been overweight prior to the onset of an eating disorder.

Anorexia and weight loss frequently occur in elderly people. The many causes range from loose dentures and poverty to drug ingestion, metabolic disease, and cancer cachexia. Robbins (1989) described the "nine d's" of weight loss in elderly patients: dentition, dysgeusia, dysphagia, diarrhea, disease (chronic), depression, dementia, dysfunction, and drugs. The most common causes are *psychiatric diseases, cancer, drugs,* and *benign upper GI disease.*

Diagnostic studies should be guided by clinical findings and may include a complete blood count, measurement of erythrocyte sedimentation rate, biochemical profile, abdominal ultrasonography, fecal occult blood test, computed tomography of the abdomen, and GI endoscopy. A positive response to a month-long trial of a dietary supplement (3000-4000 cal/day) suggests anorexia and/or depression. Questionnaires, such as the Simplified Nutritional Assessment Questionnaire (SNAQ), may be used to assess risk of weight loss in older adults (Rolland et al, 2006).

Differential Diagnosis of Weight Gain

CAUSE	NATURE OF PATIENT	NATURE OF SYMPTOMS	ASSOCIATED SYMPTOMS	PRECIPITATING AND AGGRAVATING FACTORS	AMELIORATING FACTORS	PHYSICAL FINDINGS
Physiologic factors:						
Pregnancy	Females of reproductive age	Amenorrhea				Enlarged uterus
Premenstrual fluid retention	Menstruating females	Premenstrual weight gain	Breast tenderness Swelling Finger swelling	End of menstrual cycle	End of menstruation	Swelling of extremities Tender, swollen breasts
Excessive caloric intake (most common cause of weight gain)	Patients who overeat	Gradual, progressive weight increase	*Children:* Normal linear growth, may reach puberty early *Adults:* Depression or psychological dependency on food	Increased stress (reactive hyperphagia) Environmental inducement	Decreased caloric intake Increased caloric needs	No evidence of edema Obesity generally distributed (may have proximal concentration)
Drugs	Users of: Steroids Nonsteroidal anti-inflammatory drugs Phenylbutazone Lithium Antipsychotics Antidepressants Propranolol Oral contraceptives Estrogens Anabolic steroids				Cessation of drug	

Continued

Differential Diagnosis of Weight Gain—cont'd

CAUSE	NATURE OF PATIENT	NATURE OF SYMPTOMS	ASSOCIATED SYMPTOMS	PRECIPITATING AND AGGRAVATING FACTORS	AMELIORATING FACTORS	PHYSICAL FINDINGS
Edema syndromes:						
Nephrotic syndrome		Weight increase is usually gradual	Edema Signs of deteriorating clinical status Signs of primary condition			Depends on primary disease Edema (may be pitting in legs) Periorbital edema Gallop rhythm Ascites
Congestive heart failure						
Cirrhosis (with ascites)						
Cyclic edema		Weight increase is often rapid (over 24-48 hours)				
Metabolic causes:						
Hypothyroidism		Patient unable to lose weight on previously successful plan	Constipation Intolerance of cold weather Skin is puffy, coarse, and dry			Enlarged thyroid "Hung-up" ankle jerk Coarse hair Loss of outer third of eyebrows Low, hoarse voice
Cushing's disease			Diabetes			"Buffalo hump" Hirsutism Hypertension Proximal obesity

Differential Diagnosis of Weight Loss

CAUSE	NATURE OF PATIENT	NATURE OF SYMPTOMS	ASSOCIATED SYMPTOMS	PRECIPITATING AND AGGRAVATING FACTORS	AMELIORATING FACTORS	PHYSICAL FINDINGS
Aging	Elderly	Anorexia	Occasional dyspepsia	Poverty Depression Drugs Inadequate caloric intake	Increased caloric intake	Decreased lean body mass
Depression	All ages, especially elderly	Dysphoria Anorexia	Insomnia Fatigue Decreased libido Sleep disorders	Loss of any type	Antidepressants Improved social situation	Depressed affect
Systemic diseases, especially cardiopulmonary, infectious, and metabolic		Those of underlying disease	Dyspnea Edema Fatigue Fever	Deterioration of underlying		Those of underlying disease
Eating disorders	Young women					
Medications	Users of:			Drug administration Increased dosage	Cessation of drug	
	Sedatives		Drowsiness			
	Antidepressants		Dry mouth			
	Clonidine		Drowsiness			
	Diuretics		Cramps			
	Nonsteroidal anti-inflammatory drugs		Indigestion			

Continued

Differential Diagnosis of Weight Loss—cont'd

CAUSE	NATURE OF PATIENT	NATURE OF SYMPTOMS	ASSOCIATED SYMPTOMS	PRECIPITATING AND AGGRAVATING FACTORS	AMELIORATING FACTORS	PHYSICAL FINDINGS
	Theophylline		Nausea			
	Digoxin		Nausea			
	Users of ACE inhibitors		Distortion of taste			
	Antibiotics					
	Thyroid supplements		Nervousness			
	Levodopa					
	Chemotherapeutic agents		Nausea and vomiting			
Cancer		Anorexia	Those of the cancer			Those of underlying disease
Acquired immunodeficiency syndrome	More common in young men		Recurrent infection			Adenopathy

Selected References

American Psychiatric Association: *Diagnostic and Statistical Manual of Mental Disorders*, ed 4 rev, Washington, DC, 2000, American Psychiatric Association, pp 583–595, 787.

Centers for Disease Control and Prevention: Overweight and obesity. Available at http://www.cdc.gov/obesity/index.html

Fernstrom MH: Drugs that cause weight gain, *Obes Res* 3(Suppl 4):435S-439S, 1995.

Hernandez JL, Riancho JA, Mattoras P, et al: Clinical evaluation for cancer in patients with involuntary weight loss without specific symptoms, *Am J Med* 114:631-637, 2003.

Holmes S: A difficult clinical problem: diagnosis, impact and clinical management of cachexia in palliative care, *Int J Palliat Nurs* 15:320-326, 2009.

Huffman GB: Evaluating and treating unintentional weight loss in the elderly, *Am Fam Physician* 65:640-647, 2002.

Kiess W, Boettner A: Obesity in the adolescent, *Adolesc Med* 13:181-190, 2002.

Lankisch PG, Grezmann M, Gerzmann JF, Lehnick D: Unintentional weight loss: diagnosis and prognosis: the first prospective follow-up study from a secondary referral centre, *J Intern Med* 249:41-46, 2001.

McTigue K, Hess R, Ziouras J: Obesity in older adults: a systematic review of the evidence for diagnosis and treatment, *Obesity* 14:1485-1497, 2006.

Rao G: Childhood obesity: highlights of AMA expert committee recommendations, *Am Fam Physician* 78:56-63, 2008:65–66.

Rao G: Office-based strategies for the management of obesity, *Am Fam Physician* 81:1449-1455, 2010.

Robbins L J: Evaluation of weight loss in the elderly, *Geriatrics* 44:31-34, 37, 1989.

Rolland Y, Kim M, Gammack J, et al: Office management of weight loss in older persons, *Am J Med* 119:1019-1026, 2006.

Stunkard AJ, Allison KC: Two forms of disordered eating in obesity: binge eating and night eating, *Int J Obes* 27:1-112, 2003.

Swenne I, Thurfjell B: Clinical onset and diagnosis of eating disorders in premenstrual girls is preceded by inadequate weight gain and growth retardation, *Acta Paediatr* 92:1133-1137, 2003.

Thomas DR: Distinguishing starvation from cachexia, *Clin Geriatr Med* 18:883-891, 2002.

U.S. Preventive Services Task Force: Screening and interventions to prevent obesity in adults, *Ann Intern Med* 139:933-949, 2003.

U.S. Preventive Services Task Force: Screening for obesity in children and adolescents: U.S. Preventive Services Task Force Recommendation Statement, *Pediatrics* 125:361-367, 2010.

Williams P, Goodie J, Motsinger C: Treating eating disorders in primary care, *Am Fam Physician* 77:187-197, 2008.

Index

Page numbers followed by *f* or *t* indicate figures or tables, respectively.